IMMUNOLOGY AND IMMUNE SYSTEM DISORDERS

CHRONIC FATIGUE SYNDROME

SYMPTOMS, CAUSES AND PREVENTION

IMMUNOLOGY AND IMMUNE SYSTEM DISORDERS

Additional books in this series can be found on Nova's website at:

https://www.novapublishers.com/catalog/index.php?cPath=23_29&seriesp=
Immunology+and+Immune+System+Disorders

Additional E-books in this series can be found on Nova's website at:

https://www.novapublishers.com/catalog/index.php?cPath=23_29&seriespe=
Immunology+and+Immune+System+Disorders

IMMUNOLOGY AND IMMUNE SYSTEM DISORDERS

CHRONIC FATIGUE SYNDROME

SYMPTOMS, CAUSES AND PREVENTION

EDITA SVOBODA
AND
KRISTOF ZELENJCIK
EDITORS

Nova Biomedical
Nova Science Publishers, Inc.
New York

NOTICE TO THE READER

The Publisher has taken reasonable care in the preparation of this book, but makes no expressed or implied warranty of any kind and assumes no responsibility for any errors or omissions. No liability is assumed for incidental or consequential damages in connection with or arising out of information contained in this book. The Publisher shall not be liable for any special, consequential, or exemplary damages resulting, in whole or in part, from the readers' use of, or reliance upon, this material. Any parts of this book based on government reports are so indicated and copyright is claimed for those parts to the extent applicable to compilations of such works.

Independent verification should be sought for any data, advice or recommendations contained in this book. In addition, no responsibility is assumed by the publisher for any injury and/or damage to persons or property arising from any methods, products, instructions, ideas or otherwise contained in this publication.

This publication is designed to provide accurate and authoritative information with regard to the subject matter covered herein. It is sold with the clear understanding that the Publisher is not engaged in rendering legal or any other professional services. If legal or any other expert assistance is required, the services of a competent person should be sought. FROM A DECLARATION OF PARTICIPANTS JOINTLY ADOPTED BY A COMMITTEE OF THE AMERICAN BAR ASSOCIATION AND A COMMITTEE OF PUBLISHERS.

Library of Congress Cataloging-in-Publication Data

Chronic fatigue syndrome : symptoms, causes, and prevention / editors, Edita Svoboda and Kristof Zelenjcik.
p.;cm.
Includes bibliographical references and index.
ISBN 978-1-60741-493-3 (hardcover : alk. paper)
1. Chronic fatigue syndrome. I. Svoboda, Edita. II. Zelenjcik, Kristof.
[DNLM: 1. Fatigue Syndrome, Chronic--diagnosis. 2. Fatigue Syndrome, Chronic--etiology. 3.Fatigue Syndrome, Chronic--prevention & control. WC 500 C5576 2009]
RB150.F37C486 2009
616'.0478--dc22
                                                                                                  2009027758

Published by Nova Science Publishers, Inc. ✦ *New York*

Contents

Preface

Chronic fatigue syndrome (CFS) is a complicated disorder characterized by extreme fatigue that doesn't improve with bed rest and may worsen with physical or mental activity. Chronic fatigue syndrome may occur after an infection, such as a cold or viral illness. The onset can also be during or shortly after a time of great stress, or it may come on gradually without a clear starting point or obvious cause. This book discusses new research in CFS, including the effects that CFS may have on immune system responses. The possible implications and prevention of CFS are also explored.

Chapter 1- Chronic Fatigue Syndrome/ Myalgic Encephalomyelitis (CFS/ME) is a heterogeneous multifactorial disease characterised by severe fatigue and a range of systemic symptoms resulting in an inability to function at optimal levels. The symptoms of CFS/ME vary from patient to patient; however, prolonged and disabling fatigue, impaired memory and concentration and widespread pain are typical symptoms reported by most patients. There is no known single causal factor associated with CFS/ME although development of the condition post-infection is common. CFS/ME may affect the nervous, immune, endocrine, muscular, cardiovascular and respiratory systems. The present chapter reviews research pertaining to immunological function and other related areas in CFS/ME. Research has shown that CFS/ME patients exhibit abnormalities in immune function. The T, B and Natural Killer lymphocytes are cells frequently examined in CFS/ME. Gene expression studies are providing evidence for the over expression and under expression of genes important for homeostasis. In addition, alterations in the hypothalamic-pituitary-adrenal (HPA) axis occur. This review serves as a basis for further research in the aetiology of CFS/ME.

Chapter 2- Cases of chronic fatigue syndrome/mylagic encephalomyelitis (CFS) are reported to be initiated by nine different short-term stressors, each of which increases levels of nitric oxide in the body. Elevated nitric oxide, acting through its oxidant product, peroxynitrite, initiates a local biochemical vicious cycle, the NO/ONOO- cycle, which is proposed to be the cause of CFS and related diseases. Evidence supporting this cycle mechanism in CFS comes from each of the following types of evidence: Case initiation by such stressors, the extensive evidence supporting the existence of individual cycle mechanisms, evidence showing that various cycle elements are elevated in CFS cases, evidence for a basically local mechanism in CFS and related diseases, evidence from CFS animal models, genetic evidence from genetic polymorphism studies and evidence from clinical trials of agents predicted to down-regulate the NO/ONOO-cycle. Each of the five principles underlying the NO/ONOO- cycle mechanism is supported by one or more of the above described types of evidence. The cycle involves oxidative stress, excessive nitric oxide synthase (NOS) activity, mitochondrial dysfunction, inflammatory biochemistry, excitotoxicity including excessive NMDA activity and tetrahydrobiopterin depletion. There is evidence, ranging from extensive to modest, supporting roles for each of these in CFS.

Clinical studies of treatment protocols containing 14 or more agents predicted to down-regulate the NO/ONOO- cycle appear to be effective in the treatment of CFS and related diseases. However, none of these has yet been shown to be able to cure substantial numbers of cases of CFS or related illnesses. The author discusses one such protocol and suggests an approach, previously tested only as a single agent treatment, that may strenthen these multi-agent protocols to obtain at least some of the needed cures.

Chapter 3- At least eight studies published since 1962 suggest that moderate cooling of the body (in most cases by means of cold water) can reduce fatigue in healthy subjects and in some groups of patients: fibromyalgia, multiple sclerosis, and rheumatoid arthritis. To date, there have been no studies on the effectiveness of this approach in CFS, aside from a pilot study in Australia, which used contrast water therapy in combination with nutritional and exercise interventions. Psychostimulant medications, the anti-fatigue therapy with the strongest level of clinical evidence for a number of disorders, do not appear to be effective in CFS patients.

The possible mechanisms of the anti-fatigue effect of cooling may involve the following: A) A reduction of the total level of serotonin in the brain, as evidenced by direct measurements in laboratory animals and by a drop of the plasma prolactin level in human subjects; this would be consistent with reduced fatigue according to "the serotonin hypothesis of central fatigue." B) Activation of stress-response pathways such as the hypothalamic-pituitary-adrenal axis and sympathetic nervous system. C) Systemic analgesia and reduced muscle pain in particular; this may be mediated by a spike in the plasma level of beta-endorphin, an opioid peptide, as well as by the gate control effects of sensory stimulation by cold water. D) Activation of components of the brainstem arousal system, such as raphe nuclei and locus ceruleus (most likely associated with activation of the sympathetic nervous system). This diffuse modulatory system controls the sleep/wake cycle and minor lesions correlate with severe chronic fatigue. E) Possible activation of relevant dopaminergic pathways in the brain, such as those projecting to the striatum. F) Activation of the thyroid and increased metabolic rate.

Interestingly, B, D and E resemble physiological effects of psychostimulants. Importantly, A, B, C, and possibly D, seem to be relevant to the pathophysiology of CFS and suggest that repeated moderate cooling may be beneficial for the patients. Successful application of this approach in CFS would require devising a procedure that is acceptable to patients, since regular cold showers and cold-water swimming are highly stressful. If the procedure does not involve psychological distress, inhalation of cold air, and hypothermia, then it would be expected to have little or no adverse effects on health. A lifetime experiment on rats has shown that repeated moderate cooling is most likely safe, at least in healthy subjects.

Chapter 4- Because chronic fatigue syndrome (CFS) is often diagnosed in later life of subjects who exercise frequently, exercise-induced causes of CFS are highly suspected. Muscle metabolism at rest, during, and after muscle contraction was explored in CFS patients using physiological (oxygen uptake (VO_2), arterio-venous oxygen difference) and biochemical assessment (^{31}P resonance magnetic spectroscopy, lactic acid, blood markers of oxidative stress, cytokines, and heat shock proteins, Hsp). In the majority of CFS patients, 1) muscle glycolysis is unaltered, 2) the aerobic capacity is often enhanced and about one-fourth of patients have an increased proportion of type 1 oxidative muscle fibre, 3) exercise-induced production of reactive oxygen species (ROS) is accentuated with reduction of antioxidant defences, 4) the immune response to exercise is rarely modified, 5) recent observations indicate a marked reduction of heat shock proteins (Hsp) expression in response to exercise. Because, in healthy individuals, Hsp protect the cells against the deleterious effects of ROS, it is tempting to speculate that the elevated oxidative stress in CFS patients might result from reduced Hsp expression. CFS patients have also reduced muscle excitability in response to direct stimulation (M wave) and a deregulation of the Na^+/K^+ and Ca^{2+}-ATPase pumps. M wave alterations are correlated with both the magnitude of reduced K^+ outflow from contracting muscles and accentuated oxidative stress. Thus, CFS is characterized by an altered muscle response to exercise which might result from an accentuated oxidative stress, possibly due to reduced Hsp expression.

Chapter 5- Substantial clinical overlap may exist amongst functional somatic syndromes, in general, and chronic fatigue syndrome (CFS) and fibromyalgia (FM), in particular. The underlying pathophysiology of these disorders is unclear. In this article are studies performed exploring similarities and dissimilarities between CFS and FM based on autonomic nervous functioning and electrocardiographic QT. Two methods were recently developed to assess autonomic nervous functioning via cardiovascular reactivity in response to a standardized postural challenge. The 'hemodynamic instability score' (HIS) computes blood pressure and heart rate changes along the tilt test and the resulting measurements are processed by image analysis techniques. Three studies assessed the HIS in CFS patients. Group averages of HIS were CFS = +3.72 (SD 5.02) vs. healthy = -4.62 (SD 2.26) and FM -3.25 (SD 2.63) (p <0.0001). An other technique is based on beat-to-beat heart rate and pulse transit time recordings during the tilt test, data processing by fractal and recurrence plot analysis and computing a 'Fractal & Recurrence Analysis-based Score' (FRAS). FRAS values >0.22 were specific for CFS vs. healthy subjects and FM (2 studies). A different approach, measurement of the QT interval on the surface electrocardiogram found that the corrected QT in CFS patients is relatively shortened and thereby differs from QT in FM (p <0.0001). Jointly, these records show characteristic features to the CFS dysautonomia phenotype, supporting the distinction between CFS and FM. This data may be relevant in providing objective criteria for CFS diagnosis and distinction from other functional somatic syndromes.

Chapter 6- Chronic fatigue syndrome (CFS) is an important public health problem with unique diagnostic and management challenges. Insight into the pathophysiology of CFS is elusive and treatment options are limited. With the advent of the biopsychosocial model in medicine, more recent research efforts have focused on interactions of biological and psychological factors in the development and maintenance of CFS. Stressful experiences have been identified as important risk factors of CFS, particularly when experienced early in life. In addition, psychobiological processes that may translate stress into CFS risk have been considered. This chapter, will summarize the current state of research on the role of stress in CFS. It is proposed that CFS reflects a disorder of adaptation of neural and regulatory physiological systems in response to challenge. Stress likely interacts with other vulnerability factors in determining CFS risk. Understanding the role of stress in CFS may lead towards novel strategies for prevention and treatment of this debilitating disorder.

Chapter 7- Fibromyalgia (FM) is a clinical syndrome characterized by widespread pain and abnormal sensitivity on palpation of specific tender points [1]. The pathogenesis of FM has been elusive, made difficult by the absence of distinctive biochemical or histological abnormalities. There is much debate and controversy about this condition. On the one side are those who deny the existence of fibromyalgia as a nosologic entity and consider it an artificial summation of unrelated symptoms [2, 3]. A consequence of the view that FM is but an expression of low self-esteem and unhappiness may to change our approach to this condition and deal with these patients in psychological and sociological terms. On the other side are clinicians and researchers who define fibromyalgia as a distinct clinico-pathologic disorder and suggest that it is a genetically based disease with autosomal-dominant transmission [4]. Much of the evidence that FM is the projection of an underlying physiologic disturbance relates to studies describing autonomic system dysfunction in FM patients [5-13].

A point of obfuscation in classifying patients with FM lies in the overlap of this syndrome with other functional somatic and pain syndromes: chronic fatigue syndrome, irritable bowel syndrome, Gulf War syndrome, migraine, etc [14-17]. Studies have documented common risk factors operating at the background of these syndromes as well as the presence of autonomic nervous dysfunction (Figure 1). The clinical overlap of FM and chronic fatigue syndrome (CFS) is particularly prominent and the two are mentioned frequently as a single disorder [14-16]. In a study of 163 women with primary CFS, 43% also met criteria for FM [15] and in another study, 18% of patients with FM had also been diagnosed with CFS [16].

Chapter 8- Chronic fatigue syndrome (CFS) poses many socioeconomic, psychosocial, disability and quality of life difficulties for people with CFS in Canada. The self-reported prevalence of CFS was 0.78%, 1.22% and about 201,900, 331,500 Canadians have reported having CFS in 2000 and 2005 respectively. Canadians aged 40-64 years old (57.87% in 2000, and 58.59% in 2005) were the most frequently infected. More female Canadians (71.41% in 2000, and 68.44% in 2005) were affected than males (28.59% and 31.56%). Both physical and mental fatigue caused by CFS cost the Canadian economy an estimated $3.5 billion per year, and the annual lost productivity in Canada is estimated at $2.5 billion in 2003. However, the capacity in Canada for prevention and management of CFS is limited. Currently, there are only few medical doctors using the Clinical Working Case Definition, diagnostic and treatment protocols. Therefore, there is a need for more research in the surveillance, diagnosis, treatment, and evaluation of CFS management in Canada.

Chapter9- This study provides a description and evaluation of this innovative Train-the-Trainer approach for training health care workers in the diagnosis and management of patients with CFS. Those who attended this workshop did have significant changes in their understanding of CFS as well as attitudes towards those with this illness. Following the workshops, these trainers went back to their own settings and put on workshops to train others, and through this process, several thousand individuals were presented with information about the diagnosis and management of CFS.

Chronic fatigue syndrome (CFS) is an illness characterized by prolonged, debilitating fatigue and multiple nonspecific symptoms such as headache, recurrent sore throat, muscle and joint pain, and cognitive complaints. Profound fatigue, the hallmark of the disorder, can come on suddenly or gradually and persist or recur throughout the period of illness (Fukuda et al., 1994). Unlike the short-term disability of an acute infection, CFS symptoms by definition linger for at least six months and often for years. The majority of patients report an acute onset, over a period of hours or a few days. Others report a more gradual onset, as if they have a bout of flu from which they do not completely recover. CFS is marked by a dramatic difference in the patient's pre- and post-illness activity level and stamina (Jason & Taylor, 2003). Health care professionals play an important role in diagnosing and treating patients with CFS.

Approximately a quarter of all patients seeing general practitioners complain of prolonged and incapacitating fatigue, a symptom common to many illnesses such as cancer, depression, autoimmune diseases, hormonal disorders, and infections (Friedberg & Jason, 1998). The majority of these illnesses are treatable and must be promptly identified so that timely treatment can be started. Therefore, causes of fatigue must be ruled out before a definitive diagnosis of CFS can be considered. Despite more than a decade of extensive research, the cause of CFS remains unknown and no diagnostic tests exist (Jason, Fennell, & Taylor, 2003). However, health care providers must recognize that CFS is a real and debilitating condition that can only be diagnosed through a process of elimination.

CFS is one of the nation's most prevalent, yet misunderstood, chronic illnesses. In a community based epidemiologic study by Jason and colleagues (1999), they found that about 800,000 Americans would meet the case definition for CFS, although only ten percent of those identified as having CFS in their community based sample had actually been diagnosed with this illness. The research group also identified that women, African-Americans, and Hispanics were at a greater risk for developing the illness than men, Whites, or Asian-Americans. Findings from this community-based prevalence study also indicated that rates of CFS were highest in females of lower socioeconomic status, a segment of the population that is less likely to have access to health care providers, and therefore may be less likely to seek and receive care for this disabling illness. Given the high percentage of these patients who go undiagnosed, it is clear that many patients are not receiving appropriate care for this illness. By staying abreast of new information, health care professionals can play an important role in better diagnosing this illness and providing a higher level of care to patients.

Many patients with chronic fatigue syndrome (CFS) have felt stigmatized or misunderstood by medical professionals (Looper & Kirmayer, 2004). For example, Anderson and Ferrans (1997) found that 77percent of individuals with CFS reported past negative experiences with health care providers. Another survey found that 57percent of respondents were treated badly or very badly by their doctors (David, Wessely, and Pelosi, 1991). Green, Romei, and Natelson (1999) also found that 95percent of individuals seeking medical treatment for CFS reported feelings of estrangement, and 70percent believed that others attributed their CFS symptoms to psychological causes. Asbring and Narvanen (2003) found physicians regarded the illness as less serious than the patients, and the physicians characterized the patients with CFS and Fibromyalgia as illness focused, demanding, and medicalising. Twemlow, Bradshaw, Coyne, and Lerma (1997) found that 66percent of individuals with CFS stated that they were made worse by their doctors' care. Clearly, there is a need to help sensitize health care professionals to the unique needs of patients with CFS.

It is possible that negative attitudes toward people with CFS might help explain the consistent finding that patients with CFS have mixed experiences with the health care system. Shlaes, Jason, and Ferrari (1999) developed a CFS Attitudes Test, and found that if someone believes that people with CFS are responsible for their illness, it is likely that they will also believe that people with CFS have negative personality characteristics, such as being compulsive or overly driven. It is possible that negative attitudes might be a function of past negative portrayals of CFS as either non-existent or as a function of a neurotic, overworked, stressed lifestyles (Jason et al., 1997). Any training program for health care professionals will need to deal with the negative stigma that patients with CFS feel, and attempts to change these types of negative attitudes could lead to more positive patient experiences when dealing with the health care system.

Improving patient care through the education of health care professionals has become a major initiative for The CFIDS (Chronic Fatigue Immune Dysfunction Syndrome) Association of America, the largest CFS patient and advocacy organization in the US. A Primary Care Provider Education Project was developed by the CFIDS Association to offer various learning opportunities for providers, including lecture presentations, and print, video- and Web-based self-study courses. Health care providers who were interested in educating other health care providers about CFS were offered the opportunity to attend a two-day Train-the-Trainer workshop, lead by CFS experts. After completion of this workshop, attendees were asked to return to their home regions and present one-to-two hour long programs for at least 40 of their peers, or to students in health care disciplines. Continuing education units were provided and expenses were covered for participants. This study provides a description and evaluation of this innovative Train-the-Trainer approach for training health care workers in the diagnosis and management of patients with CFS.

In: Chronic Fatigue Syndrome: Symptoms, Causes & Prevention   ISBN: 978-1-60741-493-3
Editor: E. Svoboda and K. Zelenjcik, pp. 1-25   © 2010 Nova Science Publishers, Inc.

Chapter 1

The Immune System in Chronic Fatigue Syndrome/Myalgic Encephalomyelitis

E. W. Brenu[2],
S. Marshall- Gradisnik[2] and D. Staines[1,2]
[1]Queensland Health, Gold Coast Population Health Unit, Southport, Gold Coast,
Queensland, Australia
[2]Faculty of Health Science and Medicine, Population Health and Neuroimmunology Unit,
Bond University, Robina, Queensland, Australia

Abstract

Chronic Fatigue Syndrome/ Myalgic Encephalomyelitis (CFS/ME) is a heterogeneous multifactorial disease characterised by severe fatigue and a range of systemic symptoms resulting in an inability to function at optimal levels. The symptoms of CFS/ME vary from patient to patient; however, prolonged and disabling fatigue, impaired memory and concentration and widespread pain are typical symptoms reported by most patients. There is no known single causal factor associated with CFS/ME although development of the condition post-infection is common. CFS/ME may affect the nervous, immune, endocrine, muscular, cardiovascular and respiratory systems. The present chapter reviews research pertaining to immunological function and other related areas in CFS/ME. Research has shown that CFS/ME patients exhibit abnormalities in immune function. The T, B and Natural Killer lymphocytes are cells frequently examined in CFS/ME. Gene expression studies are providing evidence for the over expression and under expression of genes important for homeostasis. In addition, alterations in the hypothalamic-pituitary-adrenal (HPA) axis occur. This review serves as a basis for further research in the aetiology of CFS/ME.

Introduction

Prolonged, excessive and incapacitating fatigue is described as Chronic Fatigue Syndrome/ Myalgic Encephalopathy (CFS/ME) [1]. The Centre for Disease Prevention and Control (CDC) describes CFS/ME as a new onset of unexplained fatigue persisting over a period of 6 months or more, during which, patients experience at least four of the following symptoms: impairments in short-term memory or concentration, sore throat, sore cervical or axillary lymph nodes, multijoint pain without the presence of swelling or redness, severe headaches, unrefreshing sleep and postexertional malaise enduring for more than 24 hours [2]. This criterion does not include psychiatric disorders such as melancholic depression, substance abuse, bipolar disorder, psychosis and eating disorders [2].

The prevalence rate of CFS/ME is between 0.2–2.6% [3]. A high proportion of this percentage is made up of females; the ratio of females to males is believed to be as high as 6:1 [4], although others place this ratio lower [5]. The incapacitating nature of this disease creates situations of unemployment amongst a majority of patients with CFS/ME [6]. Estimated rates of unemployment among CFS/ME patients in the United States are about 37% [7]. Rates of fatality of this illness are unknown and suicide is believed to be significant. However, recovery in relation to decreases in symptoms for CFS/ME has been estimated to be between 0–6% [8] with full recovery being unusual. Nisenbaum et al. [9] in a study of 59 CFS/ME patients noted that 22.5% had partial remission while 10% had complete remission with 79.2% prevalence of unrefreshing sleep and decreases in some symptoms.

Despite the extensive research in the aetiology and pathophysiology of CFS/ME no identifiable single factor or agent has been named to be responsible for the incapacitating effects created by this syndrome. Nevertheless, CFS/ME impinges on proper function of different body systems such as the nervous [10,11], endocrine [12], immune [13], respiratory and muscular systems [14]. This suggests that CFS/ME is a heterogeneous multifactorial disorder [15]. The heterogeneity of this condition can be attributed to the variation in symptoms perceived by patients at the onset of illness [16], whereas the multifactorial nature of this condition emanates from the existence of possible multiple causal factors [17].

Definitions of Chronic Fatigue Syndrome

There are other criteria for describing CFS/ME; these include the Australian, British and Canadian criteria [18,19, 20]. Slight variations exist between these definitions and the CDC 1994 definition. The British or Oxford criteria includes symptoms such as mental fatigue, psychosis and organic brain disorder [21], which suggest the presence of a psychiatric disorder [21]. Conversely, the Australian criterion disregards the presence of a new occurrence of fatigue but incorporates neuropsychiatric symptoms [21]. Similarly, the Canadian definition discounts patients exhibiting symptoms that denote the presence of mental illness [21]. The incoherent nature of these definitions necessitated the enforcement of the CDC 1994 criteria. Furthermore, the CDC 1994 case definition is continually under evaluation and amendment to create a more stringent and standardized definition of CFS/ME for both diagnostic and research purposes [22, 23].

CFS/ME and Viral and Other Infections

There are strong indications that viral infections may cause or initiate some cases of CFS/ME. Evidence for this is in relation to the number of viruses observed in serological studies patients with CFS/ME, these include Epstein-Barr virus, Human Herpes virus 6 [24] and 7 [25], Coxsackie B virus [26], Human T lymphotropic virus I and II [27], Borna disease virus [28], cytomegalovirus [29], parvovirus B19 [30], and stealth virus [31]. However, a causal rather than casual association is unknown. Nonetheless, viral infections have the capacity to disrupt immune function and can therefore compromise the activity of immune cells with lowered function thus perpetuating viral load and CFS/ME-like symptoms.

The observation that certain cases of CFS/ME are initiated by viral infections or other factors coupled with the symptom profile of patients suggests possible breakdown in other mechanisms as the immune system interacts with other physiological systems to promote homeostasis. Importantly, as the heterogeneity of CFS/ME presents itself in the cluster of symptoms observed, it is plausible that this results from impaired communication between the immune system and other systems. Hence, the purpose of this review is to examine the immune system in CFS/ME patients and its association with the nervous and neuroendocrine systems. An examination of the genetic system in relation to the immune function is also assessed in this review. A brief description of the immune system is provided beforehand to familiarize the reader with the information on immunological changes associated with CFS/ME.

Immunological System

The immunological system is comprised of the innate and adaptive immune system. At the innate level, Natural Killer (NK) lymphocytes, dendritic cells, macrophages and neutrophils are required to eliminate pathogens. These leukocytes relay information to the innate immune system via cytokine and chemokine production resulting in the recruitment of T and B lymphocytes thus enhancing the functional capacity of the immune system to eliminate infections caused by antigens and pathogens [32]. Neutrophils, T, B and NK lymphocytes are among the leukocytes that have been investigated in association with CFS/ME.

T Lymphocyte

There are two main T cell populations, cluster of differentiation (CD) four (CD4) T cells and CD8 T cells [32]. CD4 T cells are helper cells while the CD8 T cells are either cytotoxic or suppressors [33]. During T cell development in the thymus, the CD4 T cells undergo further division to differentiate into Th1 and Th2 cells [32]. The difference between these two subtypes of CD4 helper T cells pertains to the type of cytokines they produce; Th1 cells secrete pro-inflammatory like cytokines while Th2 cells secrete anti-inflammatory like cytokines [34].

B Lymphocytes

Interestingly, another subset of lymphocytes important in mediating immune response against pathogens and allergic reactions is the B lymphocytes. These lymphocytes have immunoglobulin molecules on their cell surface that allow recognition of various pathogens. An important ability of the B lymphocyte is the ability to mount effective and rapid immune response against pathogens once recognition and memory of the pathogens has been initialized. There are, therefore, a variety of immunoglobulin receptors that have specific functions and respond to different stimuli. Immunological memory is created by the immunoglobulin G (IgG); however, this is initiated once IgM has recognized the pathogen and undergone differentiation to create a specific receptor for recognition of that particular pathogen. IgE is highly proficient in allergic reaction and activates mast cell production of histamine and is also involved in the elimination of parasites [32].

Neutrophils

Neutrophils are among the phagocytic cells of the immune system. They contain phagosomes and lysomes which interact with granules present in the neutrophil for the initiation and killing of pathogens to occur. Once a pathogen is engulfed, phagocytic activity is initiated through the binding of the phagosome and the lysome to form a phagolysosome, NADPH oxidase release occurs to lyse the pathogen, the resultant effect is the production of reactive oxygen species and superoxide [35]. This collective function resolves immune invasion by bacterial or fungal pathogens. Notably neutrophils produce chemokines (IL-8) and cytokines (IL-12) required for recruiting other neutrophils and lymphocytes and initiating a type 1 inflammatory response respectively [36, 37].

Natural Killer Cells (NK)

Another significant lymphocyte is the Natural Killer (NK) cell. These cells function to eliminate virus and tumour cells while providing an adequate supply of cytokines to the immune system [38, 39]. The different types of cytokines produced by these cells include interferon-gamma (IFN-γ), tumour necrosis factor alpha (TNF-α) and granulocyte macrophage colony-stimulating factor (GM-CSF) [40]. NK cells initiate antibody dependent cellular cytotoxicity (ADCC) through the FcγRIII receptor or CD16 [41]. There are two main types of NK cells; 90% of these cells are classified as $CD56^{dim}CD16^+$ while the remaining 10% are comprised of $CD56^{bright}CD16^-$, $CD56^{dim}CD16^+$NK cells induce natural cytotoxicity and ADCC whereas $CD56^{bright}CD16^-$NK cells facilitate the production of cytokines [42].

Importantly the immune cells has a variety of cell surface molecules that enable activation and proliferation of lymphocytes and soluble proteins, these molecules act as activation markers and receptors that enable the recognition of antigens and the efficient release of cytokines at the appropriate times. Examples of these include CD45RO (memory) and CD45RA (naïve) on T cells [43, 44].

Discussion

The severe fatigue and flu-like symptoms exhibited by patients with CFS/ME suggest changes in immune response to viral, bacterial, other infections or further consequences of immune responses to these infections. Changes in immune competence in CFS/ME can be explained, at least in part, by the variation in the lymphocyte subsets, pathogen lysis, cytokine production, presence of activation markers and mitogenic responses.

CFS/ME Patients' Lymphocyte Levels

Information on lymphocyte populations in CFS/ME patients is incomplete as there may be a variation in the total numbers of lymphocytes in these individuals. In certain instances patients have been shown to demonstrate comparable levels of lymphocytes to a healthy population, while in other cases there are variations in levels of lymphocyte subsets. A substantial proportion of research on lymphocyte populations in CFS/ME has provided evidence for comparable levels of total T lymphocytes and sub-types of T lymphocytes (CD4$^+$T and CD8$^+$T cells) [45, 46, 47, 48, 49, 50, 51, 52, 53, 54, 55, 56, 57, 58, 59, 60, 61, 62, 63]. Normalization of lymphocyte numbers is sometimes associated with changes in the number of the different subtypes of lymphocytes, namely CD4$^+$ T cells, CD8$^+$ T cells and CD56^{bright}NK cells and CD56^{dim}NK cells. This is because subsets of CFS/ME patients demonstrate increased or reduced [68] numbers of CD4$^+$T cells with normal CD8$^+$T cells [59 64] while others demonstrate decreases in both CD8$^+$T cells and CD4$^+$T cells [18] and yet another set have either low [48] or high [64, 65] levels of CD8$^+$T.

B cell numbers in CFS/ME display no difference to that of the control [45, 46, 47, 52, 57, 58, 62, 66, 67, 68, 69]; however, only one study has reported increased levels of B lymphocytes in CFS/ME patients [55].

Similarly, NK cell distribution is equivocal in CFS/ME patients. Although a majority of the patients demonstrate similar levels to the healthy control population, some patients have been found to have either an increased or reduced level of NK lymphocytes [47, 46, 55, 57, 58, 59, 61, 64, 66, 68, 70, 71]. Presently, data on the subtypes of NK cells are sparse; two sets of studies have reported increases in CD56^{bright} and decreases in CD56^{dim} NK cells, others have noticed either a decreased CD56^{bright} or an increase in CD56^{dim} cells [57, 63, 64, 72].

The changes in total lymphocyte population (B cell, T cell and NK cell) in CFS/ME may occur as a result of the multifactorial and heterogeneous nature of CFS/ME. Furthermore, changes in demographics and other agents can contribute to disparities in the levels of lymphocytes. This highlights the potential for different subtypes of CFS/ME due to different causal agents or at least a variation in responses to them. Additionally, changes in lymphocytes may be dependant on the time course of the illness. Lymphocytes tend to fluctuate at different time periods during an infectious episode as such measurements of lymphocytes at different times may vary from one individual to another. Perhaps it is best to assess patients during early onset of the disease.

Lymphocyte Function

Llymphocyte response to stimulation

Mitogenic stimulation is a proven way of determining lymphocyte activation and proliferation in response to immune insults. The mitogens commonly used include phytohemagglutinin (PHA), pokeweed mitogen (PWM) and concanavalin A (ConA). Most CFS/ME patients demonstrate low levels of lymphocyte proliferation and activation in response to stimulation by PHA and PWM [64, 67, 68, 73, 74, 75]. This may explain the abnormal levels of cytokine secreted by most CFS/ME patients and the inability to either prevent or clear infections as cytokine production is a vital component of lymphocyte activation and proliferation.

Cytokine production and function

Evidence for immune pathogenesis in CFS/ME can be further supported by the disparities in the modulatory functions of cytokines. Cross talk between the immune system and other physiological and immune cells is maintained by the discharge of cytokines. The two types of cytokines produced by leukocytes are either pro (type 1/Th1) or anti-inflammatory (type 2/ Th2). Pro-inflammatory cytokines are sometimes classified as type 1 and some are produced by Th1 CD4$^+$T cells while the anti-inflammatory cytokines are type 2 and some are produced by Th2 CD4$^+$T cells [76] IL-2, TNF-α, IFN-γ, IL-12 are pro-inflammatory cytokines and   IL-6, IL-4, IL-10, IL-13 are anti-inflammatory cytokines [77, 78].

IL-2 is known to induce the production of IFN-γ and IL-4 on T cells and triggers growth and proliferation of lymphocytes and monocytes [79]. It also has analgesic effects on the function of the hypothalamic-pituitary pathway [80]. IL-6 regulates the inflammatory process by activating B, CD8 T and NK cells. Declining and elevated levels of IL-6 have been associated with inflammatory and autoimmune disorders [34, 81]. In the nervous system the involvement of IL-6 enhances differentiation and development of neural cells, thus acting as a neurotrophic factor [82, 83]. IL-12 stimulates the proliferation of CD4$^+$Th1 cells [84]. IFN-γ regulates the activation of macrophages and viral replication while conferring inhibitory effect on the CD4$^+$Th2 cells and cytokine release [85, 86]. TNF-α facilitates the recruitment of monocytes and lymphocytes to sites of infection by enhancing extravasation, permeability and adhesion of these cells to the endothelial layer [87, 88]. TNF alpha also regulates immune response in the CNS. However, the inhibitory effects of anti-inflammatory cytokines on proinflammatory cytokines can be attributed to the antagonistic effects of IL-4 and IL-10 on IL-12, IFN-γ, IL-6, IL-1 and IL-8 production, conversely, these cytokines promote the differentiation and activation of leukocytes [79, 89]. They are both recruited during neural infections [90]. In activated T cells, production of IL-12 and TNF-α, is inhibited by IL-13 [91].

Immune homeostasis is sustained when there is a balance between pro- and anti-inflammatory cytokines. Anti-inflammatory cytokines are known to prevent excessive inflammatory reactions by dampening the effects of pro-inflammatory cytokines and other immune modulators, conversely pro-inflammatory cytokines predominantly intervene during allergic reactions and immune response against pathogens [92, 93]. Dysregulation in the production of these different cytokines has been implicated in autoimmune disorders, systemic infection and fibrosis [92, 93]. The disease profile of CFS/ME denotes an involvement in cytokine dsyregulation, where there maybe a predominant shift towards an elevated production of type 2 cytokines [57, 62] or towards type 1 cytokine profile [68]. The following cytokines have been examined in CFS/ME patients; IL-1, IL-4, IL-6, IL-10, TGF-beta, IFN, IL-12 and TNF with equivocal results [46, 51, 52, 55, 57, 58, 60, 61, 62, 66, 94 95, 96].

Phagocytic activity

Phagocytosis is a poorly investigated area in CFS/ME patients; nonetheless, measurements of factors associated with phagocytosis such as nitric oxide and apoptosis have been investigated in CFS/ME patients. There is presently only one study on the state of neutrophils in CFS/ME patients. In this particular study, it was noted that neutrophils in CFS/ME patients were less viable than those in the control population, that is, the extent of neutrophil apoptosis was much higher among the CFS/ME patients [97]. Increased rate of neutrophil apoptosis was correlated to an elevated secretion of TNFR1 and TGFβ1 which heighten the susceptibility of neutrophils to undergo cell death [97]. Low levels of TNFR1 and TGFβ1 act as a protective mechanism against increased levels of apoptosis, the former is a death receptor that binds to TNF to induce apoptosis while the latter prevents the adherence of leucocytes [98]. Furthermore, these changes are also indications of cell function at the molecular level. Apoptotic genes are differentially expressed in certain CFS/ME patients as will be explained in a later section. These changes further suggest an inability of neutrophils from CFS/ME patients to induce perhaps eliminate pathogens in circulation. Additionally, increased levels of apoptosis in CFS/ME suggest distorted immune response to viruses and bacteria thus paving the way for recurring infections.

Despite the strong likelihood for the occurrence of elevated oxidative stress in CFS/ME patients, phagocytic activity and oxidative stress have not been investigated in neutrophils in these patients. Neutrophils release reactive oxygen species and free radicals through NADPH oxidation during the elimination process of pathogens [99]. Patients with neurological diseases may have increased amounts of oxidative stress and this maybe predominant expressend in neutrophils [100].

Phagocytosis by macrophages in the immune system of CFS/ME patients has also not been fully investigated. Similarly, only one study has observed changes in macrophage activity in CFS/ME patients [101]. However, changes in neutrophil function may suggest similar changes in macrophages. Additionally, the shift towards an imbalanced cytokine profile in CFS/ME involving IL-10 production in macrophages may contribute to lowered phagocytic activity [102] while high levels of nitric oxide (NO) as noted in some patients with CFS/ME may account for abnormal macrophage function [103, 104]. Interestingly NO release is associated with the activation of the *NFκB* transcription factor [105] which has been identified to be considerably upregulated in CFS/ME [106].

Cytotoxic activity

Cytotoxic activity is the predominant function of NK cells and CD8⁺T cells. Decreases in NK cytotoxic activity have been detected in CFS/ME patients [56, 64, 69, 70, 107, 108, 109]. In certain instances these decreases in function coincide with decreases in CD56^{dim}NK cells, the cytotoxic component of NK cells [56, 108]. However, others have noticed heightened or lowered numbers in CD56^{bright}NK (cells responsible for producing cytokines that enhance cytotixicity) in CFS/ME patients compared to healthy controls [56, 64]. Thus, decreases in NK activity may or may not be soley dependent on changes in the production of cytokines and lowered number of cells that exert lysis against viral cells. Decrease in cytotoxic function may alternatively be related to diminishing levels in perforin production [109]. Perforin is released in conjunction with pro-apoptotic granzymes through a granule exocytosis pathway into target cells where they stimulate apoptosis [110]. The presence of decreases in cytotoxic activity with comparable evidence for decreases in perforin production is a strong indicator for abnormal immune function and an inability to eliminate viral infection. In addition, aberrations in nitric oxide mediated NK cell activity have been identified in some CFS/ME patients [111], thus substantiating the observed changes in cytotoxic activity. Nevertheless phenotypic imbalance in NK cells distribution may alter the enhancing effects of IFN-γ on NK and CD8⁺T cells [112].

At the genomic level indications for altered cytotoxic activity is implied by the changes in *GZMA* gene [113]. *GZMA* is a required for granzyme A and perforin activity during ADCC activity initiated by CD8⁺T and NK cells through the FCγRII (CD16) [114, 115]. Hence, it is likely that changes in the expression of this gene contribute to reductions in NK cytotoxic activity.

Cytotoxic activity of CD8⁺T cells has not been directly measured in CFS/ME, nevertheless the presentation of anomalies in the expression of *GZMA* presupposes that cytotoxic activity may be compromised in CFS/ME patients. It may be necessary to further explore the cytotoxic properties of these immune cells to confirm an overall compromise in this particular lytic mechanism.

Changes in activation markers

An essential component of the immune system is the CD antigens; these intricate molecules serve a variety of important functions when present on the surface of lymphocytes. Their roles include receptors for cytokines and chemokines, adhesion molecules, co-stimulation, ligand activation and signaling for lymphocyte differentiation [43]. The significance of these molecules to CFS/ME arises from their contribution to optimal immune function at both the cellular and molecular level. During infectious episodes, there is a requirement for naïve lymphocytes to change to memory lymphocytes. This change is initiated by the presence of CD45RA⁺ and CD45RO⁺ naïve and memory antigens respectively [44]. CD45RA⁺ expression on CD4⁺T cells is meager in CFS/ME patients while CD45RO⁺ remained unchanged when compared with healthy individuals [54, 56, 64]. The consequences of these observations are not known; however, a reduction in naïve cells affects maintenance of immunological memory in the T cell population (Bell et al. 1998).

Immunological memory is a safeguard against recurrent infections and promotes efficient and rapid elimination of pathogens [116]. Although naïve cells are not rapidly recruited during an infection, they contain different signaling motifs and unspecific binding receptors that are necessary for the recognition of new infections. Therefore, decreases in these cells further suggest that the immune system is impaired in its ability to recognize and acquire memory towards new infections [116]. Hence, the maintenance of immunological memory is highly dependent on these two molecules. A lack of proper immunological memory may contribute to incidence of persistent infections noted in some cases of CFS/ME.

CD8$^+$ subset of T lymphocytes in some CFS/ME patients have marked changes in the CD11b, CD28 and CD38 antigens [51, 57, 61, 67]. The significant reductions in CD11b$^+$ and CD28$^+$ expression on the CD8$^+$T cell is a significant indication for decreases in cytotoxic T lymphocytes [51, 57, 61, 67]. Particularly, these CD antigens have been demonstrated to be preferentially present on cytotoxic CD8$^+$T lymphocyte engaged in lysis against viruses [117], that is the CD8$^+$CD28$^+$CD11b$^+$T cell [118, 119]. Changes in the production of one or the other may compromise immune function. Other activation markers such as HLA-DR and CD38 have also been shown to be increased, decreased or normal in some CFS/ME patients [51, 57, 59, 67, 69].

Gene Expression in CFS/ME

The human genome project has allowed exploration of the genomic profile of CFS/ME patients. The results from these investigations have confirmed the multifactorial and heterogeneous nature of CFS/ME. Changes in gene expression were related to genes that are important in energy metabolism, signal transduction, transcription, immunity, cellular, neuronal and development. Most of these studies were done using microarrays, PCR and a number of Pathway analysis software. It is interesting to note that each of these genes is not exclusive to one function but rather an array of other functions. The relative significance of gene expression studies to CFS/ME is not well known. This is likely related to the bi-directional effects of gene expression and CFS/ME symptomology; therefore, symptoms of CFS/ME could elicit changes in gene expression or *vice versa*. However, the relative significance of each gene is beyond the scope of this review, hence, the following section discusses genes in relation to the immunological system of CFS/ME.

The Janus kinases and signaling transducers activators of transcription (JAK/STAT) pathway is a significant immunological pathway for the activation of lymphocytes and production of soluble factors [120]. Alterations in cytokine production can prompt changes in the activation of the JAK/STAT pathways. The transcription factor *STAT5A* is activated by IL2, IL4 and IL7 and changes in *STAT5A* in CFS/ME maybe a consequence of decreases in these cytokines [113]. As indicated earlier, CFS/ME patients demonstrate either a type 1 or 2 cytokine bias, this is likely connected to downregulation of genes responsible for cytokine production. Importantly, IL7R has been shown to be decreased in expression while other cytokine genes have been shown to be increased in expression and these include *IL1RL2, IL6R, IL6ST, TNFRSF1A, TRAF3, IL10RA* and *IFNAR1* [106, 121]. *IL10RA* is an essential component of the T cell activation pathway, it also exerts inhibitory effects on T cells [122].

IL6 acts on both the adaptive and innate immune systems to counteract or provoke inflammation [123]. It regulates the JAK/STAT pathway either positively or negatively [124]. Positive activation of the JAK/STAT pathway will result in development and growth while negative activation through intense signaling of suppressors of cytokine signaling (SOCS) proteins result in inflammatory diseases [124, 125]. Therefore, changes in the expression levels of *IL6R* and *IL6ST* gene may have profound consequences on both immune-related and non-immune cells necessary for cell signaling and other physiological functions. Perhaps the changes in *JAK1* gene may be associated with changes in IL-6 gene, because JAKK1 facilitates the signal transduction of IL-6 [126].

Hypothetically, variations in the molecular expression of cytokines and cytokine receptor genes illustrate the existence of disparities in cytokine expression and imbalances as noted in some CFS/ME studies. It is well documented that anti-inflammatory cytokines have inhibitory effects on the activation pro-inflammatory genes, as pro-inflammatory cytokines promote infections [127]. Increased expression of proinflammatory genes, increase the amount of NO and inflammatory cascade disrupting cells and tissues and inadvertently causing diseased states [127]. Amplification of genes expression profiles can therefore have severe consequences on cytokine production and receptor binding properties of cells. Genes such as the *TRAF3* regulate the production of IL-10ra [128], hence and increase in this gene in the presence of alterations in *IL-10RA* may modify the concentration of IL-10 and its ability to suppress pro-inflammatory cytokines, the converse may also occur, thus initiating either a type 1 or type 2 cytokine bias.

Changes in other immune response genes have been documented for *DEFB1, PSMA3, PSMA4, CD68, CXCR5, TRAF3, CD79A, PRKCL1, CD2BP2, MAIL (NFKBIZ), IL8, CXCR4, CD47, PIK3R1, EBI2, EGR3, NFKB1, APP, CMRF35 (CD300C), ICAM2, ITGB* and *IER2* [106, 113, 129, 130, 131]. Transcription factors such as *MAIL (NFKBIZ), NFKB1* and *EGR3* control lymphocyte proliferation, apoptosis and inflammatory response [132, 133, 134]. Consequently, alterations in their expression in some CFS/ME patients may affect the ability of the lymphocyte to perform these activities in these patients. Changes in neutrophil chemotaxis and T cell activity are perhaps attributable to defaults in chemokine receptor genes *IL8, CXCR4* and *CXCR5* [135, 136]. Chemotaxis is an essential component of the immune response through which leukocytes in circulation are mobilized to sites of infection using chemicals released by chemokines and other interleukins. *TRAIL* increases neutrophil apoptosis as such overexpression of this gene may also explain the increases in neutrophil apoptosis noticed in CFS/ME patients [137]. Furthermore, *TRAIL* may effectively lyse Th1 cells under certain conditions [138], this is significant to the observation of a type 2 cytokine shift in CFS/ME patients. Other genes such as *DEFB1* have an involvement in the elimination of bacteria and infectious diseases [139]. *CD68* is expressed by macrophage and is known to be associated with insulin levels and adipose tissue inflammation [140]. Conversely the *CD47* modulates the function of dendritic, T cells and recognition of antigen presenting cells by lymphocytes [141], while B cell receptor function is regulated by *CD79a* expression [142]. Signaling and activation pathways disregulation in lymphocytes may be linked to over-expression of *CD2BP2, CMRF35* and *PIK3R1* gene [143, 144, 145]. Similarly, NK activity and recruitement to sites of infection is heightened by *ICAM-2* [146]. The manifestation of viral infections preceding some instance of CFS/ME can however be confirmed by the increase in the expression of *EBI2* [147].

Perhaps, another contribution to the impaired cytokine profile is the observation of decreased expression of IL-17F produced by the Th17, a novel subset of T helper cells known to have a role in autoimmune diseases [148]. Importantly IL-6 promotes the differentiation of Th17 cells in order for it to participate in the pro-inflammatory mehcanism [149, 150]. This involvement of IL-6 and Th17 is therefore highly important to immune cytokine balance and the elimination of disease; any perceived shifts in the expression of *IL-6R* and *IL-6ST* may affect the efficiency of trans-signalization and alter the inflammatory process. Consequently there could be an increase in viral load and other related fatigue symptoms.

Interactions between the Immune System and Other Systems in CFS/ME

Immune-neuroendocrine interactions

The immune system interacts with various other systems to maintain physiological homeostasis. These interactions are necessary to preserve the expression of cells, hormones and cytokines. The intricate network formed between the immune system and the neuroendocrine system plays a significant role in physiological homeostasis. This complex network is thought to be distorted in CFS/ME patients.

Alterations in neuroendocrine-immune interactions maybe related to deteriorations in the hypothalamic-pituitary-adrenal (HPA) axis. In some CFS/ME patients a decreased pattern of reactivity in the HPA axis occurs [152, 153]. Furthermore changes in the glucocorticoid receptor gene sequence (*NR3C1*), highlights the changes in HPA axis [153]. Modifications in the HPA system may arise as a result from poor communication between the immune and neuroendocrine signaling molecules and receptors. Most immune cells have receptors for various hormones on their cell surfaces while the endocrine system is also able to produce soluble proteins that bind immune cells and *vice versa* [154, 155]. Moreover, alterations in HPA axis can be explained by the responsiveness of certain hormones. For example the responsiveness of adrenocortico-trophic hormone (ACTH) is significantly reduced in some cases of CFS/ME patients [156] importantly distorted ACTH response is evident in the presence of corticosteroid releasing hormone (CRH), arginine vasopressin and naloxone [157, 158, 159].

Neuroendocrine-immune interaction in CFS/ME patients maybe distorted due to the inability of the immune system to respond to the regulatory effects of the neuroendocrine system [160]. This maybe associated with an inability of T cells to respond to the inhibitory effects of the endocrine system and diminished response of IL-10 and TNF-α to β_2-adrenergic agonist [160]. Decreases in receptors and lowered signal transduction events at the intracellular level may potentially promote this adverse effect [160]. However, lack of communication between cytokines and hormones in the form of an unresponsive pattern of IL-12 and IL-4 to dexamethasone but heightened susceptibility of TNF-α and IL-6 to glucocorticoids [161, 162]. However changes in the *IL-10R* in CFS/ME patients, likely results in diminished responsiveness to other hormones [106, 130]. Furthermore, the dysfunction in the HPA axis may emanate from discrepancies in communication between neurons and cytokines produced by the immune system and may consequently prompt depletion in the production of glucocorticoids and reduced responsiveness to other cytokines [163]. Changes in cortisol [164] and acetylcholine [165] may occur in CFS/ME, however, these vary from patient to patient and maybe dependent on the time of day on which the measurements were made.

It maybe plausible to suggest that shifts in cytokine profile may account for the perceived dysregulation in the HPA axis in CFS/ME patients. Changes in cytokine profile either severely alter neuronal stimulation or modify the release of neurotransmitters and hormones and thus reduce the responsiveness of the immune system to the endocrine system and to infections, hence promoting CFS/ME like symptoms. In addition changes in cytokine expreeion at the molecular level may also be a contributory factor. Alterations especially in genes related to IL-10, IL-6, IL-7, TNF and IFN can significantly affect this immune neuroendocrine interaction in CFS/ME [106]. The link between the genomic expression of cytokines and the consequences of this on the immune system and neuroendocrine system has not been clearly established, however, it may be speculated that changes in the expression pattern of these genes combined with other associated factors contribute to the pathogenesis of the disease.

Interaction between the immune system and the nervous system

Fatigue, impaired memory and concentration, pain and headaches are suggestive of a dysfunctional central nervous system in the pathogenesis of CFS/ME. This may be due to antagonistic effects and reduced levels of immune cells participation in the nervous system signaling pathways. Although the CNS is generally regarded as immune-privileged, the involvement of the immune system in various parts of the brain confers a protective mechanism against infection in the nervous system [166]. This occurs in the presence of leucocytes, microglia and soluble proteins which induce lysis of pathogens and restore damaged brain tissue [166]. The presence of T lymphocytes and pro-inflammatory cytokines in the brain and central nervous system serves as another protective mechanism against neural immune insults; furthermore, the neural networks in the brain in turn regulate the function of the immune system. There is, therefore, a cross communication between these two systems. In CFS/ME patients may demonstrate low levels of granulocyte-macrophage colony stimulating factor with increased levels of IL-8 and IL-10 in their spinal fluid [167]. The consequence of this is reduced immune response against bacterial and other related infections and the perceived neurological symptoms such as neuropathic pain. Additionally IL-6, TNF-α, IL-2 and IFN-γ have been associated with mood changes, distorted sleep patterns and fatigue in CFS/ME patients. These findings are consistent with gene expression studies where the *IL-6R* and *IL-6ST* both implicated in the function of the nervous system have demonstrated changes in expression [106].

Conclusion

Immunological aberrations are well proven in CFS/ME and are quite diverse in scope and severity. These aberrations have not been adequately explained to date in terms of aetiological pathogenesis. The problem may be one of dysregulation of immunological response to infection or one of an autoimmune response, possibly associated with environmental insults. Whether a definite shift in type 1/type 2 cytokine ratios occurs is still a matter for further investigation.

Indications of deficits in neurological and endocrine function amy exist as a consequence of poor communication between the immune products and these two systems. Changes in the function of the immune system and the lack of efficient networking from other systems may arise from genetic changes in immunological mechanisms. Perhaps some environmental triggers during the course of life of a CFS/ME patient overwhelm the genomic system resulting in changes in the level of expression of genes linked to immunological function and possibly function of other bodily systems. However, changes in the immune, neurological or endocrine system can affect the level of expression of genes. The former and latter triggers or changes initiate the abnormalities noticed in number and function of cells of the immune system. Considering that lymphocytes and soluble proteins impact other systems of the body, changes at the molecular level will also affect other systems such as the neurological and endocrine systems in CFS/ME patients. Possibly these collective effects disrupt physiological homeostasis resulting in CFS/ME-like symptoms described by patients.

Regardless of the number of studies that have investigated CFS/ME, the results are inconclusive as they do not point to a single defining cause or pathway for the disorder. Further studies are needed to fully understand the underlying pattern of immune activity in CFS/ME due to the varying factors that may affect the function of the immune system at both the molecular and cellular level. Novel pathways of immune regulation could be involved in the pathogenesis of CFS/ME and, therefore, need to be explored to provide a more concise and conclusive understanding of this disease. These pathways are likely to be complex, multi-system and powerful, involving the interplay of the endocrine, neurological and other systems. It is possible that these pathways mediate the functions of all leukocytes in various parts of the body thus exerting negative effects on a variety of body systems. CFS/ME affects body systems other than the immune system. This may be because of the multifaceted function of the immune system and its influence on other systems possibly resulting from infections.

Additionally, certain neuropeptides may contribute to the disparities in the immune system as they exert protective effects on some lymphocytes and alter the activity of others. This may explain the imbalances in cytokine production, either towards a Th1/type 1 or a Th2/type 2 pattern, in CFS/ME patients. The expression of certain genes possibly plays a role in the variations in cytokines production. These genes may either activate or down regulate specific pathways associated with cytokine production and function. However changes in their expression or mutations in their sequence alter their expression and result in disproportionate levels of cytokines production that severely alters immune, endocrine and neurological function. Further research is required to investigate these assumptions. Disparities in some of the data could support the concept of several types of CFS/ME expressing some variation in symptoms. Although some studies have sought to prove and institute these distinctions, further research needs to establish the basis for subtypes and whether they have a genetic component. This ultimately may provide a link between the expression of immune genes and the function of the immunological system.

References

[1]   Lewis, G; Wessely, S. The epidemiology of fatigue: more questions than answers. J Epidemiol Community Health. 1992 Apr, 46(2), 92-97.

[2]   Fukuda, K; Straus, SE; Hickie, I; Sharpe, MC; Dobbins, JG; Komaroff, A. The chronic fatigue síndrome: A comprehensive approach to its definition and study. Ann Intern Med. 1994 Dec,121(12), 953-959

[3]   Harvey, SB; Wadsworth, M; Wessely, S; Hotopf, M. Etiology of Chronic Fatigue Syndrome: Testing popular hypotheses using a national birth cohort study. *Psychosom Med*. 2008,70, 488-495

[4]   Devanur, LD; Kerr, JR. Chronic Fatigue Syndrome: Review. *J Clin Virol*. 2006, 37, 139-150.

[5]   Willson, A; Hickie, I; Hadzi-Pavlovic, D; Wakefield, D; Parker, G; Straus, SE; Dale, J; McCluskey, D; Hinds, G; Brickman, A; Goldenberg, D; Demitrack, M; Blakely, T; Wessley, S; Sharpe, M, Lloyd, A. What is chronic fatigue syndrome? Heterogeneity within an international multicentre study. *Aust N Z J Psychiatry*. 2001 Aug, 35(4), 520-7.

[6]   Lloyd, AR; Pender, H The economic impact of chronic fatigue syndrome. *Med J Aust*. 1992 Nov 2;157(9), 599-601

[7]   Cairns, R; Hotopf, M. A systematic review describing the prognosis of chronic fatigue syndrome. *Occup Med (Lond)*. 2005 Jan, 55(1), 20-31. Review

[8]   Hotopf, M; Wessely, S. Stress in the workplace: unfinished business. *J Psychosom Res*. 997 Jul, 43(1), 1-6.

[9]   Nisenbaum, R; Jones, JF; Unger, ER; Reyes, M; Reeves, WC. A population-based study of the clinical course of chronic fatigue syndrome. *Health and Qual of Life Outcomes*. 2003, 1(49), 1-9

[10] de Lange, FP; Kalkman, JS; Bleijenberg, G; Hagoort, P; van der Werf, SP; van der Meer, JW; Toni, I. Neural correlates of the chronic fatigue syndrome--an fMRI study. *Brain*. 2004 Sep, 127(Pt 9), 1948-57

[11] Siemionow, V; Fang, Y; Calabrese, L; Sahgal, V; Yue, GH. Altered central nervous system signal during motor performance in chronic fatigue syndrome. *Clin Neurophysiol*. 2004 Oct, 115(10), 2372-81

[12] Cleare, AJ; O'Keane, V; Miell, JP. Levels of DHEA and DHEAS and responses to CRH stimulation and hydrocortisone treatment in chronic fatigue syndrome. *Psychoneuroendocrinology*. 2004 Jul, 29(6), 724-32.

[13] Lyall, M; Peakman, M; Wessely, S. A systematic review and critical evaluation of the immunology of chronic fatigue syndrome. *J Psychosom Res*. 2003 Aug, 55(2), 79-90

[14] Fulcher, KY; White, PD. Strength and physiological response to exercise in patients with chronic fatigue syndrome. *J Neurol Neurosurg Psychiatry*. 2000 Sep, 69(3), 302-7.

[15] Afari, N; Buchwald, D. Chronic fatigue syndrome: a review. *Am J Psychiatry*. 2003 Feb, 160(2), 221-36

[16] Wilson, A; Hickie, I; Hadzi-Pavlovic, D; Wakefield, D; Parker, G; Straus, SE; Dale, J; McCluskey, D; Hinds, G; Brickman, A; Goldenberg, D; Demitrack, M; Blakely, T; Wessely, S; Sharpe, M; Lloyd, A. What is chronic fatigue syndrome? Heterogeneity within an international multicentre study. *Aust N Z J Psychiatry*. 2001 Aug, 35(4), 520-7.

[17] Salit, IE. Precipitating factors for the chronic fatigue syndrome. *J Psychiatr Res*. 1997 Jan-Feb, 31(1), 59-65

[18] Lloyd, AR; Hickie, I; Boughton, CR; Spencer, O; Wakefield, D. Prevalence of chronic fatigue syndrome in an Australian population. *Med J Aust*. 1990 Nov 5, 153(9), 522-8

[19] Sharpe, MC; Archard, LC; Banatvala, JE; Borysiewicz, LK; Clare, AW; David, A; Edwards, RH; Hawton, KE; Lambert, HP; Lane, RJ; McDonald, EM; Mowbray, JF; Pearson, DJ; Peto TEA; Preedy, VR; Smith, AP; Smith, DG; Taylor, DJ; Tyrrell, DA; Wessely, S; White, PD. report--chronic fatigue syndrome: guidelines for research. *J R Soc Med*. 1991 Feb, 84(2), 118-21

[20] Carruthers, BM; Jain, AK; De Meirleir, KL; Peterson, DL; Klimas, NG; Lerner, AM; Bested, AC; Flor-Henry, P; Joshi, P; Powles, ACP; Sherkey, JA; van de Sande, MI. Myalgic Encephalomyelitis/Chronic Fatigue Syndrome: Clinical Working Case Definition; Diagnostic and Treatment Protocols. *J Chronic Fatigue Syndr*. 2003, 11(1), 7-36

[21] Wyller, VB. The chronic fatigue syndrome--an update. *Acta Neurol Scand Suppl*. 2007, 187, 7-14

[22] Reeves, WC; Lloyd, A; Vernon, SD; Klimas, N; Jason, LA; Bleijenberg, G; Evengard, B; White, PD; Nisenbaum, R; Unger, ER; International Chronic Fatigue Syndrome Study Group. Identification of ambiguities in the 1994 chronic fatigue syndrome research case definition and recommendations for resolution. *BMC Health Serv Res*. 2003 Dec 31, 3(1), 25

[23] Jones, JF; Maloney, EM; Boneva, RS; Jones, AB; Reeves, WC. Complementary and alternative medical therapy utilization by people with chronic fatiguing illnesses in the United States. *BMC Complement Altern Med*. 2007 Apr 25, 7, 12.

[24] Nicolson, GL; Gan, R; Haier, J. Multiple co-infections (Mycoplasma; Chlamydia; human herpes virus-6) in blood of chronic fatigue syndrome patients: association with signs and symptoms. *APMIS*. 2003 May, 111(5), 557-66.

[25] Di Luca, D; Zorzenon, M; Mirandola, P; Colle, R; Botta, GA; Cassai, E. Human herpesvirus 6 and human herpesvirus 7 in chronic fatigue syndrome. *J Clin Microbiol*. 1995 Jun, 33(6), 1660-61

[26] Miller, G. Molecular approaches to epidemiologic evaluation of viruses as risk factors for patients who have chronic fatigue syndrome. *Rev Infect Dis*. 1991 Jan-Feb, 13 Suppl 1, S119-22

[27]   DeFreitas, E; Hilliard, B; Cheney, PR; Bell, DS; Kiggundu, E; Sankey, D; Wroblewska, Z; Palladino, M; Woodward, JP; Koprowski, H. Retroviral sequences related to human T-lymphotropic virus type II in patients with chronic fatigue immune dysfunction syndrome. *Proc Natl Acad Sci U S A*. 1991 Apr 1, 88(7), 2922-6

[28]   Nakaya, T; Takahashi, H; Nakamur, Y; Kuratsune, H; Kitani, T; Machii, T; Yamanishi, K; Ikuta, K. Borna disease virus infection in two family clusters of patients with chronic fatigue syndrome. *Microbiol Immunol*. 1999, 43(7), 679-89

[29]   Martin, WJ; Zeng, LC; Ahmed, K; Roy, M. Cytomegalovirus-related sequence in an atypical cytopathic virus repeatedly isolated from a patient with chronic fatigue syndrome. *Am J Pathol*. 1994 Aug, 145(2), 440-51

[30]   Kerr, JR; Bracewell, J; Laing, I; Mattey, DL; Bernstein, RM; Bruce, IN; Tyrrell, DA. Chronic fatigue syndrome and arthralgia following parvovirus B19 infection. *J Rheumatol*. 2002 Mar, 29(3), 595-602.

[31]   Martin, WJ. Detection of RNA sequences in cultures of a stealth virus isolated from the cerebrospinal fluid of a health care worker with chronic fatigue syndrome. Case report. *Pathobiology*. 1997, 65(1), 57-60.

[32]   Murphy, K; Travers, P; Walport, M. *Janeway's Immunobiology*. 7th ed. London:Garland Science Taylor & Francis group;2008

[33]   Freedman, MS; Ruijs, TC; Blain, M; Antel, JP. Phenotypic and functional characteristics of CD8$^+$ cells: a CD11b$^-$CD28$^-$ subset mediates noncytolytic functional suppression. *Clin Immunol Immunopathol;* 1991 Aug, 60(2), 254-267.

[34]   Sredni-Kenigsbuch, D. TH1/TH2 cytokines in the central nervous system. *Int J Neuosci*. 2002 Jun, 112(6), 665-703

[35]   Segal, AW. How neutrophils kill microbes. *Annu. Rev. Immunol*. 2005, 23, 197-223

[36]   Baggiolini, M; Dewald, B; Moser, B. Interleukin-8 and related chemotactic cytokines-CXC and CC chemokines. *Adv Immunol*. 1994, 55, 97-179

[37]   Mackay, C; Lanzavecchia, A; Sallusto, F. Chemoattractant receptors and immune responses. *The Immunologist*. 1999, 7, 112-118

[38]   Hamerman, JA; Ogasawara, K; Lainer, LL. NK cells in innate immunity. *Curr Opin Immunol*. 2005, 17, 29-35.

[39]   Farag, SS; Fehniger, TA; Ruggeri, L; Velardi, A; Caligiuri, MA. Natural killer cell receptors: new biology and insights into the graft-versus-leukaemia effect. *Am Soc Hematol*. 2002, 100(6), 1935-1947.

[40]   Viver, E; Tomasello, E; Baratin, M; Walzer, T; Ugolini, S. Functions of natural killer cells. *Nature Immunol*. 2008 May, 9(5), 503-510

[41]   Cooper, MA; Fehniger, TA; Caligiuri, MA. The biology of human natural killer cell subsets. *Trends Immunol*. 2002 Nov, 22(11), 633-640

[42]   Freud, AG; Caligiuri, MA. Human natural killer cell development. *Immuol Rev*. 2006 Dec;214, 56-72

[43]   Reddy, M; Eirikis, E; Davis, C; Davis, HM; Prabhakar, U. Comparative analysis of lymphocyte activation marker expression and cytokine secretion profile in stimulated human peripheral blood mononuclear cell cultures: an in vitro model to monitor cellular immune function. *J Immunol Methods*. 2004 Oct, 293(1-2), 127-142

[44] Rothstein ,DM; Sohen, S. Daley, JF; Schlossman, SF; Morimoto, C. CD4+ CD45RA+ and CD4+ CD45RA- T cell subsets in man maintain distinct function and CD45RA expression persists on a subpopulation of CD45RA+ cells afer activation with Con A. *Cell Immunol* 1990, 129, 449-67.

[45] Peterson, PK; Shepard, J; Macres, M; Schenck, C; Crosson, J; Rechtman, D; Lurie, N. A controlled trial of intravenous immunoglobulin G in chronic fatigue syndrome. *Am J Med.* 1990, 89(5), 554-60

[46] Chao, CC; Janoff, EN; Hu, SX; Thomas, K; Gallagher, M; Tsang, M; Peterson, PK. Altered cytokine release in peripheral blood mononuclear cell cultures from patients with chronic fatigue syndrome. *Cytokine* 1991, 3(4), 292-8

[47] Miller, NA; Camichael, HA; Calder, BD; Behan, PO; Bell, EJ; MaCartney, RA; Hall, FC. Antibody to coxsackie B virus in diagnosing postviral fatigue syndrome. *Br Med J.* 1991, 302(6769), 140-3

[48] Hickie, I; Lloyd, A; Wakefield, D. Immunological and psychological dysfunction in patients receiving immunotherapy for chronic fatigue syndrome. *Aust NZ J Psychiatry.* 1992, 26(2), 249-56

[49] Milton, JD; Morris, AG; Christmas, SE; Edwards, RHT. Interferon production by mononuclear cells from patients with chronic fatigue syndrome-a controlled cross sectional study. *J Rheumatol.* 1994, 21(8), 1527-31

[50] Gupta, S; Vayuvegula, B. A comprehensive immunological analysis in chronic fatigue syndrome. *Scand J Immunol.* 1991, 33(3), 319-27

[51] Landay, Al; Jessop, C; Lennette, ET; Levy, JA. Chronic fatigue syndrome: clinical condition associated with immune activation. *Lancet.* 1991, 338(8769), 707-12

[52] Linde, A; Anderson, B; Svenson, SB; Ahrne, H; Carlsson, M; Forsberg, P; Hugo, H; Karstorp, A; Lenikei, R; Lindwall, A; Loftenius, A; Sall, C; Anderson, J. Serum levels of lymphokines and soluble cellular receptors in primary Epstein-Barr virus infection and in patients with chronic fatigue syndrome. *J Infect Dis* 1992, 165(6), 994-1000

[53] Lloyd, A; Hickie, I; Hickie, C; Dwyer, J Wakefield, D. Cell-mediated immunity in patients with chronic fatigue syndrome; healthy control subjects and patients with major depression. *Clin Exp Immunol.* 1992, 87(1), 76-9

[54] Tirelli, U; Pinto, A; Marotta, G; Crovato, M; Quaia, M; De Paoli, P; Galligioni, E; Santini, G. Clinical and immunological study of 205 patients with chronic fatigue syndrome: a case series from Italy. *Arch Intern Med.* 1993, 153(1), 116-7

[55] Rasmussen, Ak; Nielsen, H; Andersen, V; barington, T; Bendtzen, K; Hansen, MB; Nielsen, L; Pedersen, BK; Wiik, A. Chornic fatigue syndrome-a controlled cross sectional study. *J Rheumatol.* 1994, 21(8), 1527-31

[56] Tirelli, U; Marotta, G; Importa, S; Pinto, A. Immunological abnormalities in patients with CFS. *Scand J Immunol.* 1994, 40(6), 601-608

[57] Swanink, C; Vercoulen, J; Galama, J; Roos, M; Meycard, L; van der Ven,-Jongekrigg, J; de Nijis, R; Bleijenberg, G; Fennis, J; Miedma, F; vander Meer, J. Lymphocyte subsets; apoptosis and cytokines in patients with CFS. *J Infect Dis.* 1996, 3(4), 292-8

[58] Mawle, AC; Nisenbaum, R; Dobbins, JG; Gary, HE; Stewart, JA; Reyes, M; Steele, L; Schmid, DS; Reeves, WC. Immune response associated with chronic fatigue syndrome: a case control study. *J Infect Dis* 1997, 175(1), 136-41

[59] Peakman, M; Deale, A; Field, R; Mahalingam, M; Wessely, S. Clinical improvement in chronic fatigue syndrome is not associated with lymphocyte subset function or activation. *Clin Immunol Immunopathol.* 1997, 82(1), 83-91

[60] Visser, J; Blauw, B; Hinloopen, B; Brommer, E; De Kloet, ER; Kluft, C; Nagelkerken, L. CD4 T lymphocytes from patients with chronic fatigue syndrome have decreased interferon-gamma production and increased sensitivity to dexamenthasone. *J Infect Dis* 1998, 177(2), 451-4

[61] La Manaca, JJ; Sisto, SA; Zhou, XD; Ottenweller, JE; Cook, S; Peckerman, A; Zhang, Q; denny, TN; Gause, WC; Natelson, BH. Immunological response in chronic fatigue syndrome following a graded exercise test to exhaustion. *J Clin Immunol.* 1999, 19(2), 135-42

[62] Skowera, A; Cleare, A; Blair, D; Bevis, L; Wessely, SC; Peakman, M. High levels of type 2 cytokine-producing cells in chronic fatigue syndrome. *Clin Exp Immunol.* 2004 Feb, 135(2), 294-302

[63] Robertson, MJ; Schacterle, RS; Mackin, GA; Wilson, SN; Bloomingdale, KL; Ritz, J; Komaroff, AL. Lymphocyte subset differences in patients with chronic fatigue syndrome; multiple sclerosis and major depression. *Clin Exp Immunol.* 2005 Aug, 141(2), 326-32.

[64] Klimas, N; Salvato, F; Morgain, R; Fletcher, MA. Immunologic abnormalities in chronic fatigue syndrome. *J Clin Micro* 1990, 28(6), 1403-1410.

[65] Patarca, R; Klimas, NG; Lugtendorf, S; Antoni, M; Fletcher, MA. Dysregulated expression of tumor necrosis factor in chronic fatigue syndrome: interrelations with cellular sources and patterns of soluble immune mediator expression. *Clin Infect Dis.* 1994 Jan, 18 Suppl 1, S147-53

[66] Natelson, BH; LaManca, JJ; Denny, TN; Vladutiu, A; Oleske, J; Hill, N; Bergen, MT; Korn, L; Hay, J. Immunologic parameters in chronic fatigue syndrome; major depression; and multiple sclerosis. *Am J Med.* 1998 Sep 28, 105(3A), 43S-49S

[67] Hassan, IS; Bannister, BA; Akbar, A; Weir, W; Bofill, M. A study of the immunology of the chronic fatigue syndrome: correlation of immunologic parameters to health dysfunction. *Clin Immunol Immunopathol.* 1998 Apr; 87(1), 60-7

[68] Roberts, TK; McGregor, NR; Dunstan, RH; Donohoe, M; Murdoch, RN; Hope, D; Zhang, S; Butt, HL; Watkins, JA; Taylor, WG. Immunological and haematological parameters in patients with chronic fatigue syndrome. *J Chronic Fatigue Syndr.* 1998, 4(4), 51-65

[69] Barker, E; Fujimura, SF; Fadem, MB; Landay, AL; Levy, JA. Immunologic abnormalities associated with chronic fatigue syndrome. *Clin Infect Dis.* 1994 Jan, 18 Suppl 1, S136-41.

[70] See, DM; Tilles, JG. Alpha interferon treatment of patients with chronic fatigue syndrome. *Immunol Invest* 1996, 25(1-2), 153-64

[71] Morrison, LJA; Behan, WHM; Behan, PO. Changes in natural killer cell phenotype in patients with post-viral fatigue syndrome. *Clin Exp Immunol.* 1991, 83, 441-446.

[72] Masuda, A; Nozoe, SI; Matsuyama, T; Tanaka, H. Psychobehavioral and immunological characteristics of adult people with chronic fatigue and patients with chronic fatigue syndrome. *Psychosom Med.* 1994, 56, 512-518.

[73] Jones, JF; Streib J; Baker, S; Herberger, M. Chronic fatigue syndrome: I. Epstein-Barr virus immune response and molecular epidemiology. *J Med Virol.* 1991 Mar, 33(3), 151-8.

[74] Lloyd, AR; Wakefield, D; Boughton, CR; Dwyer, JM. Immunological abnormalities in the chronic fatigue syndrome. *Med J Aust.* 1989 Aug 7, 151(3), 122-4.

[75] Lutgendorf, SK; Antoni, MH; Ironson, G; Fletcher, MA; Penedo, F; Baum, A; Schneiderman, N; Klimas, N. Physical symptoms of chronic fatigue syndrome are exacerbated by the stress of Hurricane Andrew. *Psychosom Med.* 1995 Jul-Aug, 57(4), 310-23

[76] Lucey, DR; Clerici, M; Shearer, GM. Type 1 and type 2 cytokine dysregulation in human infectious; neoplastic; and inflammatory diseases. *Clin Microbiol Rev.* 1996 Oct, 9(4), 532-62.

[77] Coussens, LM; Werb, Z. Inflammation and cancer. *Nature.* 2002 Dec 19-26, 420(6917), 860-7.

[78] Chung, KF. Cytokines in chronic obstructive pulmonary disease. Eur Respir J Suppl. 2001

[79] Van Meir, EG. Cytokines and tumors of the central nervous system. *Glia.* 1995 Nov, 15(3), 264-88.

[80] Jiang, CL; Lu, CK. Interleukin-2 and its effects in the central nervous system. *Biol Sig Recep.* 1998, 1.7, 148-156.

[81] Salvi, M; Girasole, G; Pedrazzoni, M; Passeri, M; Giuliani, N; Minelli, R; Braverman, LE; Roti, E. Increased serum concentrations of interleukin-6 (IL-6) and soluble IL-6 receptor in patients with Graves' disease. *J Clin Endocrinol Metab.* 1996 Aug, 81(8), 2976-2979

[82] Frei, K; Malipiero, U; Lesit, TP; Zinkernagel, RM; Schwab, ME; Fontana, A. On the cellular source and function of interleukin 6 produced in the central nervous system in viral disease. *Eur J Immunol.*1989, 19, 689-694.

[83] Wagner, JA. Is IL-6 both a cytokine and a neurotrophic factor? *J Exp Med.* 1996, 183, 2417-2419

[84] Manetti, R; Parronchi, P; Giudizi, MG; Piccinni, MP; Maggi, E; Trinchieri, G. Natural Killer cell stimulatory factor [interleukin12 [12]] induces T helper type1 [Th1]-specific immune responses and inhibits the development of IL-4 producing Th cells. *J Exp Med.* 1993, 177, 1199-1204.

[85] Farrar, MA; Schrieher, RD. The molecular cell biology of interferon-γ and its receptor. *Annu of RevImmunol.* 1993, 11, 571-611.

[86] Boehm, U; Klamp, T; Groot, M; Howard, JC. Cellular responses to interferon-γ. *Annu Rev Immunol.* 1997, 15, 749-795.

[87] Pohlman, TH; Stanness, KA; Beauty, PG; Ochs, HD & Harlan, JM. 1986. An endothelial cell surface factor(s) induced in vitro by lipopolysaccharide interleukin 1; and tumor necrosis factor-alpha increase neutrophil adherence by CDw 18-dependent mechanism. *J Immunol.* 136, 4558-4563

[88] Brett, J; Gerlach, H; Nawroth, P; Steinberg, S; Godman, G; Stem, D. Tumor necrosis factor cachectin increases permeability of endothelial cell monolayers by a mechanism involving regulatory G protein. *J Exp Med.* 1989 Jun, 169(6), 1977-1991.

[89] Romagnani, S. Human, Th1 and Th2 subsets: "eppuur si muove". *Eur Cytokine Netw.* 1994 Jan-Feb, 5(1), 7-12.

[90] Mizuno, T; Sawada, M; Marunouchi, T; Suzumra, A. Production of interleukin-10 by Mouse glial cells in culture. *Biochem Biophys Res Commun.* 1994 Dec, 205(3), 1907-1910

[91] Cosentino, G; Soprana, E; Thienes, CP; Siccardi, AG; Viale, G; Vercelli, D. IL-13 down-regulates CD14 expression and TNF-alpha secretion in normal human monocytes. *J Immunol.* 1995 Sep 15, 155(6), 3145-51

[92] Keane, MP; Strieter, RM. The importance of balanced pro-inflammatory and anti-inflammatory mechanisms in diffuse lung disease. *Respir Res.* 2002, 3, 5.

[93] Opal, SM; DePalo, VA. Anti-inflammatory cytokines. *Chest.* 2000 Apr, 117(4), 1162-72

[94] Lloyd, A; Gandevia, S; Brockman, A; Hales, J; Wakefield, D. Cytokine production and fatigue in patients with chronic fatigue syndrome and healthy control subjects in response to exercise. *Clin Infect Dis.* 1994, 18(Suppl.1), S142-6

[95] Patarca, R; Klimas, N; Garca, M; Walters, M; Dumbroski, D; Pons, H; Fletcher, M. Dysregulated expression of soluble immune mediator responses in a subset of patients with CFS: cross-sectional categorisation of patients by immune status. *J Chronic Fatigue Syndr* 1995, 1(1), 81-96

[96] Buchwald, D; Wener, MH; Pearlman, T; Kith, P. Markers of inflammation and immune activation in chronic fatigue syndrome. *J Rheumatol.* 1997, 24(2), 372-6

[97] Kennedy, G; Spence, V; Underwood, C; Belch, JJ. Increased neutrophil apoptosis in chronic fatigue syndrome. *J Clin Pathol.* 2004 Aug, 57(8), 891-3.

[98] Seely, AJ; Swartz, DE; Giannias, B; Christou, NV. Reduction in neutrophil cell surface expression of tumor necrosis factor receptors but not Fas after transmigration: implications for the regulation of neutrophil apoptosis. *Arch Surg.* 1998 Dec, 133(12), 1305-10

[99] Segal, AW. How neutrophils kill microbes. *Annu. Rev. Immunol.* 2005, 23, 197-223

[100] Vitte, J; Michel, BF; Bongrand, P; Gastaut, JL. Oxidative stress level in circulating neutrophils is linked to neurodegenerative diseases. *J Clin Immunol.* 2004 Nov, 24(6), 683-92

[101] Prieto, J; Subirá, ML; Castilla, A; Serrano, M. Naloxone-reversible monocyte dysfunction in patients with chronic fatigue syndrome. *Scand J Immunol.* 1989 Jul, 30(1), 13-20

[102] Ganea, D; Delgado, M. Neuropeptides as modulators of macrophage functions. Regulation of cytokine production and antigen presentation by VIP and PACAP. *Archivum Immunologiae et Therapiae Experimentalis.* 2001, 49, 101-110

[103] Nijs, J. Chronic fatigue syndrome: intracellular immune deregulations as a possible etiology for abnormal exercise response. *Medical Hypotheses.* 2004. May, 62(5), 759-765

[104] Maes, M; Mihaylova, I; Kubera, M; Bosmans, E. Not in the mind but in the cell: increased production of cyclo-oxygenase-2 and inducible NO synthase in chronic fatigue syndrome. *Neuro Endocrinol Lett.* 2007. Aug, 28(4), 463-469

[105] Makarov, SS. NF-κB in rheumatoid arthritis: a pivotal regulator of inflammation; hyperplasia; and tissue destruction. *Arthritis Res.* 2001. March, 3, 200-2006

[106] Kerr, JR; Petty, R; Burke, B; Gough, J; Fear, D; Sinclair, LI; Mattey, DL; Richards, SC; Montgomery, J; Baldwin, DA; Kellam, P; Harrison, TJ; Griffin, GE; Main, J; Enlander, D; Nutt, DJ; Holgate, ST. Gene expression subtypes in patients with chronic fatigue syndrome/myalgic encephalomyelitis. *J Infect Dis.* 2008 Apr, 197(8), 1171-1184.

[107] Aoki, T; Miyakoshi, H; Usuda, Y; Herberman, RB. Short analytical review: Low NK syndrome and its relationship to chronic fatigue syndrome. *Clin Immunol Immunopathol.* 1993, 69(3), 253-265.

[108] Masuda, A; Nozoe, SI; Matsuyama, T; Tanaka, H. Psychobehavioral and immunological characteristics of adult people with chronic fatigue and patients with chronic fatigue syndrome. *Psychosom Med.* 1994 Nov-Dec, 56(6), 512-8

[109] Maher, KJ; Klimas, NG; Fletcher, MA. Chronic fatigue syndrome is associated with diminished intracellular perforin. *Clin & Exp Immunol* 2005, 142(3), 505-511.

[110] Scott, GB; Meade, JL; Cook, GP. Profiling killers; unravelling the pathways of human natural killer cell function. *Brief Funct Genomic Proteomic.* 2008 Jan, 7(1), 8-16.

[111] Ogawa, M; Nishiuira, T; Yoshimura, M; Horikawa, Y; Yoshida, H; Okajima, Y; Matsumura, I; Ishikawa, J; Nakao, H; Tomiyama, Y; Kanakura, Y; Matsuzawa, Y. Decreased nitric oxide-mediated natural killer cell activation in chronic fatigue syndrome. *European Journal of Clin Investi.* 2006, 28(11), 937-943.

[112] Tsutsui, H; Nakanishi, K; Matsui, K; Higashino, K; Okamura, H; Miyazawa, Y; Kaneda, K. IFN-gamma-inducing factor up-regulates Fas ligand-mediated cytotoxic activity of murine natural killer cell clones. *J. Immunol.* 1996, 157(9), 3967-3973

[113] Saiki, T; Kawai, T; Morita, K; Ohta, M; Saito, T; Rokutan, K; Ban, N. Identification of marker genes for differential diagnosis of chronic fatigue syndrome. *Mol Med.* 2008 Sep-Oct, 14(9-10), 599-607

[114] Lahmers, KK; Hedges, JF; Jutila, MA; Deng, M; Abrahamsen, MS; Brown, WC. Comparative gene expression by WC1$^+$ γδ and CD4$^+$αβ T lymphocytes; which respond to Anaplasma marginale demonstrates higher expression of chemokines and other myeloid cell-associated gene by WC1$^+$ γδ T cells. *J Leuko Biol.* 2006, 80, 939-952.

[115] Madueno, JA; Munzo, E; Blazquez, V; Gonzalez, R; Aparicio, P; Pena, J. The CD26 antigen is copules to protein tyrosine phosphorylation and implicated in CD16-meadiated lysis in natural killer cells. *Scand J Immunol.* 1993, 37(4), 425-429.

[116] Hall, SR; Heffernan, BM; Thompson, NT; Rowan, WC. CD4$^+$CD45RA$^+$ and CD4$^+$CD45RO$^+$ T cells differ in their TCR-associated signalling responses. *Euro J Immunol.* 1999, 29, 2098-2106

[117] Fiorentini, S; Licenziati, S; Alessandri, G; Castelli, F; Caligaris, S; Bonafede, M; Grassi M; Garrafa, E; Balsari, A; Turano, A; Caruso, A. CD11b expression identifies CD8+CD28+ T lymphocytes with phenotype and function of both naïve/memory and effector cells. *J Immunol.* 2001 Jan, 166, 900-907.

[118] Koide, J; Englleman, EG. Differences in surface phenotype and mechanism of action between alloantigen-specific CD8$^+$ cytotoxic and suppressor T cell clones. *J Immunol.* 1990; 144, 32-40.

[119] Freedman, MS; Ruijs, TC; Blain, M; Antel, JP. Phenotypic and functional characteristics of CD8$^+$ cells: a CD11b$^-$CD28$^-$ subset mediates noncytolytic functional suppression. *Clin Immunolo Immunopathol.* 1991, 60, 254-267.

[120] Imada, K; Leonard, WJ. The Jak-STAT pathway. Mol Immunol. 2000 Jan-Feb;37(1-2), 1-11

[121] Whistler, T; Jones, JF; Unger, ER; Vernon, SD. Exercise responsive genes measured in peripheral blood of women with chronic fatigue syndrome and matched control subjects. *BMC Physiol.* 2005 Mar 24, 5(1), 5

[122] Moore, KW; Waal Malefyt, R; Coffman, RL; Garra, A. Interleukin 10 and the interleukin-10 receptor. *Ann Rev Immunol.* 2001, 19, 638-765

[123] Kamimura, D; Ishihara, K; Hirano, T. IL-6 signal transduction and its physiological roles: the signal orchestration model. Rev Physiol Biochem Pharmacol. 2003, 149, 1-38.

[124] Kristiansen, OP; Mandrup-Poulsen, T. Interleukin-6 and Diabetes the good; the bad; or the indifferent? *Diabetes.* 2005, 54, S114-S124.

[125] Rawlings, JS; Rosler, KM; Harrison, DA. The JAK/STAT signalling pathway. *J Cell Sci.* 2004, 117, 1281-1283

[126] Guschin, D; Rogers, N; Briscoe, J; Witthuhn, B; Watling, D; Horn, F; Pellegrini, S; Yasukawa, K; Heinrich, P; Stark, GR; Kerr, IM. A major role for the protein tyrosine kinase JAK1 in JAK/STAT signal transduction pathway in response to interleukin-6. *EMBO J.* 1995, 14, 1421-1429

[127] Dinarello, CA. Proinflammatory Cytokines. *Chest.* 2000, 118, 503-508

[128] Gao, J; Killedar, S; Cornelius, JG; Nguyen, C; Cha, S; Peck, AB. Sjögren's syndrome in the NOD mouse model is an interleukin-4 time-dependent; antibody isotype-specific autoimmune disease. *J Autoimmun.* 2006 Mar, 26(2), 90-103

[129] Powell, R; Ren, J; Lewith, G; Barclay, W; Holgate, S; Almond, J. Identification of novel expressed sequences; up-regulated in leucocytes of chronic fatigue syndrome patients. *Clin Exp Allergy.* 2003 Oct, 33(10), 1450-1456.

[130] Kaushik, N; Fear, D; Richards, SC; McDermott, CR; Nuwaysir, EF; Kellam, P; Harrison, TJ; Wilkinson, RJ; Tyrrell, DA; Holgate, ST; Kerr, JR. Gene expression in peripheral blood mononuclear cells from patients with chronic fatigue syndrome. *J Clin Pathol.* 2005, 58(8), 826-832

[131] Vernon, SD; Shukla, SK; Conradt, J; Unger, ER; Reeves, WC. Analysis of 16S rRNA gene sequences and circulating cell-free DNA from plasma of chronic fatigue syndrome and non-fatigued subjects. *BMC Microbiol.* 2002 Dec 23, 2, 39

[132] Yamamoto, M.; Yamazaki, S.; Uematsu, S.; Sato, S.; Hemmi, H.; Hocino, K.; Kaisho, T.; Kuwata, H; Takeuchi, O; Takeshige, K. Regulation of Toll/IL-1 receptor-mediated gene expression by the inducible nuclear protein IkappaBzeta. *Nature.* 2004, 430, 218-222.

[133] Beinke, S; Ley, SC. Functions of NF-κB1 and NF-κB2 in immune cell biology. *J Biochem.* 2004, 382, 393-409.

[134] Inoue, A.; Omoto, Y; Yamaguchi, Y; Kiyama, R; Hayashi, SI. Transcription factor EGR3 is envolved in the estrogen-signaling pathway in breast cancer cells. *J Mol Endocrinol.* 2004 Jun, 32(3), 649-661.

[135] Kuwahara, I; Lillehoj, EP; Lu, W; Singh, I; Isohama, Y; Miyata, T; Kim, KC. Neutrophil elastase induces IL-8 gene transcription and protein release through p38/NF-κB activation via EGFR transactivation in a lung epithelial cell line. *Am J Physiol Lung Cell Mol Physiol.* 2006 Sep, 291(3), L407-L416

[136] Yung, R; Mo, R; Grolleau-Julius, A; Hoeltzel, M. The effect of aging and caloric restrictioin in murine CD8⁺T cell chemokine receptor gene expression. *Immun Ageing.* 2007 Nov, 4, 8

[137] Renshaw, SA; Parmar, JS; Singleton, V; Rowe, SJ; Dockrell, DH; Dower, SK; Bingle, CD; Chilvers, ER; Whyte, MK. Acceleration of human neutrophil apoptosis by TRAIL. *J Immunol.* 2003 Jan 15, 170(2), 1027-33

[138] Zhang, X; Brunner, T; Carter, L; Dutton, RW; Rogers, P; Bradley, L; Sato, T; Reed, JC; Green, D; Swain, SL. Unequal death in T helper cell (Th)1 and Th2 effectors: Th1 but not Th2; effectors undergo rapid Fas/FasL-mediated apoptosis. *J Exp Med.* 1997, 185, 1837-1849

[139] Jurevic, RJ; Bai, M; Chadwick, RB; White, TC; Dale, BA. Single-nucleotide polymorphisms (SNPs) in human beta-defensin 1, high-throughput SNP assays and association with Candida carriage in type I diabetics and nondiabetic controls. *J Clin Microbiol.* 2003 Jan, 41(1), 90-6.

[140] Gil, A; María Aguilera, C; Gil-Campos, M; Cañete, R. Altered signalling and gene expression associated with the immune system and the inflammatory response in obesity. *Br J Nutr.* 2007 Oct, 98 Suppl 1, S121-6.

[141] Sarfati, M; Fortin, G; Raymond, M; Susin, S. CD47 in the immune response: role of thrombosponding and SIRP-alpha reverse signaling. *Curr Drug Targets.* 2008 Oct, 9(10), 842-50

[142] Barrow Alexander David, 1; Trowsdale; John. The extended human leukocyte receptor complex: diverse ways of modulating immune responses. *Immunol Rev.* 2008 Aug, 224(1), 98-123.

[143] Heinze, M; Kofler, M; Freund, C. Investigating the functional role of CD2BP2 in T cells. *Int Immunol.* 2007 Nov, 19(11), 1313-8

[144] Clark, GJ; Rao, M; Ju, X; Hart, DN. Novel human CD4⁺ T lymphocyte subpopulations defined by CD300a/c molecule expression. *J Leukoc Biol.* 2007 Nov;82(5), 1126-35

[145] Deane, JA; Fruman, DA. Phosphoinositide 3-kinase: diverse roles in immune cell activation. 2004, 22, 563-98

[146] Gahmberg, CG; Valmu, L; Tian, L; Kotovuori, P; Fagerholm, S; Kotovuori, A; Kantor, C; Hilden, T. Leukocyte adhesion- a funfamental process in leukocyte physiology. *Braz J Med Biol Res.* 1999 May, 32(5), 511-7

[147] Rosenkilde, MM; Benned-Jensen, T; Andersen, H; Holst, PJ; Kledal, TN; Luttichau, HR; Larsen, JK; Christensen, JP; Schwartz, TW. Molecular pharmacological phenotyping

[148] Metzger, K; Frémont, M; Roelant, C; De Meirleir, K. Lower frequency of IL-17F sequence variant (His161Arg) in chronic fatigue syndrome patients. *Biochem Biophys Res Commun.* 2008 Nov 7, 376(1), 231-3.

[149] Harrington, LE; Hatton, RD; Mangan, PR; Turner, H; Murphy, TL; Murphy, KM; Weaver, CT. Interleukin 17-producing CD4+ effector T cells develop via a lineage

distinct from the T helper type 1 and 2 lineages. *Nat Immunol*. 2005 Nov, 6(11), 1123-32.

[150] Park, H; Li, Z; Yang, XO; Chang, SH; Nurieva, R; Wang, YH; Wang, Y; Hood, L; Zhu, Z; Tian, Q; Dong, C. A distinct lineage of CD4 T cells regulates tissue inflammation by producing interleukin 17. *Nat Immunol*. 2005 Nov, 6(11), 1133-41.

[151] Demitrack, MA; Dale, JK; Straus, SE. Laue, L; Listwak, SJ; Kruesi, MJ; Chrousos, GP; Gold, PW. Evidence for impaired activation of the hypothalamic-pituitary-adrenal axis in patients with chronic fatigue syndrome. *Clin Endocrinol Metab*. 1991, 73, 1224-1234.

[152] Jerjes, WK; Taylor, NF; Peters, TJ; Wessely, S; Cleare, AJ. Urinary cortisol and cortisol metabolite excretion in chronic fatigue syndrome. *Psychosom Med*. 2006 Jul-Aug, 68(4), 578-82

[153] Rajeevan, MS; Smith, AK; Dimulescu, I; Unger, ER; Vernon, SD; Heim, C; Reeves, WC. Glucocorticoid receptor polymorphisms and haplotypes associated with chronic fatigue syndrome. *Genes Brain Behav*. 2008, 6(2), 167-176.

[154] Blalock, JE. The syntax of immune-neuroendocrine communication. *Immunol Today*. 1994 Nov;15(11), 504-11

[155] Wilder, RL. Neuroendocrine-immune system interactions and autoimmunity. *Annu Rev Immunol*. 1995, 13, 307-38'

[156] Di Giorgio, A; Hudson, M; Jerjes, W; Cleare, AJ. 24-hour pituitary and adrenal hormone profiles in chronic fatigue syndrome. *Psychosom Med*. 2005 May-Jun, 67(3), 433-40

[157] Altemus, M; Dale, JK; Michelson, D; Demitrack, MA; Gold, PW; Straus, SE. Abnormalities in response to vasopressin infusion in chronic fatigue syndrome. *Psychoneuroendocrinology*. 2001 Feb, 26(2), 175-88.

[158] Scott, LV; Medbak, S; Dinan, TG. The low dose ACTH test in chronic fatigue syndrome and in health. *Clin Endocrinol (Oxf)*. 1998 Jun, 48(6), 733-7.

[159] Scott LV; Dinan TG. The neuroendocrinology of chronic fatigue syndrome: focus on the hypothalamic-pituitary-adrenal axis. *Funct Neurol*. 1999 Jan-Mar, 14(1), 3-11.

[160] Kavelaars, A; Kuis, W; Knook, L; Sinnema, G; Heijnen, CJ. Disturbed neuroendocrine-immune interactions in chronic fatigue syndrome. *J Clin Endocrinol Metab*. 2000 Feb, 85(2), 692-6.

[161] Visser, JT; De Kloet, ER; Nagelkerken, L. Altered glucocorticoid regulation of the immune response in the chronic fatigue syndrome. *Ann N Y Acad Sci*. 2000, 917, 868-75.

[162] Gaab, J; Hüster, D; Peisen, R; Engert, V; Heitz, V; Schad, T; Schürmeyer, T; Ehlert, U. Assessment of cortisol response with low-dose and high-dose ACTH in patients with chronic fatigue syndrome and healthy comparison subjects. *Psychosomatics*. 2003. Mar-Apr, 44(2), 113-9.

[163] Gerrity, TR; Papanicolaou, DA; Amsterdam, JD; Bingham, S; Grossman, A; Hedrick, T; Herberman, RB; Krueger, G; Levine, S; Mohagheghpour, N; Moore, RC; Oleske, J; Snell, CR; CFIDS Association of America. Immunologic aspects of chronic fatigue syndrome. Report on a Research Symposium convened by The CFIDS Association of

America and co-sponsored by the US Centers for Disease Control and Prevention and the National Institutes of Health. *Neuroimmunomodulation*. 2004,11(6), 351-7

[164] Moorkens, G; Berwaerts, J; Wynants, H; Abs, R. Characterization of pituitary function with emphasis on GH secretion in the Chronic Fatigue Syndrome. *Clin Endocrinol.* 2000, 53, 99-106

[165] Spence, VA; Khan, F; Kennedy, G; Abbot, NC; Belch, JJF. Acetylcholine mediated vasodilatation in the microcirculation of patients with chronic fatigue syndrome. *Prostaglandins Leukot Essent Fatty Acids* 2004, 70, 403-407

[166] Graber, JJ. Dhib-Jalbut, S. 2008. Protective autoimmunity in the nervous system. Pharmacology and therapeutics; [Epub ahead of print]

[167] Natelson, BH; Weaver, SA; Tseng, CL; Ottenweller, JE. Spinal fluid abnormalities in patients with chronic fatigue syndrome. *Clin Diagn Lab Immunol.* 2005 Jan, 12(1), 52-5.

In: Chronic Fatigue Syndrome: Symptoms, Causes & Prevention   ISBN: 978-1-60741-493-3
Editor: E. Svoboda and K. Zelenjcik, pp. 27-56   © 2010 Nova Science Publishers, Inc.

Chapter 2

The NO/ONOO-Vicious Cycle Mechanism as the Cause of Chronic Fatigue Syndrome/Myalgic Encephalomyelitis

Martin L. Pall[*]

Professor Emeritus of Biochemistry and Basic Medical Sciences, Washington State
University, and Research Director,
The Tenth Paradigm Research Group Washington, USA

Abstract

Cases of chronic fatigue syndrome/mylagic encephalomyelitis (CFS) are reported to be initiated by nine different short-term stressors, each of which increases levels of nitric oxide in the body.   Elevated nitric oxide, acting through its oxidant product, peroxynitrite, initiates a local biochemical vicious cycle, the NO/ONOO- cycle, which is proposed to be the cause of CFS and related diseases. Evidence supporting this cycle mechanism in CFS comes from each of the following types of evidence: Case initiation by such stressors, the extensive evidence supporting the existence of individual cycle mechanisms, evidence showing that various cycle elements are elevated in CFS cases, evidence for a basically local mechanism in CFS and related diseases, evidence from CFS animal models, genetic evidence from genetic polymorphism studies and evidence from clinical trials of agents predicted to down-regulate the NO/ONOO-cycle. Each of the five principles underlying the NO/ONOO- cycle mechanism is supported by one or more of the above described types of evidence. The cycle involves oxidative stress, excessive nitric oxide synthase (NOS) activity, mitochondrial dysfunction, inflammatory biochemistry, excitotoxicity including excessive NMDA activity and tetrahydrobiopterin depletion. There is evidence, ranging from extensive to modest, supporting roles for each of these in CFS.

Clinical studies of treatment protocols containing 14 or more agents predicted to down-regulate the NO/ONOO- cycle appear to be effective in the treatment of CFS and

[*] E-mail: martin_pall@wsu.edu; Tel: 503-232-3883

related diseases. However, none of these has yet been shown to be able to cure substantial numbers of cases of CFS or related illnesses. The author discusses one such protocol and suggests an approach, previously tested only as a single agent treatment, that may strenthen these multi-agent protocols to obtain at least some of the needed cures.

Introduction

Chronic fatigue syndrome (CFS) and such related multisystem illnesses as multiple chemical sensitivity (MCS), fibromyalgia (FM) and post-traumatic stress disorder (PTSD) are all thought to be caused by a biochemical vicious cycle mechanism now called the NO/ONOO- cycle [1-14]. Cases of these illnesses are initiated by any of several diverse short-term stressors, each of which has the ability to increase nitric oxide levels in the body [1,6,9,13], Table 1.

Cases of CFS are most commonly initiated by viral or bacterial infections, with the viruses including coxsackie, Epstein-Barr, rubella, varicella, parvovirus, Borna and Ross River viruses [1,4]. West Nile virus should probably be added to this list, since substantial numbers of severe infections with that virus are reported to develop chronic CFS-like symptoms [15]. Such initiating stressors as viral, bacterial and protozoan infections and also exposure to ionizing radiation act to increase nitric oxide levels by inducing the inducible nitric oxide synthase, iNOS [1,4,13], whereas each of the stressors that initiate cases of MCS (Table 1) as well as some others [1,10], act via increased NMDA activity which acts, in turn, through calcium-dependent stimulation of nNOS and eNOS activity. So the common feature is not the specific nitric oxide synthase (NOS) isozyme involved, let alone the pathway of such NOS stimulation, but rather the consequent increase in nitric oxide. The consequent chronic illness initiated by such largely short-term nitric oxide level increases is thought to be produced by the NO/ONOO- cycle (Figure 1), a cycle that may be initiated largely via peroxynitrite, a potent oxidant formed by the diffusion-limited reaction of nitric oxide and superoxide (OO·-) [1,4,6,10].

Each of the arrows diagrammed in Figure 1 represents one or more mechanisms by which one of the elements of the cycle produces increases in another such element [1,6]. The combination of these mechanisms produces, therefore, a series of interacting cycles that is known as the NO/ONOO- cycle, based on the structure of nitric oxide (NO) and peroxynitrite (ONOO-), pronounced no, oh no! Other elements of the cycle include superoxide, oxidative stress (an imbalance between oxidants and antioxidants), intracellular calcium levels, NF-κB activity (an important transcription factor stimulated by both oxidants (including peroxynitrite and many free radicals) and by intracellular calcium, certain inflammatory cytokines shown in the upper right corner box, iNOS, nNOS and eNOS activity and various mechanisms increasing superoxide levels (Figure 1.) [see ref. 1,6]. In addition, certain receptors occurring in neuronal and also some non-neuronal cells, the vanilloid (TRPV1) receptors and the NMDA receptors are thought to have important roles, as well [1-3,6,10,12]. There are 22 distinct mechanisms proposed to be involved in these arrows, of which 19 are well accepted, established biochemistry and physiology [1]. Of the other three, the actions of nitric oxide and peroxynitrite on the electron transport chain of the mitochondrion and the action of oxidants in increasing TRPV1 activity, these three are now considerably better documented [10] then they were when the Figure 1. cycle was previously proposed [1,6]. Furthermore, other members of the TRP receptor family, including the TRPA1 receptors and TRPM2 receptors are also stimulated by correlates of oxidative stress [10], suggesting that they may play similar roles, as well.

Consequently, it may be seen from the above, that there is a massive amount of evidence supporting the specific mechanisms of the NO/ONOO- cycle diagrammed in Figure 1 and the only thing that is truly original is the assumption that these mechanisms fit together in the way one might assume when placing them into juxtaposition with each other.

Despite the complexity of the Figure 1 cycle diagram, there are two distinct parts of the NO/ONOO- cycle that are not apparent from it [1,2,10,13]:

1. There are several specific mechanisms that produce mitochondrial/energy metabolism dysfunction. These include the attack by peroxynitrite on several important mitochondrial proteins, acting by disrupting iron-sulfur clusters and by nitration of tyrosine residues; stimulation of poly ADP-ribosylation of chromosomal proteins by peroxynitrite-generated single strand nicks in DNA, leading in turn to depletion of NAD/NADH pools; oxidation of cardiolipin molecules in the inner mitochondrial membrane, initiated by elevated superoxide levels in the mitochondrion, leading in turn to lowered complex I, III and IV activity; inhibition of cytochrome oxidase (complex IV) activity by nitric oxide. Each of these will produce lowered oxygen utilization in the tissues, something reported to occur in CFS. Such mitochondrial/energy metabolism dysfunction will act as part of the NO/ONOO- cycle by increasing NMDA activity and probably by increasing intracellular calcium levels, with the latter being a consequence of lowered calcium-ATP activity, an activity essential to the lowering of intracellular calcium levels.

2. Peroxynitrite oxidizes a compound known as tetrahydrobiopterin (BH4), a compound that acts as a cofactor for the nitric oxide synthases and also has a role in the production of catecholamines and serotonin/melatonin. The consequent BH4 deficiency produces a partial uncoupling of the nitric oxide synthases, such that uncoupled enzymes generate superoxide instead of nitric oxide [13]. Such BH4 depletion in tissues with high NOS activity will produce adjacent NOS enzymes generating nitric oxide and superoxide which will react rapidly with each other to form more peroxynitrite. This may serve as an inner vicious cycle within the larger NO/ONOO- cycle, such that increasing BH4 levels and lowering peroxynitrite levels may be essential to effectively treating NO/ONOO- cycle diseases by down-regulating the NO/ONOO- cycle.

The elevated peroxynitrite/BH4 depletion couplet will be expected to lower nitric oxide levels while increasing peroxynitrite levels. It follows that agents that lower this couplet activity, may actually increase nitric oxide levels while producing clinical improvements in the patients [13]. It is even possible that the action of this couplet may produce NO/ONOO-cycle illnesses where the whole body production of nitric oxide may not be elevated in comparison with controls. The two published studies of nitric oxide production in CFS support the view that such production is elevated but that is not necessarily predicted to occur in all NO/ONOO- cycle diseases.

A diagram containing these additional aspects of the cycle is shown in Figure 2. We have here the reciprocal interactions between peroxynitrite (abbreviated PRN) and BH4 depletion. Also the depletion of ATP pools and its roles in the cycle are diagrammed as well. In the upper left hand corner, it is suggested that not only the TRPV1 (vanilloid) receptor has a role here, but other member of the transfer receptor potential (TRP) family including TRPA1 and TRPM2 may have roles as well [9,10].

Five Principles

There are five principles underlying the NO/ONOO- cycle mechanism, the first two of which have already been discussed [taken from the authors web site and also refs. 1,6,10]:

1. Cases can be initiated by short-term stressors that increase nitric oxide and/or other cycle elements.
2. The chronic phase of illness is produced by the NO/ONOO- cycle. It is predicted, therefore, that the cycle elements will be elevated in the chronic phase of illness.
3. The symptoms and signs of illness must be generated by one or more elements of the cycle.
4. The basic mechanism of the cycle is local and will be localized to different tissues in different individuals. The reason for this primarily local nature is that the three compounds involved, nitric oxide, superoxide and peroxynitrite, have limited half lives in biological tissues. And the mechanisms of the cycle, those various arrows, act at the level of individual cells. This allows for great variations tissue distribution from one patient to another, producing a huge spectrum of illness. The point here is not that there are no systemic changes – clearly antioxidant depletion, neuroendocrine and immune system changes and actions of some inflammatory cytokines will be systemic. But rather this primarily local nature gives much inherent variation due to the tissue localization of the basic mechanism [see Chapter 4 ref.1]. A correlate of the local basic nature of the cycle is that different NO/ONOO- cycle diseases will differ from one another in what tissue or tissues must be impacted by the cycle in order to be diagnosed as a specific cycle-caused disease.

5. NO/ONOO- cycle diseases should be treated by down-regulating the NO/ONOO- cycle biochemistry, rather than by symptomatic relief. In other words, we should treat the cause, rather than the symptoms.

These five principles are important in three distinct ways. Firstly, they collectively produce an essentially complete model of any NO/ONOO- cycle disease. Secondly, the fit to each of the five principles for a particular disease or illness provides a distinct type of evidence for the causality of the cycle. Such diverse evidence for causality, such as may be provided by the fit to all five principles, is essential to provide a robust structure of evidence, suggesting that the cycle is the cause of a specific disease. Accordingly, the third important way in which the five principles are important is as follows: The fit to each of the five serves as a criterion for deciding whether a specific disease/illness is a good candidate for inclusion under the NO/ONOO- cycle paradigm. As such, the five principles function for the NO/ONOO- cycle a bit like Koch's postulates function for possible infectious diseases.

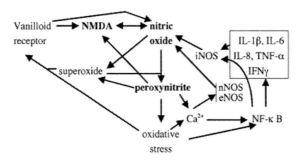

Figure 1. Vicious (NO/ONOO-) cycle diagram. Each arrow represents one or more mechanisms by which the variable at the foot of the arrow can stimulate the level of the variable at the head of the arrow. It can be seen that these arrows form a series of loops that can potentially continue to stimulate each other. An example of this would be that nitric oxide can increase peroxynitrite which can stimulate oxidative stress which can stimulate NF-□ B which can increase the production of iNOS which can, in turn increase nitric oxide. This loop alone constitutes a potential vicious cycle and there are a number of other loops, diagrammed in the figure that can collectively make up a much larger vicious cycle. The challenge, according to this view, in these illnesses is to lower this whole pattern of elevations to get back into a normal range. You will note that the cycle not only includes the compounds nitric oxide, superoxide and peroxynitrite but a series of other elements, including the transcription factor NF-□ B, oxidative stress, inflammatory cytokines (in box, upper right), the three different forms of the enzymes that make nitric oxide (the nitric oxide synthases iNOS, nNOS and eNOS), and two neurological receptors the vanilloid (TRPV1) receptor and the NMDA receptor. The figure and legend are taken from the author's web site with permission.

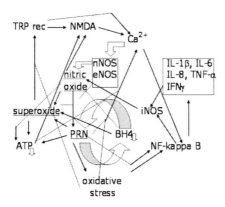

Figure 2. A more complete NO/ONOO- cycle diagram. Central to the figure are the reciprocal interactions between peroxynitrite, abbreviated as PRN and tetrahydrobiopterin (BH4) depletion. Also indicated is the ATP depletion produced by peroxynitrite, superoxide and nitric oxide. And in the upper left corner, TRP represents the three TRP receptors, TRPV1, TRPA1 and TRPM2, each of which is stimulated via distinct mechanisms by oxidative stress. Each arrow in the figure represents one or more mechanisms by which one element of the cycle stimulates another element of the cycle. Figure and legend is taken from the author's web site with permission.

CFS and the First Two Principles

We've already discussed the first principle and how it fits well for CFS. Each of the nine short-term stressors implicated in the initiation of cases of CFS (Table 1) can increase the levels of nitric oxide in regions of the body impacted by them. So we have a very good fit for the first principle.

To look for fit to the second principle, we must look for where the various elements of the cycle have been studied in CFS. CFS has been extensively reported in 13 different studies to have elevated markers of oxidative stress [reviewed in 1,14,16] and two additional such studies have been reported more recently [17,18], clearly showing that oxidative stress is one of the most extensively documented properties of CFS. It also has extensive evidence for mitochondrial dysfunction [reviewed in 1,4], leading to lowered oxygen utilization in the tissues [19-21] and lactate accumulation in the cerebrospinal fluid [22].

One specific mechanism described above for the mitochondrial dysfunction, is the generation of cardiolipin oxidation by elevated superoxide levels in the mitochondrion and there is evidence that this occurs in CFS. Hokama and his colleagues [23,24] have reported that a ciguatera epitope occurs in the blood of people with CFS and some other diseases and has also reported that the same epitope occurs in commercial grade cardiolipin [24]. Such commercial grade cardiolipin is almost certainly highly oxidized because cardiolipin contains essentially all highly oxidizable linoleic acid residues, suggesting that the ciguatera epitope is none other than a peroxidation product of cardiolipin. It may be inferred from these observations that CFS patients probably have elevated levels of superoxide in the mitochondria, leading to elevated cardiolipin peroxidation.

There are two studies, one of them my own, reporting that nitric oxide levels are elevated in CFS [25,26]. The importance of this is emphasized by the apparent clinical responses to the potent nitric oxide scavenger, the form of vitamin B_{12} known as hydroxocobalamin [1,11,27].

There have been multiple studies reporting elevated levels of inflammatory cytokines in CFS [reviewed in refs. 1,4,28]. I discuss further evidence, below, for an important causal role for inflammatory responses in CFS from animal model studies, from the effectiveness of an antiinflammatory therapeutic agent and from gene expression studies.

There are clinical observations strongly suggesting that there is excessive excitotoxicity in CFS, including excessive NMDA activity [26,29-31]. In the closely related diseases, FM and MCS, the evidence for excessive NMDA activity is much more extensive [reviewed in 1,4,6,10].

Two recent studies have reported elevated NF-κB activity in CFS, while mistakenly calling it NF-kappa beta [32,33]. These two studies ascribed the induction of iNOS and certain inflammatory cytokines to increased NF-κB activity, as I had done much earlier [4]. And while TRPV1 activity has not been studied in CFS, it has been shown to be elevated in MCS as well as the comorbid illness irritable bowel syndrome [reviewed in 1,9,10].

And, finally although BH4 depletion has not been studied directly in CFS, there is evidence that will be discussed below that agents known to be able to help restore BH4 pools, are helpful in the therapy of CFS. Furthermore autism patients, which many have argued are similar to CFS patients, have been shown in three clinical trials to be helped by BH4 nutritional supplements [reviewed in chapter 14, ref. 1].

Table 1: The stressors implicated in the initiation of these illnesses are summarized.
Illness Stressors Implicated in Initiation of Illness

Chronic fatigue syndrome	**Viral infection, bacterial infection, organophosphorus pesticide exposure**, carbon monoxide exposure, ciguatoxin poisoning, physical trauma, severe psychological stress, toxoplasmosis (protozoan) infection, ionizing radiation exposure
Multiple chemical sensitivity	**Volatile organic solvent exposure, organophosphorus/carbamate pesticide exposure**, organochlorine pesticide exposure, pyrethroid exposure; hydrogen sulfide; carbon monoxide; mercury
Fibromyalgia	**Physical trauma (particularly head and neck trauma), viral infection**, bacterial infection, severe psychological stress, pre-existing autoimmune disease
Post-traumatic stress disorder	**Severe psychological stress**, physical (head) trauma

Animal Models

There are limited animal model studies of CFS and these also have shown elevation of certain NO/ONOO- cycle elements.

A mouse model of CFS is initiated to apparent fatigue by treatment with a bacterial extract [34-36] that increases nitric oxide levels [37,38]. It is characterized by elevated inflammatory cytokines [34,35] and also mitochondrial dysfunction in regions of the brain [36]. Other apparent CFS animal models also implicated increased inflammatory cytokines [39,40].

In another mouse model of CFS, chronic fatigue was correlated with elevated markers of oxidative stress [41-43]. A number of antioxidants were found to be useful in treatment [41-43], suggesting that oxidative stress has a substantial causal role.

Thus the available data on these animal models properties appear to be consistent with a NO/ONOO- cycle mechanism.

Genetic Studies

Genes that produce an increased susceptibility for a disease can often provide very useful information regarding possible biological mechanism. Several such studies have been published on CFS, so it is important to look at them to determine whether they are consistent with the NO/ONOO- cycle mechanism. Let's look at the various examples of genetic roles with this question in mind.

Studies of an Australian family by Torpy and coworkers have shown that a gene for defective cortisol binding protein causes a strong predisposition for developing CFS [44-46]. It was also associated with orthostatic intolerance, a common correlate of CFS and related illnesses. Defective cortisol binding protein is expected to produce a lowered ability to respond to cortisol. A study of genes influencing the hypothalamic-pituitary adrenal axis, which may act through changed cortisol production, were also found to influence the prevalence of unexplained chronic fatigue [47]. Since cortisol and other glucocorticoids are known to lower the induction of iNOS [reviewed in 4], these studies are consistent with a role for nitric oxide in initiating cases of CFS. A role for cortisol is also supported by a recent study of single nucleotide polymorphisms in the glucocorticoid receptor gene [48], where several such alleles were associated with increased risk for CFS.

Alleles of a serotonin transporter gene producing increased serotonin transport and therefore lowered extracellular serotonin was also found to produce increased susceptibility to developing CFS [49]. The authors suggested that this polymorphism may act to produce lowered cortisol production [49]. The serotonin receptor HTR2A was implicated in CFS, because the promoter region polymorphism, -1438G/A was associated with increased prevalence of CFS and also unexplained fatigue [50]. However the interpretation for this is unclear because the data on whether this polymorphism produces increased or decreased promoter activity is mixed [50]. So at this point, it is difficult to interpret the serotonin related genetic activity for CFS.

Vladutiu and Natelson [51] found a polymorphism in the angiotensin converting enzyme (ACE) that was associated with unexplained fatigue in the Gulf War veterans. ACE is known to act by generating angiotensin II. Angiotensin II is known to act to produce tetrahydrobiopterin (BH4) depletion [52-54], leading to partial uncoupling of the nitric oxide synthases and increased superoxide production [52-54]. Thus this study provides some support for a role for two elements of the NO/ONOO- cycle, BH4 depletion and superoxide.

Carlo-Stella et al. [55] reported that pro-inflammatory alleles in the TNF-α gene and the IFN-γ gene were associated with CFS. Metzger et al. [56] reported that a pro-inflammatory allele in the IL-17 gene was also associated with CFS. Both of these studies, then, implicate inflammatory responses as having causal roles in CFS, and ref.55 implicates two specific inflammatory cytokines suggested to be involved in the NO/ONOO- cycle.

Boles and coworkers [57,58] have shown that maternally inherited mitochondrial mutations can produce CFS or, at least, CFS-like symptoms, along with a much broader spectrum of symptoms. These results suggest that mitochondrial/energy metabolism dysfunction can have a causal role in producing CFS, another observation compatible with the the NO/ONOO- cycle mechanism.

Another observation that may also be compatible with a role of energy metabolism, is that Ehlers-Danlos syndrome may play a causal role in cases of CFS and orthostatic intolerance [59]. Ehlers-Danlos is a genetic defect in the structure of collagen and many cases of Ehlers-Danlos syndrome produce vascular dysfunction and therefore possible tissue hypoxia and deficient oxidative phosphorylation [59-61]. It follows that this observation may possibly be interpreted as being due to a role of normal energy metabolism in preventing cases of CFS.

In summary, then, the various genetic studies provide evidence for an important role of such NO/ONOO- cycle elements as inflammatory biochemistry, mitochondrial/energy metabolism dysfunction and BH4 depletion and consequent increased superoxide production. The role of cortisol can be interpreted as being due to the role of cortisol in limiting iNOS induction and may act in this way to influence another cycle element. So these observations seem to be quite compatible with a NO/ONOO- cycle mechanism, although we clearly need considerably more study of the genetics of CFS.

Generation of Shared Symptoms and Signs

The third principle of the NO/ONOO- cycle is that symptoms or signs of illness must each be generated by one or more elements of the cycle.

Table 2. Explanations for Symptoms and Signs

Symptom/Sign	Explanation based on elevated nitric oxide/peroxynitrite theory
energy metabolism /mitochondrial dysfunction	Inactivation of several proteins in the mitochondrion by peroxynitrite; inhibition of some mitochondrial enzymes by nitric oxide and superoxide; NAD/NADH depletion; cardiolipin oxidation
oxidative stress	Peroxynitrite, superoxide and other oxidants
PET scan changes	Energy metabolism dysfunction leading to change transport of probe; changes in perfusion by nitric oxide, peroxynitrite and isoprostanes; increased neuronal activity in short-term response to chemical exposure
SPECT scan changes	Depletion of reduced glutathione by oxidative stress; perfusion changes as under PET scan changes
Low NK cell function	Superoxide and other oxidants acting to lower NK cell function
Other immune dysfunction	Sensitivity to oxidative stress; chronic inflammatory cytokine elevation
Elevated cytokines	NF-κB stimulating of the activity of inflammatory cytokine genes
Anxiety	Excessive NMDA activity in the amygdala
Depression	Elevated nitric oxide leading to depression; cytokines and NMDA increases acting in part or in whole via nitric oxide.
Rage	Excessive NMDA activity in the periaqueductal gray region of the midbrain
Cognitive/learn-ing and memory dysfunction	Lowered energy metabolism in the brain, which is very susceptible to such changes; excessive NMDA activity and nitric oxide levels and their effects of learning and memory
Multiorgan pain	All components of cycle have a role, acting in part through nitric oxide and cyclic GMP elevation
Fatigue	Energy metabolism dysfunction
Sleep disturbance	Sleep impacted by inflammatory cytokines, NF-κB activity and nitric oxide
Orthostatic intolerance	Two mechanisms: Nitric oxide-mediated vasodilation leading to blood pooling in the lower body; nitric oxide-mediated sympathetic nervous system dysfunction
Irritable bowel syndrome	Sensitivity and other changes produced by excessive vanilloid and NMDA activity, increased nitric oxide
Intestinal permeabilization leading to food allergies	Permeabilization produced by excessive nitric oxide, inflammatory cytokines, NF-κB activity and peroxynitrite; peroxynitrite acts in part by stimulating poly(ADP)-ribose polymerase activity

Taken from the author's web site with permission. It should be noted that while each of these are plausible mechanisms and, in most cases well-documented mechanisms under some pathophysiological circumstances, in most cases their role in generating these symptoms in these multisystem illnesses is not established.

Many symptoms and signs of CFS are also shared by other multisystem illnesses proposed to also be NO/ONOO- cycle diseases, notably fibromyalgia, multiple chemical sensitivity and post-traumatic stress disorder. A list of such shared symptoms and signs, along with plausible mechanisms by which they may be generated by cycle elements, is shown in Table 2. One point should be emphasized – these are plausible mechanisms not established mechanisms in CFS.

Specific Signs and Symptoms for CFS and Where to Look for a Specific Biomarker Test

According to the NO/ONOO- cycle model, the difference between one NO/ONOO- cycle disease/illness and another, lies in the tissue or tissues that must be impacted by the cycle in order to meet the diagnostic criteria for that specific disease. An example of such specific tissue involvement may be found in FM, where it appears likely that the thalamus must be impacted in order to generate the widespread excessive pain that is the most characteristic symptom in FM [1,6].

What is the critical tissue that must be impacted in CFS and what impact does such impact have? I don't know the answer to the first part of this question but I do think I know the answer to the second part. The most characteristic symptom in CFS is thought to be what has been called post-exertional malaise [62-64]. Here, all of the symptoms of CFS are increased following excessive exercise. So the thing that is most characteristic of CFS is the inability to deal effectively with exercise and possibly certain other stressors. This also suggests that in order to develop a specific biomarker test for CFS, we should not look to the various systemic biochemical changes which may be in common with many other diseases, but rather we should look to one or more differences in response to exercise.

When I was discussing this issue with Dr. Paul Cheney, he suggested that the differences he sees with his CFS patients in response to exercise is their cortisol response. When normal people exercise, their cortisol levels go up [65,66]. This is not surprising, given that cortisol is used in the body to adjust to quite a number of stressors. What Cheney told me is that when his CFS patients exercise, cortisol levels either stay the same or drop. Similar cortisol responses to exercise in CFS patients have been reported by Ottenweller et al. [67], suggesting this may be a common, possibly universal feature of CFS patients.

It should be noted that hypothalamic-pituitary-adrenal axis dysfunction occurs in CFS, FM, MCS and PTSD, all proposed NO/ONOO- cycle diseases, as well as in many other chronic inflammatory diseases [Chapter 3 in ref. 1], so some changes in the control of cortisol release are not specific for CFS. These may, rather, reflect some aberration produced by oxidative stress or some other general correlate of these diseases. However, there is some published evidence, that CFS may have a more specific change in cortisol regulation not found in FM patients [68-70].

It may be argued that because of the role of cortisol and other glucocorticoids in lowering iNOS induction, as discussed above, that the failure to up-regulate cortisol levels following exercise may lead to an inappropriate increase in iNOS levels, leading in turn to increased nitric oxide levels and NO/ONOO- cycle activity. In this way, the across the board increase in symptoms in CFS patients following exercise ("post-exertional malaise"), may be explained as a consequence of the up-regulation of the basic mechanism causing CFS.

An up-regulation of the NO/ONOO- cycle biochemistry in response to exercise may explain the observations of Melvin Ramsay in his pioneering observations on CFS. Ramsay reported that those who persist in working after coming down with CFS until they collapse have the poorest prognosis [71]. Somewhat similarly, Harvey et al. [72] suggested that "Continuing to be active despite increasing fatigue may be a crucial step in the development of CFS." A possible causal relationship between hypocortisol responses in CFS and post-exertional malaise was proposed by Baschetti et al. [73], who reviewed several studies of cortisol control in CFS. Baschetti et al. [73] also noted that many people diagnosed on the Oxford criteria do not have the hypocortisol response to exercise and therefore may not have true chronic fatigue syndrome.

These considerations suggest that a search for specific biomarker tests for CFS, should focus on changes in response to exercise that may be specific for CFS patients, that is not shared either by normals or by others suffering from different diseases. There have been a number of studies showing that in addition to cortisol, CFS patients respond to exercise in ways that are different from the responses of normal controls. Jammes et al. [74] reported that oxidative stress markers increased more in CFS patients after exercise than in normal controls, consistent with a NO/ONOO- cycle elevation. La Manca et al. [75] found much larger cognitive deficits after exercise in CFS patients than in normal controls. There may be a number of responses to exercise that may be appropriate as specific biomarker tests for CFS. The ones that may be the best, from the standpoint of the NO/ONOO- cycle mechanism, may be cortisol levels or responses of NO/ONOO- cycle elements.

Before leaving this topic, however, there is an additional issue that may be understood as possibly being a consequence of changed cortisol control in CFS. Peckerman et al. [77,78] and Cheney [79] have reported that many CFS patients have cardiac dysfunction including left ventricular function. There is no understanding, to my knowledge, of how these cardiac changes may be produced as a consequence of the CFS pathophysiology. However, there is evidence that lowered cortisol levels can produce cardiac dysfunction, including lowered left ventriculal function [80-86]. It seems likely that the need for cortisol in the heart may be expected to be particularly important during and immediately following exercise due to the stresses placed on the heart by exercise. It may be suggested, therefore, that the cardiac dysfunction seen in many CFS patients may be caused by their lowered cortisol production during and following exercise.

Local Nature of the CFS Mechanism

The stunning variation of symptoms seen from one CFS patient to another has created substantial difficulties in coming up with a simple case definition/set of diagnostic criteria for CFS [62,63,76]. It is difficult to expain this variation without either postulating a dozen or more "causes" or, alternatively and much more simply, a single local mechanism with variation in tissue distribution, from one patient to another.

Direct evidence for such variation of impact on local tissues has been seen in brain scan studies of CFS patients, where such tissue variation can be directly observed. I will only discuss two such studies here, both magnetic resonance imaging (MRI) studies from the Natelson group. In one of these [87], CFS patients had much higher frequencies of abnormal scans, but the scan patterns from one patient to another were highly variable. In a second study [88], there were again highly variable scans among patients. Those with the most severe cognitive dysfunction had substantial frontal lobe impact.

Both of these studies provide substantial evidence for a local mechanism, with the second suggesting that specific region impact may be responsible for the generation of specific symptoms. This is not the only suggested role of a specific region of the brain in the generation of specific symptoms in this group of illnesses. Impact on the thalamus is likely to generate the widespread excessive pain in fibromyalgia and the anxiety and panic attack symptoms that are common symptoms with these illnesses may be due to impact on the amygdala [1,6].

Similar variations in brain scans have also been seen in such related illnesses as FM, MCS and PTSD [1].

There is also evidence from variations in gene expression from one CFS patient to another, suggesting variable tissue distribution. The most apparently relevant of such gene expression studies is the recently published study of Kerr et al. [89]. In that study, CFS patients were divided into different subtypes based on their gene expression patterns. These also corresponded, at least to some extent to variations is symptomatic patterns. Based on the gene expression patterns [89], different patients differed in terms of gene expression for genes linked to cognitive, musculoskeletal, anxiety/depression, neurological, gastrointestinal and hematological function. Each of these can be interpreted in terms of gene expression relating to different regions of the body. While it is unclear to me why lymphocytes and other white blood cells should have increased gene expression for genes related to, for example, neurological function, it is difficult to avoid the inference that impact on regions of the body must lead to increased gene expression for genes whose functions are linked to those regions of the body. So this study supports the interpretation that there appear to be regional variation among patients of a basically local mechanism, leading, in turn, to classification of different patients to different subtypes.

Gene Expression Studies: Evidence for Role of Cycle Elements

There have been a number of additional gene expression studies of CFS. Several of these provide substantial evidence for the involvement of mechanisms that are part of the NO/ONOO- cycle.

For example, several of these studies provide evidence for changes in gene expression of genes that function on energy metabolism and mitochondrial function [89-92], suggesting an important role of mitochondrial dysfunction in CFS. Several studies also provide evidence for chronic inflammatory responses in CFS [93-95], supporting another aspect of the

NO/ONOO- cycle. The data of Kaushik et al. provide evidence for a role of neuronal dysfunction including possible excitotoxicity [90].

To my knowledge, there has not been any analysis of the gene expression data to determine whether they provide evidence for elevated NF-κB activity or activity of other transcriptional factors that are known to be activated by oxidants and oxidative stress. So we do have evidence from gene expression studies of CFS, supporting roles for elements of the NO/ONOO- cycle but we are still in the early stages of analyzing the available data for consistency with the predictions of the NO/ONOO- cycle.

Therapy: Avoiding Infections, Excessive Exercise, Allergens and Other Stressors

The fifth principle is that NO/ONOO- cycle diseases should be treated by lowering the cycle biochemistry. There are two aspects to this approach: Avoiding stressors that will otherwise up-regulate the NO/ONOO- cycle biochemistry and using agents that lower the cycle biochemistry. Both are important and this section considers the first of these. Among the stressors that are important in exacerbating CFS are infections and there is a large literature reporting that infections can not only initiate cases of CFS, but that infections can exacerbated cases as well. Among the infectious agents that are implicated in chronic infections of CFS cases, are Borrelia (Lyme disease) and other tick-born infectious agents, mycoplasma, Chlamydia and herpes viruses including HHV-6. In some instances, these may have initiated the CFS cases but in others, an opportunistic infectious role may be more plausible. The general question is whether these can be treated by treatments that help restore normal immune function or whether it is necessary to use antibiotic treatments to effectively treat CFS?

Other stressors that will commonly up-regulate the NO/ONOO- cycle biochemistry include exercise triggering post-exertional malaise, as discussed above and exposure food or other allergens in the many CFS patients that suffer from such allergies.

Stressors that up-regulate the NO/ONOO- cycle biochemistry in related illnesses, such as MCS or PTSD, notably chemical exposure or psychological stress, may also have roles in some CFS cases.

Clearly there is a lot of variation in the impact of various stressors among CFS cases and these lead to variations in the optimal strategy for treatment among cases, as well.

Therapy: Agents That Lower NO/ONOO-Cycle Biochemistry

In Chapter 15, ref.1, there were 30 different agents/classes of agents listed and available currently that were predicted to lower different aspects of the NO/ONOO- cycle biochemistry and others have become apparent since that chapter was written. Of these agents/classes of agents, we have clinical trial studies on sixteen of them in CFS and/or FM and all 16 have been reported to be helpful in treatment (Table 3). These studies not only provide evidence supporting the NO/ONOO- cycle mechanism as a whole, but also provide evidence for a substantial causal role for several specific aspects of the cycle mechanism.

Table 3.

Agent or class	Mechanism	Comments
Vitamin C (ascorbic acid)	Chain breaking antioxidant; lowers NF-kappa B activity; reported to scavenge peroxynitrite and also help restore tetrahydrobiopterin (BH4) levels by reducing an oxidized derivative of BH4	May require high doses to be effective with the latter two mechanisms; this may be the basis of so called "megadose therapy" for vitamin C; clinical trials on CFS and MCS used high dose IV ascorbate
Magnesium	Lowers NMDA activity and may be useful in improving energy metabolism and ATP utilization	Magnesium is the agent that is most widely studied and found to be useful in the treatment of the multisystem illnesses
Fish oil (long chain omega-3 fatty acids)	Lowers iNOS induction; lowers production of inflammatory eicosonoids; important for brain function	Highly susceptible to lipid peroxidation and may, therefore be depleted; four studies reported improvements in clinical trials, 3 with CFS and one with FM
Flavonoids	Chain breaking antioxidants; some scavenge peroxynitrite, some scavenge superoxide; some reported to induce SOD; All three types are found in FlaviNox; some flavonoids may also act to help restore BH4 levels; lower NF-kappa B activity	Ginkgo extract tested in CFS; anthocyanidin flavonoids in FM; other flavonoids tested in CFS animal model
NMDA antagonists	Lower NMDA activity	Four different antagonists reported to be effective in the treatment of fibromyalgia; anecdotal reports of effectiveness for MCS
Agents that indirectly lower excitotoxicity including NMDA activity		Only clinical trials done with pregabalin for fibromyalgia, but other members of this class often used clinically
Acetyl L-carnitine/ carnitine	Helps transport fatty acids into mitochondria; may be important here not only directly for energy metabolism but also to restore the oxidized fatty acid residues that may be produced in the cardiolipin of the inner membrane	May also help lower reductive stress; two trials in CFS
Ecklonia cava extract	Polyphenolic chain breaking antioxidant; reported to help scavenge both peroxynitrite and superoxide; based on its reported properties, it may also help restore BH4 levels	Appears to stay in the body much longer than do the flavonoids, a useful property; reported to be helpful in a clinical trial study of fibromyalgia
Reductive stress relieving agents	These include S-adenosyl methionine (SAM or SAMe), trimethylglycine (betaine), carnitine and choline	SAM reported to be effective in multiple clinical trials with FM and CFS patients; betaine widely used clinically
Hydroxocobalamin form of vitamin B-12	Potent nitric oxide scavenger, lowers nitric oxide levels	Limited intestinal transport; often taken by IM injection or as a nasal spray or inhalant; clinical trial with CFS-like illnesses; widely used for treatment of CFS, FM and MCS
Folic acid	Relatively high doses will lower the partial	Reacts with oxidants and therefore may

	uncoupling of the nitric oxide synthases by helping to restore tetrahydrobiopterin (BH4)	be depleted due to the NO/ONOO- cycle
Algal supplements	Probably act as antioxidants	
Hyperbaric oxygen	May act to help restore cytochrome oxidase activity by competing with nitric oxide	My impression is that this approach needs to be used with substantial care – too high or prolonged dosage can cause damage
Trimethyl glycine (betaine), S-adenosyl methionine (SAM), choline, carnitine	Lower reductive stress; also helps with the generation of S-adenosyl methionine (SAM)	While lowering reductive stress may be the main concern, SAM generation may also be of concern; the enzyme methionine synthase is inhibited by nitric oxide and inactivated under conditions of oxidative stress, thus leading to lowered SAM and lowered methylation
Coenzyme Q10 (ubiquinone)	Important in mitochondrial function; important antioxidant, especially in mitochondrion; reported to scavenge peroxynitrite	Optimal dosage may vary considerably among different individuals; suggest taking early in day
D-ribose, RNA or inosine	Two important functions: Provides adenosine for restoring adenine nucleotide pools after energy metabolism dysfunction; when catabolized, the purine bases generate uric acid, a peroxynitrite scavenger	Each of these may act somewhat similarly; however only D-ribose has been tested in a clinical trial and reported to be effective; each of these agents has distinct drawbacks

Modified from the author's web site, used with permission. References provided in Chapter 15, ref.1, except as follows [96-102]. In a number of cases, only one of a class of agents has been tested via clinical trial with CFS and/or FM.

As can be seen from Table 3, of these 16 classes of agents, at least four have antioxidant properties, providing evidence that oxidative stress has an important causal role in generating these illnesses. Some of these agents either act as NMDA antagonists, or act indirectly to lower NMDA activity, thus providing strong evidence for a causal role of excessive NMDA activity. Carnitine/acetyl carnitine, coenzyme Q10 and possibly hyperbaric oxygen are likely to act to help improve mitochondrial function, thus providing evidence for a substantial causal role of mitochondrial/energy metabolism dysfunction.

The potent nitric oxide scavenger, hydroxocobalamin is a form of vitamin B_{12}, raising the question of whether it is acting here primarily as a nitric oxide scavenger or to allay a B_{12} deficiency. In the published clinical trial study [27], there was no correlation between initial B_{12} levels and the clinical response. Furthermore, much higher doses are needed to get good clinical responses here than are needed to treat a B_{12} deficiency [Chapter 6, ref.1]. It seems unlikely, therefore, that hydroxocobalamin is acting to allay a B_{12} deficiency. The potent action of hydroxocobalamin as a nitric oxide scavenger is well established, such that hydroxocobalamin has been used in experimental settings to establish a role for nitric oxide in biological processes [11, Chapter 6, ref.1]

There is also weaker evidence for two other aspects of the NO/ONOO- having a causal role. The long chain omega-3 fatty acids in fish oil are well established to have antiinflammatory aspects, so that their reported efficacy provides some evidence for an inflammatory causal role. High dose vitamin C and high dose folate supplements help restore BH4 levels, suggesting a causal role of BH4 depletion, but again, there are other possible interpretations for their action, so the evidence for BH4 depletion being causal in CFS, from clinical trial data alone, must be viewed as relatively weak. Interestingly in autism, which some view as being similar to CFS, there are three clinical trial studies all reporting that BH4 supplements produce statistically significant improvements [Chapter 14, ref.1].

The evidence for roles of oxidative stress, mitochondrial dysfunction and excitotoxicity including excessive NMDA activity from clinical trial data are relatively strong. We have weaker but still suggestive data for roles of excessive nitric oxide, chronic inflammatory biochemistry and BH4 depletion from such clinical trial data. It is difficult to see how these various cycle elements can be implicated from clinical trial data alone, unless the NO/ONOO- cycle or something very similar to it is the central causal mechanism in CFS and FM. When you add the various other types of evidence, supporting roles for each of these cycle elements in CFS that were reviewed above, the case for the NO/ONOO- cycle being the central causal mechanism in CFS becomes very substantial.

Treatment Protocols with Multiple Agents Lowering NO/ONOO-Cycle Biochemistry

In Chapter 15, ref.1, five treatment protocols are discussed that include at least 14 agents/classes of agents and have been tried with CFS, FM and/or MCS. Of these, only two, those of Teitelbaum and Nicolson, have been tested in clinical trials and found to be effective. The other three, Cheney's, Petrovic's and the one I worked on with Dr. Grace Ziem only have clinical observations of apparent effectiveness. Nevertheless, it appears that these are considerably more effective than are the individual agents that make them up, suggesting that an approach using multiple agents may be an attractive one for the treatment of presumed NO/ONOO- cycle diseases. The reader can get more information on those protocols from Chapter 15, ref.1.

I will discuss here, an additional protocol, this one containing 22 different agents predicted to down-regulate various aspects of the NO/ONOO- cycle, with each of these agents being nutritional supplements available to persons in the U.S., Canada and the EU. This nutritional support protocol was designed by me for the Allergy Research Group, using four supplement combinations that are newly formulated and three others that were already being sold by the Allergy Research Group. The components of this protocol, and indeed the entire nutritional support protocol, is not sold to treat or cure any disease.of the 22 different types of supplements included, 11 are listed in Table 3 and are follows:

> Trimethylglycine (betaine)
> Coenzyme Q10
> RNA
> Folic acid (folate)
> Hydroxocobalamin (B_{12})
> Ecklonia cava extract
> Acetyl-L-carnitine
> Flavonoids
> Fish oil

> ➢ Magnesium
> ➢ Vitamin C

The other 11 are described in Table 4.

The reader needs to be skeptical about my descriptions of apparent responses to the nutritional support protocol provided below for three distinct reasons:

1. These descriptions are all based on feedback from physicians and other health care providers as well as from anecdotal reports from individuals with these multisystem illnesses who have tried this protocol.
2. There have been *no* clinical trials of this protocol.
3. I receive a small royalty for the design of four of these supplement combinations, and *so I have a conflict of interest here.* The reader needs to keep that in mind.

Suggested dosage for Allergy Research Group nutritional support protocol, follows. My suggestion is that people interested in taking this protocol, introduce one combination at a time, for three days before introducing the next. The idea here is that if any of the seven supplement combinations are not well tolerated, it can be dropped by the individual. Some individuals, particularly in the MCS group, do not tolerate individual supplements and there is at least one type of person who does not tolerate most of them.

1. #75930 CoQ-Gamma E with Tocotrienols & Carotenoids: one capsule per day in the morning. Those with body weights over 100 lbs should add a second capsule at mid-day.
2. #75780 FlaviNox: one capsule, four times per day, three preferably with or after meals. Those with body weights over 120 lbs, should add a second capsule with each of three meals.
3. #75940 MVM-A Antioxidant Protocol, multivitamin mineral supplement with added acetyl L-carnitine: one capsule, four times per day, three preferably with or after meals. Those with body weights over 120 lbs, should add a second capsule, with breakfast and with dinner.
4. #75960 NAC Enhanced Antioxidant Formula: one each twice per day, with or after breakfast and supper.
5. #71250 or #73870 Super EPA (fish oil): one per day in the morning after breakfast. Those with body weights over 100 lbs, should add a second capsule at mid-day, taken with or after lunch.
6. #75910 FibroBoost (*Ecklonia cava* extract): one each twice per day, with or after breakfast and supper.
7. #70010 Buffered Vitamin C: one capsule, four times per day, preferably three with or after meals.

It is suggesting that the three products that are to be taken four times per day, be taken at the same times, with three being taken with or after the three meals of the day and the fourth taken at bedtime.

Table 4. Additional agents, not explicitly discussed in Table 3, that are included in the Allergy Research Group nutritional support protocol.

Vitamin B6, including pyridoxal phosphate	multiple functions, most relevant may be to stimulate glutamate decarboxylase activity, limit excitotoxicity
Niacin, including nicotinic acid and nicotinamide	Helps restore NAD/NADH pools after poly-ADP ribosylation leads to pool depletion; important for energy metabolism
Thiamine	Is depleted by oxidants; essential for two steps in pentose phosphate shunt and is needed, therefore to help provide NADPH for glutathione reductase
Riboflavin including 5'-phosphate	Depletion can limit glutathione reductase activity
Carotenoids including natural β-carotene, lycopene, lutein	Helps scavenge peroxynitrite, especially in biological membranes
Natural vitamin E, including γ-tocopherol and the tocotrienols	γ-tocopherol thought to have special role in scavenging NO2 radical (from peroxynitrite); tocotrienols may have special role in protecting from excitotoxicity and/or mitochondrial oxidation
Taurine	thought to lower excitoxicity by stimulating gabaergic activity
Zinc, manganese, copper	Modest doses used; may increase superoxide dismutase activity
α-lipoic acid	Multiple antioxidant roles on reduction to dihydrolipoic acid; helps restore reduced glutathione pools
N-acetyl cysteine	Helps restore reduced glutathione pools; modest doses used to prevent or lower possible excitotoxicity
Selenium as seleno-L-methionine	Important antioxidant; a variety of organic selenium compounds are peroxynitrite scavengers; selenium levels often low in multisystem illnesses

Modified from the author's web site with permission.

Description of Responses (and Again, Skepticism Should be Maintained)

Something like 80 to 85% of individuals trying this protocol report distinct improvements, with roughly similar percentages for CFS, FM and MCS sufferers. This is somewhat surprising given that most medical care providers feel that the MCS cases are the most difficult to treat and there are reports in the literature that perhaps 10% of CFS and FM patients see a full recovery but there are no similar reports for the MCS group. In most cases a wide variety of symptoms show improvement. Improvements where seen are maintained—that is relapses among those staying on the protocol are rare. However, stressors do cause a distinct worsening of symptoms but that worsening is not sustained when the stressor is no longer present.

In some cases, there are remarkable improvements, even among those who have been ill for two decades or more. And such remarkable improvements even occur in those who have been severely ill. Where people respond well to this nutritional support protocol, they typically respond within a month or less, although I suggest that people who tolerate it well, stay on it for three months even when they do not respond in less than a month, as some take longer to respond. However, others show much more modest improvements and there are some who show no clear-cut improvement.

A low percentage do not tolerate most of the protocol. Some, perhaps all of these have high levels of mercury. The probable reason for this inability to tolerate is that α-lipoic acid is present in four of the seven components, and α-lipoic acid is capable of mobilizing mercury in the body. It seems likely, therefore, that those with high levels of mercury will have to undergo extensive mercury detoxification in order to go back on the protocol.

In addition to the a low percentage with mercury toxicity problems, there are others (perhaps 10–15%) who tolerate most of the protocol but do not respond in any distinct fashion to it, either positively or negatively. I speculate that these may be people with major issues caused by intransigent chronic infections or possibly chemically sensitive individuals who are continually exposed to chemicals. Still others may have problems continual exposure to environmental molds or with food allergens. However, this is speculation that must be questioned.

In general, most individuals with CFS, MCS or FM respond well to the protocol, even those who have been ill for two or more decades and those who have been severely ill. The fact that all three of these respond roughly equally well to the protocol suggests a that the NO/ONOO- cycle is a common mechanism for all three. However, with some having been on the protocol for a year or more at this point, we are not seeing the cures that might have been anticipated. This nutritional support protocol is limited to agents that can be sold over-the-counter and limited to nutritional supplements, so there may be ways of improving it, a number of which are discussed in Chapter 15, ref.1.

How Can We Obtain Substantial Numbers of Cures?

The simple answer to this question is that I don't know yet, but there is an approach that is feasible and plausible that should be tried, in my judgment. First let's ask why we are not seeing substantial numbers of cures?

In principle, there are three possible answers to this, assuming that the NO/ONOO- cycle mechanism is central to the etiology of these diseases:

1. The first is that there are aspects of the cycle that we do not yet understand and that therefore cannot effectively treat. This is certainly possible since the cycle has become much more complex since I first proposed it [4]. Additional aspects of the cycle have been added as a function of important observations on these multisystem diseases. They have also been added as I have researched the basic chemistry, biochemistry and physiology of various potential cycle elements. Thus new mechanisms, the arrows in Figures 1 and 2, have been added as it has been possible to document them. Obviously if we are missing something essential in our understanding of the cycle, we don't know how to deal with it.

2. The second possibility is that many of the sufferers have to deal with stressors that are up-regulating the cycle and are not adequately avoiding these stressors. The

three of these that may be most important for the CFS group are chronic infections, allergens including food allergens and exercise leading to post-exertional malaise.

3.   The third possibility is that there is one (or perhaps more) aspect of the cycle that we are not effectively down-regulating, that may be so important to the cycle that it is preventing our obtaining such cures. It is this third possibility that is the focus of the rest of this section.

I have argued above, that the most central part of the cycle is the central couplet, the reciprocal interactions between peroxynitrite and BH4. Recall that peroxynitrite oxidizes BH4, leading to BH4 depletion and partial uncoupling of the nitric oxide synthases, causing them to generate both superoxide and nitric oxide, which react with each other to form more peroxynitrite (see Figure 2.). This central couplet, acting as a vicious cycle within the larger NO/ONOO- cycle may well be the core of the cycle and therefore the most important part of the cycle to down-regulate. We do have agents in the Allergy Research Group protocol predicted to down-regulate both ends of this couplet, but it is not clear that they are effective *in vivo* at the doses one normally uses.

My candidate for an agent to down-regulate this central couplet is high dose, intravenous (IV) ascorbate (vitamin C). This so-called megadose therapy approach is attractive for four different reasons:

1.   It has been reported to be effective in clinical trials for both CFS [103-106] and MCS [107]. I am also aware of physicians who have used it in their treatment of both of these diseases, and reported very substantial apparent effectiveness. My suggestion is to use it with a wide ranging protocol designed to down-regulate various aspects of the NO/ONOO- cycle, rather than on its own, but the apparent effectiveness of it as a single agent is certainly encouraging.

2.   Ascorbate scavenges peroxynitrite and its breakdown products, although it is not very effective at the usual blood levels obtained from the use of oral supplements [108-112]. Because IV ascorbate can generate blood levels on the order of 30 times or more compared with those typically obtained from oral supplements [113,114], it is expected to be much more effective at these high levels.

3.   When BH4 is oxidized by peroxynitrite it is first converted to the one electron oxidation product, BH3 [111,112], which is itself unstable. However BH3 can be reduced back to BH4 by ascorbate [111,112] and with the high levels generated by high dose IV ascorbate, may be expected to be fairly efficiently reduced before it is converted to other, higher level oxidation products. Thus high dose, IV ascorbate may be expected to allow recovery of much of the BH4 that was oxidized by peroxynitrite.

4.   High dose ascorbate produced by such IV infusion leads to the generation of substantial amounts of hydrogen peroxide in the body [115,116] and hydrogen peroxide has been shown to induced the enzyme GTP cyclohydolase I [117-119]. GTP cyclohydrolase I is the first and rate limiting enzyme in the *de novo* pathway for the synthesis of BH4. Thus high dose IV ascorbate will be expected to increase the availability of BH4 by stimulating its synthesis via the *de novo* pathway.

As one might expect from a combination of these three mechanisms, there is evidence that high dose ascorbate increases availability of BH4 [120,121].

In summary, there are three mechanisms by which high dose IV ascorbate is predicted to down-regulate the couplet that appears to be most central to the NO/ONOO- cycle. This same treatment appears to be effective in clinical trial studies in the treatment of CFS and MCS. It is, consequently, my best candidate for an addition to protocols containing wide-ranging agents down-regulating various aspects of the NO/ONOO- cycle, to hopefully obtain substantial numbers of cures of NO/ONOO- cycle diseases.

Summary: CFS as a NO/ONOO-Cycle Disease

There are a number of types of evidence that provide support for a NO/ONOO- cycle mechanism for CFS:

1. It is supported by a pattern of evidence where nine diverse short-term stressors reported to initiate cases of CFS can all act to increase nitric oxide levels.
2. It is supported by the large amount of data supporting the existence of and biological impact of specific cycle mechanisms in animals and humans.
3. It is supported by plausible mechanisms by which cycle elements can generate symptoms and signs often found in cases of CFS.
4. The basic local nature is supported by the stunning variation in symptoms seen among different CFS patients, the variations in brain tissue distribution seen in brain scan studies and the variations in gene expression reported in different CFS patients.
5. It is supported by animal model data.
6. It is supported by the fact that other, related illnesses, including FM and MCS also can be explained through a NO/ONOO- cycle mechanism.
7. It is supported by studies of genes that help determine susceptibility to CFS.
8. It is supported by clinical trial and clinical observation studies of agents that are reported to be helpful in the CFS and/or FM illnesses.

The last two types of evidence (7 and 8), provide evidence for a role for several different aspects of the NO/ONOO- cycle mechanism. Notably, oxidative stress, mitochondrial/energy metabolism dysfunction, elevated nitric oxide levels, inflammatory biochemistry, excitotoxicity including excessive NMDA activity and BH4 depletion. It is difficult to see how this group of mechanisms could be involved in CFS, unless the NO/ONOO- cycle or something very similar to it is the central cause of CFS.

It is my opinion that the NO/ONOO- cycle mechanism has already led to approaches that can produce substantial improvements in the large majority of cases of CFS and other related multisystem illnesses, and that modification of these approaches will probably lead to cures for many such sufferers. But then, I have always been an optimist when it comes to these diseases.

References

[1] Pall, M. L. (2007) Explaining "Unexplained Illnesses": Disease Paradigm for Chronic Fatigue Syndrome, Multiple Chemical Sensitivity, Fibromyalgia, Post-Traumatic Stress Disorder, *Gulf War Syndrome and Others.* Harrington Park (Haworth) Press, Bighamton, NY.

[2] Pall, M. L. (2002) NMDA sensitization and stimulation by peroxynitrite, nitric oxide and organic solvents at the mechanism of chemical sensitivity in multiple chemical sensitivity. *FASEB J 16,* 1407-1417.

[3] Hill, H. U., Huber, W., Müller, K. (2008) Multiple Chemikalien Sensibilität. Shaker-Verlag, Aachen.

[4] Pall, M. L. (2000). Elevated, sustained peroxynitrite levels as the cause of chronic fatigue syndrome. *Med Hypotheses, 54,* 115-125.

[5] Pall, M. L. (2001). Common etiology of posttraumatic stress disorder, fibromyalgia, chronic fatigue syndrome and multiple chemical sensitivity via elevated nitric oxide/peroxynitrite. *Med Hypotheses, 57,* 139-145.

[6] Pall, M. L. (2006). The NO/ONOO- cycle as the cause of fibromyalgia and related illnesses: Etiology, explanation and effective therapy. In: New Research in Fibromyalgia, John A. Pederson, Ed., pp 39-59, Nova Science Publishers, Inc., Hauppauge, NY.

[7] Pall, M. L. (2007). Nitric oxide synthase partial uncoupling as a key switching mechanism for the NO/ONOO- cycle. *Med Hypotheses, 69,* 821-825.

[8] Pall, M. L. & Satterlee J. D. (2001). Elevated nitric oxide/peroxynitrite mechanism for the common etiology of multiple chemical sensitivity, chronic fatigue syndrome, and posttraumatic stress disorder. *Ann N Y Acad Sci, 933,* 323-329.

[9] Pall, M. L. & Anderson J. H. (2004). The vanilloid receptor as a putative target of diverse chemicals in multiple chemical sensitivity. *Arch Environ Health, 59,* 363-372.

[10] Pall M. L. (2009). Multiple chemical sensitivity: toxicological questions and mechanisms. General and Applied Toxicology, 3rd Edition, Bryan Ballantyne, Timothy C. Marrs, Tore Syversen, Eds., Wiley & Sons, New York, in press.

[11] Pall, M. L. (2001). Cobalamin used in chronic fatigue syndrome therapy is a nitric oxide scavenger. J Chronic Fatigue Syndr, 8, 39-45.

[12] Pall, M. L. (2003). Elevated nitric oxide/peroxynitrite theory of multiple chemical sensitivity: central role of N-methyl-D-aspartate receptors in the sensitivity mechanism. Environ Health Perspect, 111, 1461-1464.

[13] Pall, M. L. (2008). Post-radiation syndrome as a NO/ONOO(-) cycle, chronic fatigue syndrome-like disease. *Med Hypotheses, 71,* 537-541.

[14] Smirnova, I. V. & Pall, M. L. (2003). Elevated levels of protein carbonyls in sera of chronic fatigue syndrome patients. *Mol Cell Biochem, 248,* 93-95.

[15] Carson, P. J., Konweko, P., Wold, P., et al. (2006). Long-term clinical and neuropsychological outcomes of West Nile virus infection. *Clin Infect Dis, 43,* 723-730.

[16] Kennedy, G., Spence, V. A., McLaren, M., Hill, A., Underwood, C. & Belch, J. J. (2005). Oxidative stress levels are raised in chronic fatigue syndrome and are associated with clinical symptoms.*Free Radic Biol Med, 39,* 584-589.

[17] Richards, R. S., Wang, L. & Jelinek, H. (2007). Erythrocyte oxidative damage in chronic fatigue syndrome. *Arch Med Res, 38,* 94-98.

[18] Miwa, K. & Fujita, M. (2008). Increased oxidative stress suggested by low serum vitamin E concentrations in patients with chronic fatigue syndrome. Int J Cardiol [Epub ahead of print].

[19] McCully, K. K., Natelson, B. H., Iotti, S., Sisto, S., Leigh, J. S. Jr. (1996). Reduced oxidative muscle metabolism in chronic fatigue syndrome. *Muscle Nerve, 19,* 621-625.

[20] McCully, K. K. & Natelson, B. H. (1999). Impaired oxygen delivery to muscle in chronic fatigue syndrome. *Clin Sci (Lond), 97,* 603-608.

[21] Farquhar, W. B., Hunt, B. E, Taylor, J. A., Darling, S. E. & Freeman, R. (2002). Blood volume and its relation to peak O(2) consumption and physical activity in patients with chronic fatigue. *Am J Physiol Heart Circ Physiol, 282,* H66-H71.

[22] Mathew. S. J., Mao. X., Keegan. K. A., Levine. S. M., Smith. E. L., Heier. L. A., Otcheretko. V., Coplan. J. D. & Shungu. D. C. (2008). Ventricular cerebrospinal fluid lactate is increased in chronic fatigue syndrome compared with generalized anxiety disorder: an in vivo 3.0 T (1)H MRS imaging study. *NMR Biomed,* [Epub ahead of print].

[23] Hokama, Y., Uto, G. A., Palafox, N. A., Enlander, D., Jordan, E. & Cocchetto, A. (2003). Chronic phase lipids in sera of chronic fatigue syndrome (CFS), chronic ciguatera fish poisoning (CCFP), hepatitis B, and cancer with antigenic epitope resembling ciguatoxin, as assessed with MAb-CTX. *J Clin Lab Anal, 17,* 132-139.

[24] Hokama, Y., Empey-Campora, C., Hara, C., Higa, N., Siu, N., Lau, R., Kuribayashi, T. & Yabusaki, K. (2008). Acute phase phospholipids related to the cardiolipin of mitochondria in the sera of patients with chronic fatigue syndrome (CFS), chronic Ciguatera fish poisoning (CCFP), and other diseases attributed to chemicals, Gulf War, and marine toxins. *J Clin Lab Anal, 22,* 99-105.

[25] Pall, M. L. (2002). Levels of nitric oxide synthase product citrulline are elevated in sera of chronic fatigue syndrome patients. *J Chronic Fatigue Syndr, 10(3/4),* 37-41.

[26] Kurup, R. K. & Kurup, P. A. (2003). Hypothalamic digoxin, cerebral chemical dominance and myalgic encephalomyelitis. *Int J Neurosci, 113,* 683-701.

[27] Ellis, F. R. & Nasser, S. (1973). A pilot study of vitamin B12 in the treatment of tiredness. *Br J Nutr, 30,* 277-283.

[28] Spence, V. A., Kennedy, G., Belch, J. J., Hill, A. & Khan, F. (2007). Low grade inflammation and arterial wave reflection in patients with chronic fatigue syndrome. *Clin Sci (Lond), 114,* 561-566.

[29] Carpman, V. (1995). CFIDS treatment: the Cheney clinics strategic approach. *CFIDS Chronicle Spring*, 38-45.

[30] Hoh, D. (1998). Treatment at the Cheney clinic. *CFIDS Chronicle, 11,* 13-14.

[31] Goldstein, J. A. (2004). Tuning the Brain: Principles and Practice of Neurosomatic Medicine. Haworth Medical Press, Binghamton, NY.

[32] Maes, M., Mihaylova, I., Kubera, M. & Bosmans, E. (2007). Not in the mind but in the cell: increased production of cyclo-oxygenase-2 and inducible NO synthase in chronic fatigue syndrome. *Neuro Endocrinol Lett, 28,* 463-469.

[33] Maes, M., Mihaylova, I. & Bosmans, E. (2007). Not in the mind of neurasthenic lazybones but in the cell nucleus: patients with chronic fatigue syndrome have increased production of nuclear factor kappa beta. *Neuro Endocrinol Lett, 28,* 456-462.

[34] Chao, C. C., DeLaHunt, M., Hu, S., Close, K. & Peterson, P. K. (1992). Immunologically mediated fatigue: a murine model. *Immunopathol Clin Immunol, 64,* 161-165.

[35] Sheng, W. S., Hu, S., Lamkin, A., Peterson, P. K. & Chao, C. C. (1996). Susceptibility to immunologically mediated fatigue in C57BL/6 versus Balb/c mice. *Clin Immunol Immunopathol, 81,*161-167.

[36] Sheng, W. S., Lin, J. C., Apple, F., Hu, S., Peterson, P. K. & Chao, C. C. (1999). Brain energy stores in C57BL/6 mice after C. parvum injection. *Neuroreport, 10,* 177-181.

[37] Smith, S. R., Manfra, D., Davies, L., Terminelli, C., Denhardt, G. & Donkin, J. (1997). Elevated levels of NO in both unchallenged and LPS-challenged C. parvum-primed mice are attributable to the activity of a cytokine-inducible isoform of iNOS. *J Leukoc Biol, 61,* 24-32.

[38] Rees, D. D., Cunha, F. Q., Assreuy, J., Herman, A. G. & Moncada, S. (1995). Sequential induction of nitric oxide synthase by Corynebacterium parvum in different organs of the mouse. *Br J Pharmacol, 114,* 689-693.

[39] Katafuchi, T., Kondo, T., Take, S. & Yoshimura, M. (2006). Brain cytokines and the 5-HT system during poly I:C-induced fatigue. *Ann N Y Acad Sci, 1088,* 230-237.

[40] Dantzer, R. & Kelley, K. W. (2007). Twenty years of research on cytokine-induced sickness behavior. *Brain Behav Immun, 21,* 153-160.

[41] Singh, A., Naidu, P. S., Gupta, S. & Kulkarni, S. K. (2002). Effect of natural and synthetic antioxidants in a mouse model of chronic fatigue syndrome. *J Med Food, 5,* 211-220.

[42] Singh, A., Garg, V., Gupta, S. & Kulkarni, S. K. (2002). Role of antioxidants in chronic fatigue syndrome in mice. *Indian J Exp Biol. 40,* 1240-1244.

[43] Singal, A., Kaur, S., Tirkey, N. & Chopra, K. (2005). Green tea extract and catechin ameliorate chronic fatigue-induced oxidative stress in mice. *J Med Food, 8,* 47-52.

[44] Torpy, D. J., Bachmann, A. W., Grice, J. E., Fitzgerald, S. P., Phillips, P. J., Whitworth, J. A. & Jackson, R. V. (2001). Familial corticosteroid-binding globulin deficiency due to a novel null mutation: association with fatigue and relative hypotension. *J Clin Endocrinol Metab, 86,* 3692-3700.

[45] Torpy, D. J., Bachmann, A. W., Gartside, M., Grice, J. E., et al. (2004) Association between chronic fatigue syndrome and the corticosteroid-binding globulin gene ALA SER224 polymorphism.*Endocr Res, 30,* 417-429.

[46] Torpy, D. J. & Ho, J. T. (2007). Corticosteroid-binding globulin gene polymorphisms: clinical implications and links to idiopathic chronic fatigue disorders. *Clin Endocrinol (Oxf) 67,* 161-167.

[47] Smith, A. K., White, P. D., Aslakson, E., Vollmer-Conna, U. & Rajeevan, M. S. (2006). Polymorphisms in genes regulating the HPA axis associated with empirically delineated classes of unexplained chronic fatigue. *Pharmacogenomics, 7,* 387-394.

[48] Rajeevan, M. S., Smith, A. K., Dimulescu, I., Unger, E. R., Vernon, S. D., Heim, C. & Reeves, W. C. (2007). Glucocorticoid receptor polymorphisms and haplotypes associated with chronic fatigue syndrome. *Genes Brain Behav, 6,* 167-176.

[49] Narita, M, Nishigami, N., Narita, N., et al. (2003). Association between serotonin transporter gene polymorphism and chronic fatigue syndrome. *Biochem Biophys Res Commun, 311,* 264-266.

[50] Smith, A. K., Dimulescu, I., Falkenberg, V. R., et al. (2008). Genetic evaluation of the serotonergic system in chronic fatigue syndrome. *Psychoneuroendocrinology, 33,* 188-197.

[51] Vladutiu, G. D. & Natelson, B. H. (2004). Association of medically unexplained fatigue with ACE insertion/deletion polymorphism in Gulf War veterans. *Muscle Nerve, 30,* 38-43.

[52] Kase, H., Hashikabe, Y., Uchida, K., Nakashini, N. & Hattori, Y. (2005). Supplementation with tetrahydrobiopterin prevents the cardiovascular effects of angiotensin II-induced oxidative and nitrosative stress. *J Hypertens, 23,* 1375-1382.

[53] Oak, J. H. & Cai, H. (2007). Attenuation of angiotensin II signalling recouples eNOS and inhibits nonendothelial NOX activity in diabetic mice. *Diabetes, 56,* 118-126.

[54] Yamamoto, E., Kataoka, K., Shintaku, H., et al. (2007). Novel mechanism and role of angiotensin II induced vascular endothelial injury in hypertensive diastolic heart failure. *Arterioscler Thromb Vasc Biol, 27,* 2569-2575.

[55] Carlo-Stella, N., Badulli, C., De Silvestri, A., et al. (2006). A first cytokine polymorphism in CFS: Positive association of TNF-857 and IFNgamma 874 rare alleles. *Clin Exp Rheumatol, 24,* 179-182.

[56] Metzger, K., Frémont, M., Roelant, C. & De Meirleir, K. (2008). Lower frequency of IL-17F sequence variant (His161Arg) in chronic fatigue syndrome patients. *Biochem Biophys Res Commun, 376,* 231-233.

[57] Boles, R. G., Burnett, B. B., Gleditsch, K., et al. (2005). A high predisposition to depression and anxiety in mothers and other matrilineal relatives of children with presumed maternally inherited mitochondrial disorders. *Am J Med Genet B Neuropsychiatr Genet, 137B,* 20-24.

[58] Higashimoto, T., Baldwin, E. E., Gold, J. I. & Boles, R. G. (2008). Reflex sympathetic dystrophy: complex regional pain syndrome type I in children with mitochondrial disease and maternal inheritance. *Arch Dis Child, 93,* 390-397.

[59] Rowe, P. C., Barron, D. F., Calkins, H., Maumenee, I. H., Tong, P. Y. & Geraghty, M. T. (1999). Orthostatic intolerance and chronic fatigue syndrome associated with Ehlers-Danlos syndrome. *J Pediatr, 135,* 494-499.

[60] Germain, D. P. (2006). The vascular Ehlers-Danlos syndrome. *Curr Treat Options Cardiovasc Med 8,* 121-127.

[61] Pepin, M., Schwarze, U., Superti-Furga, A. & Byers, P. H. (2000). Clinical and genetic features of Ehlers-Danlos syndrome type IV, the vascular type. *N Engl J Med 342*, 673-680.

[62] Jason, L. A., Torres-Harding, S. R., Jurgens, A. & Helgerson, J. (2004). Comparing the Fukuda et al. Criteria and the Canadian Case Definition for Chronic Fatigue Syndrome. *J Chronic Fatigue Syndr, 12(1),* 37-52.

[63] Carruthers, B. M., Jain, K. L., De Meirleir, D. L., et al. (2003) Myalgic Encephalomyelitis/ Chronic Fatigue Syndrome: Clinical Working Case Definition, Diagnostic and Treatment Protocols. *J Chronic Fatigue Syndr, 11(1),* 7-115.

[64] Jason, L. A., Corradi, K., Gress, S., Williams, S. & Torres-Harding, S. (2006). Causes of death among patients with chronic fatigue syndrome. *Health Care Women Int, 27,* 615-626.

[65] Mastorakos, G. & Pavlatou, M. (2005). Exercise as a stress model and the interplay between the hypothalamus-pituitary-adrenal and the hypothalamus-pituitary-thyroid axes. *Horm Metab Res, 37,* 577-584.

[66] McMurray, R. G. & Hackney, A. C. (2005). Interactions of metabolic hormones, adipose tissue and exercise. *Sports Med, 35,* 393-412.

[67] Ottenweller, J. E., Sisto, S. A., McCarty, R. C. & Natelson, B. H. (2001). Hormonal responses to exercise in chronic fatigue syndrome. *Neuropsychobiology, 43,* 34-41.

[68] Demitrack, M. A. & Crofford, L. J. (1998). Evidence for and pathophysiologic implications of hypothalamic-pituitary-adrenal axis dysregulation in fibromyalgia and chronic fatigue syndrome. *Ann N Y Acad Sci, 840,* 684-697.

[69] Crofford, L. J., Young, E. A., Engleberg, N. C., et al. (2004). Basal circadian and pulsatile ACTH and cortisol secretion in patients with fibromyalgia and/or chronic fatigue syndrome. *Brain Behav Immun, 18,* 314-325.

[70] Adler, G. K., Mansfredsdottir, V. F. & Rackow, R. M. (2002). Hypothalamic-pituitary-adrenal axis function in fibromyalgia an chronic fatigue syndrome. *The Endrocrinologist, 12,* 513-522.

[71] Ramsay, M. A. (1988). Myalgic Encephalomyelitis and Postviral Fatigue State: The Saga of Royal Free Disease, 2nd Edition. London, Gower.

[72] Harvey, S. B., Wadsworth, M., Wessely, S. & Hotopf, M. (2008). Etiology of chronic fatigue syndrome: testing popular hypotheses using a national birth cohort study. *Psychosom Med, 70,* 488-495.

[73] Baschetti, R. (2005). Chronic fatigue syndrome, exercise, cortisol and lymphadenopathy. *J Intern Med, 258,* 291-292.

[74] Jammes, Y., Steinberg, J. G., Mambrini, O., Brégeon, F. & Delliaux, S. (2005). Chronic fatigue syndrome: assessment of increased oxidative stress and altered muscle excitability in response to incremental exercise. *J Intern Med, 257,* 299-310.

[75] LaManca, J. J., Peckerman, A., Sisto, S. A., DeLuca, J., Cook, S. & Natelson, B. H. (2001). Cardiovascular responses of women with chronic fatigue syndrome to stressful cognitive testing before and after strenuous exercise. *Psychosom Med 63,* 756-764.

[76] Fukuda, K., Straus, S. E., Hickie, I., Sharpe, M. C., Dobbins, J. G. & Komaroff, A. (1994). The chronic fatigue syndrome: a comprehensive approach to its definition and

study. International Chronic Fatigue Syndrome Study Group. *Ann Intern Med 121,* 953-959.

[77] Peckerman, A., LaManca, J. J. Dahl, K. A., et al. (2003). Abnormal impedance cardiography predicts symptom severity in chronic fatigue syndrome. *Am J Med, 326,* 55-60.

[78] Peckerman, A., LaManca, J. J., Qureshi, B., et al. (2003). Baroreceptive reflex and integrative stress responses in chronic fatigue syndrome. *Psychosom Med, 65,* 889-895.

[79] http://phoenix-cfs.org/Cardio%20IVa%20Superoxide.htm

[80] Aoyama, T., Matsui, T., Novikov, M., et al. (2005). Serum and glucocorticoid-responsive kinase-1 regulates cardiomyocyte survival and hypertrophic response. *Circulation, 111,* 16523-1659.

[81] Narayanan, N., Yang, C., Xur, A. (2004). Dexamethasone treatment improves sarcoplasmic reticulum function and contractile performance in aged myocardium. *Mol Cell Biochem, 266,* 31-36.

[82] Chiu, C. Z., Nakatani, S., Zhang, G., et al. (2005). Prevention of left ventricular remodeling by long-term corticosteroid therapy in patients with cardiac sarcoidosis. *Am J Cardiol, 95,* 143-146.

[83] Iga, K., Hori, K. & Gen, H. (1992). Deep negative T waves associated with reversible left ventricular dysfunction in acute adrenal crisis. *Heart Vessels, 7,* 107-111.

[84] Allolio, B., Ehses, W., Steffen, H. M. & Muller, R. (1994). Reduced lymphocyte beta 2-adreoreceptor density and impaired diastolic left ventricular function in patients with glucocorticoid deficiency. *Clin Endocrinol, 40,* 769-775.

[85] Boachour, G., Tirot, P., Varache, N., et al. (1994). Hemodynamic changes in acute adrenal insufficiency. *Intensive Care Med, 20,* 138-141.

[86] Emir, M., Ozisik, K., Cagli, K., et al. (2005). Beneficial effect of methylprednisone on cardiac myocytes in a rat model of severe brain injury. *Tohoku J Exp Med, 207,* 119-124.

[87] Natelson, B. H., Cohen, J. M., Brassloff, I. & Lee, H. J. (1993). A controlled study of brain magnetic resonance imaging in patients with the chronic fatigue syndrome. *J Neurolo Sci, 15,* 213-217.

[88] Lange, G., DeLuca, J., Maldjian, J. A., Lee, H., Tiersky, L. A. & Natelson, B. H. (1999). Brain MRI abnormalities exist in a subset of patients with chronic fatigue syndrome. *J Neurol Sci, 171,* 3-7.

[89] Whistler, T., Unger, E. R., Nisenbaum, R. & Vernon, S. D. (2003). Integration of gene expression, clinical and epidemiological data to characterize chronic fatigue syndrome. *J Transl Med, 1(1),*10.

[90] Kaushik, N., Fear, D., Richards, S. C., et al. (2005). Gene expression in peripheral blood mononuclear cells from patients with chronic fatigue syndrome. *J Clin Pathol, 58,* 826-832.

[91] Saiki, T., Kawai, T., Morita, K., Ohta, M., Saito, T., Rokutan, K. & Ban, N. (2008). Identification of marker genes for differential diagnosis of chronic fatigue syndrome. *Mol Med, 14,* 599-607.

[92] Whistler, T., Taylor, R., Craddock, R. C., Broderick, G., Klimas, N., Unger, E. R. (2006). Gene expression correlates unexplained fatigue. *Pharmacogenomics*, *7*, 395-405.

[93] Aspler, A. L., Bolshin, C., Vernon, S. D. & Broderick, G. (2008). Evidence of inflammatory immune signaling in chronic fatigue syndrome: A pilot study of gene expression in peripheral blood. *Behav Brain Funct Sep, 26,* 4:44.

[94] Fuite, J., Vernon, S. D. & Broderick, G. (2008). Neuroendocrine and immune network re-modeling in chronic fatigue syndrome: An exploratory analysis. Genomics Sep 30. [Epub ahead of print].

[95] Fang, H., Xie, Q., Boneva, R., Fostel, J., Perkins, R. & Tong, W. (2006). Gene expression profile exploration of a large dataset on chronic fatigue syndrome. *Pharmacogenomics, 7*, 429-440.

[96] Crofford, L. J., Rowbotham, M. C., Mease, P. J., Russell, I. J,, Dworkin, R. H., Corbin, AE, et al. (2005) Pregabalin for the treatment of fibromyalgia syndrome: results of a randomized, double-blind, placebo-controlled trial. *Arthritis Rheum, 52*, 1264-1273.

[97] Bierman, R. (2008). Ecklonia Cava Extract: Superior Polyphenol and Super-Antioxidant for Our Time. *Townsend Lett Doctors Patients,* Jan 2008.

[98] Gilula, M. F. (2007). Cranial electrotherapy stimulation and fibromyalgia. *Expert Rev Med Devices, 4,* 489-495.

[99] In Focus (2007) http://www.nutricology.com/In-Focus-April-2007-Ecklonia-Cava-sp-52.html

[100] Teitelbaum, J. E., Johnson, C. & St Cyr J. (2006). The use of D-ribose in chronic fatigue syndrome and fibromyalgia: a pilot study. *J Altern Complement Med, 12,* 857-862.

[101] Malaguarnera, M., Gargante, M. P., Cristaldi, E., et al. (2008). Acetyl L-carnitine (ALC) treatment in elderly patients with fatigue. *Arch Gerontol Geriatr, 46,* 181-190.

[102] Gebhart, B. & Jorgenson, J. A. (2004). Benefit of ribose in a patient with fibromyalgia. *Pharmacotherapy, 24*, 1646-1648.

[103] Kodama, M. & Kodama, T. (2006). Four problems with the clinical control of interstitial pneumonia, or chronic fatigue syndrome, using the megadose vitamin C infusion system with dehydroepiandrosterone-cortisol annex. *In Vivo, 20,*285-291.

[104] Kodama, M., Kodama, T. (2005). The clinical course of interstitial pneumonia alias chronic fatigue syndrome under the control of megadose vitamin C infusion system with dehydroepiandrosterone-cortisol annex. *Int J Mol Med, 15,*109-116.

[105] Kodama M., Kodama T., Murakami, M. (1996). The value of the dehydroepiandrosterone-annexed vitamin C infusion treatment in the clinical control of chronic fatigue syndrome (CFS). II. Characterization of CFS patients with special reference to their response to a new vitamin C infusion treatment. *In Vivo, 10,* 585-

[106] Kodama, M., Kodama, T. & Murakami, M. (1996). The value of the dehydroepiandrosterone-annexed vitamin C infusion treatment in the clinical control of chronic fatigue syndrome (CFS). I. A Pilot study of the new vitamin C infusion treatment with a volunteer CFS patient. *In Vivo, 10,* 575-584.

[107] Heuser, G. & Vojdani, A. (1997). Enhancement of natural killer cell activity and T and B cell function by buffered vitamin C in patients exposed to toxic chemicals: the role of protein kinase-C. *Immunopharmacol Immunotoxicol, 19,* 291-312.

[108] Ferroni, F., Maccaglia, A., Pietraforte, D., Turco, L. & Minetti, M. (2004). Phenolic antioxidants and the protection of low density lipoprotein from peroxynitrite-mediated oxidations at physiologic CO_2. *J Agric Food Chem, 52,* 2866-2874.

[109] Sakihama, Y., Tamaki, R., Shimoji, H., Ichiba, T., Fukushi, Y., Tahara, S. & Yamasaki, H. (2003). Enzymatic nitration of phytophenolics: evidence for peroxynitrite-independent nitration of plant secondary metabolites. *FEBS Lett, 553,* 377-380.

[110] Whiteman, M., Ketsawatsakul, U. & Halliwell, B. (2002). A reassessment of the peroxynitrite scavenging activity of uric acid. *Ann N Y Acad Sci, 962,* 242-259.

[111] Patel, K. B., Stratford, M. R., Wardman, P., Everett, S. A. (2002). Oxidation of tetrahydrobiopterin by biological radicals and scavenging of the trihydrobiopterin radical by ascorbate. *Free Radic Biol Med, 32,* 203-211.

[112] Kuzkaya, N., Weissmann, N., Harrison, D. G. & Dikalov, S. (2003). Interactions of peroxynitrite, tetrahydrobiopterin, ascorbic acid, and thiols: implications for uncoupling endothelial nitric-oxide synthase. *J Biol Chem, 278,* 22546-22554.

[113] Padayatty, S. J., Sun, H., Wang, Y., Riordan, H. D., Hewitt, S. M., Katz, A., Wesley, R. A. & Levine, M. (2004). Vitamin C pharmacokinetics: implications for oral and intravenous use. *Ann Intern Med, 140,* 533-537.

[114] Duconge, J., Miranda-Massari, J. R., Gonzalez, M. J., Jackson, J. A., Warnock, W. & Riordan, N. H. (2008). Pharmacokinetics of vitamin C: insights into the oral and intravenous administration of ascorbate. *P R Health Sci J, 27,* 7-19.

[115] Chen, Q., Espey, M. G., Krishna, M. C., Mitchell, J. B., Corpe, C. P., Buettner, G. R., Shacter, E. & Levine, M. (2005). Pharmacologic ascorbic acid concentrations selectively kill cancer cells: action as a pro-drug to deliver hydrogen peroxide to tissues. *Proc Natl Acad Sci USA, 102,* 13604-13609.

[116] Clément, M. V., Ramalingam, J., Long, L. H., Halliwell, B. (2001). The in vitro cytotoxicity of ascorbate depends on the culture medium used to perform the assay and involves hydrogen peroxide. *Antioxid Redox Signal, 3,* 157-163.

[117] Shimizu, S., Shiota, K., Yamamoto, S., Miyasaka, Y., Ishii, M., et al. (2003). Hydrogen peroxide stimulates tetrahydrobiopterin synthesis through the induction of GTP-cyclohydrolase I and increases nitric oxide synthase activity in vascular endothelial cells. *Free Radic Biol Med, 34,* 1343-1352.

[118] Ishii, M., Shimizu, S., Wajima, T., Hagiwara, T., Negoro, T., Miyazaki, A., Tobe, T. & Kiuchi, Y. (2005). Reduction of GTP cyclohydrolase I feedback regulating protein expression by hydrogen peroxide in vascular endothelial cells. *J Pharmacol Sci, 97,*299-302.

[119] Kalivendi, S., Hatakeyama, K., Whitsett, J., Konorev, E., Kalyanaraman, B. & Vásquez-Vivar, J. (2005). Changes in tetrahydrobiopterin levels in endothelial cells and adult cardiomyocytes induced by LPS and hydrogen peroxide--a role for GFRP? *Free Radic Biol Med, 38,* 481-491.

[120] Baker, T. A., Milstien, S. & Katusic, Z. S. (2001). Effect of vitamin C on the availability of tetrahydrobiopterin in human endothelial cells. *J Cardiovasc Pharmacol, 37*, 333-338.

[121] d'Uscio, L. V., Milstien, S., Richardson, D., Smith, L. & Katusic, Z. S. (2003). Long-term vitamin C treatment increases vascular tetrahydrobiopterin levels and nitric oxide synthase activity. *Circ Res, 92*, 88-95.

In: Chronic Fatigue Syndrome: Symptoms, Causes & Prevention   ISBN: 978-1-60741-493-3
Editor: E. Svoboda and K. Zelenjcik, pp. 57-88   © 2010 Nova Science Publishers, Inc.

Chapter 3

The Anti-Fatigue Effect of Moderate Cooling: The Evidence, Physiological Mechanisms, and Possible Implications for the Prevention or Treatment of CFS

Nikolai A. Shevchuk

Molecular Radiobiology Division, Department of Radiation Oncology, Virginia
Commonwealth University School of Medicine, Richmond, VA 23298.

Abstract

At least eight studies published since 1962 suggest that moderate cooling of the body (in most cases by means of cold water) can reduce fatigue in healthy subjects and in some groups of patients: fibromyalgia, multiple sclerosis, and rheumatoid arthritis. To date, there have been no studies on the effectiveness of this approach in CFS, aside from a pilot study in Australia, which used contrast water therapy in combination with nutritional and exercise interventions. Psychostimulant medications, the anti-fatigue therapy with the strongest level of clinical evidence for a number of disorders, do not appear to be effective in CFS patients.

The possible mechanisms of the anti-fatigue effect of cooling may involve the following: A) A reduction of the total level of serotonin in the brain, as evidenced by direct measurements in laboratory animals and by a drop of the plasma prolactin level in human subjects; this would be consistent with reduced fatigue according to "the serotonin hypothesis of central fatigue." B) Activation of stress-response pathways such as the hypothalamic-pituitary-adrenal axis and sympathetic nervous system. C) Systemic analgesia and reduced muscle pain in particular; this may be mediated by a spike in the plasma level of beta-endorphin, an opioid peptide, as well as by the gate control effects of sensory stimulation by cold water. D) Activation of components of the brainstem arousal system, such as raphe nuclei and locus ceruleus (most likely associated with activation of the sympathetic nervous system). This diffuse modulatory system controls the sleep/wake cycle and minor lesions correlate with severe chronic fatigue. E) Possible activation of relevant dopaminergic pathways in the brain, such as those projecting to the striatum. F) Activation of the thyroid and increased metabolic rate.

Interestingly, B, D and E resemble physiological effects of psychostimulants. Importantly, A, B, C, and possibly D, seem to be relevant to the pathophysiology of CFS and suggest that repeated moderate cooling may be beneficial for the patients. Successful application of this approach in CFS would require devising a procedure that is acceptable to patients, since regular cold showers and cold-water swimming are highly stressful. If the procedure does not involve psychological distress, inhalation of cold air, and hypothermia, then it would be expected to have little or no adverse effects on health. A lifetime experiment on rats has shown that repeated moderate cooling is most likely safe, at least in healthy subjects.

1. Introduction

Therapeutic use of cold water has a long history, for example, cold water affusions and cold baths were used for the treatment of fever in Europe two centuries ago [1]. Around that time, Scottish physician James Currie noticed that immersion in cold water could act as a central nervous system stimulant [1]. More recently, in the 1960s, two studies investigated specifically the effect of body cooling on mental and physical fatigue [2,3]. The first study (Pratusevich and Shustruiskaia, 1962) showed that exposure to cold air with or without physical exercise can reduce mental fatigue in children [2]. The other study (Roundy and Cooney, 1968) demonstrated that abdominal cold packs and cold showers can reduce physical fatigue in adults [3]. After that, there seems to be a long gap in literature in this field and the effects of systemic cooling on fatigue were revisited only at the beginning of the 21th century by a series of studies that included both healthy subjects and some groups of patients [4-6]. It should be noted that there were also several published studies on the effects of local cooling on muscle fatigue in the 1950s- 70s [7-11].

The recent studies of systemic cooling were prompted in part by the observation that in some groups of patients (e.g. multiple sclerosis), fatigue can increase significantly in a warm environment [12]. This lead to the development of the cooling suit, which is applied to the torso and parts of the head and can reduce the core body temperature of a patient by 0.5-1.0 degrees Celsius by means of a circulating cooled liquid [13]. Two studies that used a small sample of multiple sclerosis patients (8-20 participants) showed that the cooling suit can reduce fatigue both in a warm and in a thermoneutral environment [4,13]. It was concluded that the cooling suit can significantly improve quality of life of multiple sclerosis patients (the majority of whom are heat-sensitive) [4]. Another series of studies investigated physiological effects of winter swimming, a practice that is rather widespread in Scandinavian countries [5,14,15]. After participants in the initial studies reported improved mood and reduced tiredness [14,15], Huttunen et al. (2004) set out to specifically investigate the effects of winter swimming on mood and fatigue [5]. In that study, a mixed group of volunteers (both healthy subjects and some patients with somatic disorders) used winter swimming 4 times per week for 4 months starting in October. The study showed statistically significant reduction of fatigue in the experimental group compared to the control group (no treatment) [5]. The experimental group included patients with rheumatoid arthritis and fibromyalgia, the disorders that are often associated with the symptom of chronic fatigue. These patients reported reduced fatigue as a result of winter swimming, although these results most likely were not statistically significant because the size of each patient group was too small. The authors concluded that winter swimming can improve general well-being in healthy subjects and in some patients [5]. Although that study did not report adverse effects on health among the participants, winter swimming should be used with caution because it can easily cause hypothermia and the associated negative effects as described in more detail in Section 4 below. One of the more recent studies included 3 healthy participants who used cold affusions and cold showers (15-20°C) on a regular basis, one of them for as long as 19 years at the time of publication [16]. These subjects reported that cold hydrotherapy can reduce fatigue caused by physical exercise or by a febrile illness [16].

There seem to be no published studies on the effects of body cooling on patients with chronic fatigue syndrome (CFS). An unpublished observational study was conducted in Australia in the 1990s that included over a hundred CFS patients over a period of several years (Dr. Andriya M. Martinovic, Bidgerdii Community Health Service, Blackwater, QLD, Australia, unpublished data). Cold showers were part of complex protocol that included a visit to a steam room immediately before a cold shower (1-3 hot/cold cycles per session, the contrast water therapy session was repeated daily), and also a program of physical exercise and nutritional changes designed to modify essential fatty acid metabolism [17]. Average duration of enrollment in the study was 4-6 months and some patients reported improvement of physical functioning, although it would be difficult to attribute the clinical change to cold showers specifically.

It should be noted that many of the above-mentioned reports contain a small number participants and the results are not statistically significant. In summary, it can be concluded that the existing empirical data seem promising and further research is needed to confirm the anti-fatigue effect of whole-body cooling.

2. Body Cooling and Athletic Performance

Interestingly, the anecdotal evidence of reduced muscle fatigue as a result of local or systemic cooling has prompted some researchers to investigate whether this approach can improve athletic performance. Various studies have reported the effect of local muscle cooling on total work completed, fatigability, and power output of athletes [7-11,18,19]. Some reports showed reduced or unchanged power output [7,20-22], while others showed an improvement [18,19]. Two reports by Verducci (1999 and 2002) showed that cooling of relevant muscles by local application of ice can reduce fatigability and increase total power output in weight lifters and baseball pitchers [18,19]. Some investigators believe that there is an optimal muscle temperature that results in the greatest total work completed, which is thought to be around 27°C (reviewed in [18]). Studies suggest that both lower and higher temperatures result in smaller amounts of work completed by the muscle [8,10,23,24]. With respect to power output as a function of muscle temperature, there is no consensus among researchers in this field. Some studies suggest that heating of skeletal muscle can increase power output [20,25-27], while others show that heating has no effect on performance whereas cooling can reduce power output [7,22].

As for systemic cooling, two studies showed that precooling of the body before exercise [24,28] or exercising in a moderately cold environment, around 10°C [23], can increase the total work completed and delay the onset of fatigue. A recent paper by Vaile *et al.* has shown that head-out cold-water immersion (15°C for 15 min) repeated daily after bouts of exercise improved performance in twelve cyclists [6]. The authors report that this cooling approach resulted in a statistically significant improvement of both power output and total work completed by the cyclists. The control interventions were hot water immersion and passive recovery. Interestingly, contrast water therapy, i.e. alternating 1-min immersion in hot and cold water (7 cycles) within 14 minutes, has shown a similar performance-enhancing effect compared to cold water immersion [6]. The study design was a multiple-period crossover and each of the four interventions was tested for five consecutive days. The authors conclude that some types of hydrotherapy can improve recovery from exercise-induced fatigue and that their results support the use of cold water immersion and contrast water therapy as performance-enhancing techniques for athletes. It is worth mentioning that these techniques have been used by many athletes for some time now, without firm scientific evidence to support this practice [6].

All of the empirical observations discussed above raise the question of the mechanism behind the anti-fatigue effect of cooling, which is the subject of the next section.

3. Possible Mechanisms of the Anti-Fatigue Effect of Cooling

As described in more detail in the subsections below, possible mechanisms of the reduction of fatigue by body cooling can be the following: A) A reduction of the total level of serotonin in the brain, as evidenced by direct measurements in laboratory animals and by a drop of the plasma prolactin level in human subjects; this would be consistent with reduced fatigue according to "the serotonin hypothesis of central fatigue." B) Activation of stress-response pathways such as the hypothalamic-pituitary-adrenal axis and sympathetic nervous system. C) Systemic analgesia and reduced muscle pain in particular; this may be mediated by a spike in the plasma level of beta-endorphin, an opioid peptide, as well as by the gate control effects of sensory stimulation by cold water. D) Activation of components of the brainstem arousal system, such as raphe nuclei and locus ceruleus (most likely associated with activation of the sympathetic nervous system). This diffuse modulatory system controls the sleep/wake cycle and minor lesions correlate with severe chronic fatigue. E) Possible activation of relevant dopaminergic pathways in the brain, such as those projecting to the striatum. F) Activation of the thyroid and increased metabolic rate. G) Normalization of elevated body temperature, since hyperthermia (including fever) is usually associated with fatigue.

3.a. Cerebral Serotonin and Fatigue

Studies of animal models of exercise-induced fatigue have shown that prolonged exercise (to near-exhaustion) results in an elevated extracellular level of serotonin in certain areas of the brain, particularly in the hippocampus and frontal cortex, which led to the formulation of "the serotonin hypothesis of central fatigue" [29-35]. Since central serotonin is known to play a role in sleep, lethargy and loss of motivation, it was hypothesized that accumulation of serotonin in certain areas of the brain may cause fatigue [29]. In particular, it is known that one of the most common side effects of drugs that can increase extracellular level of serotonin in the brain is drowsiness (and sometimes also fatigue) [36,37]. These drugs include serotonin-releasing agents such as d-fenfluramine (a now defunct anti-obesity drug) and selective serotonin reuptake inhibitors (SSRIs) such as antidepressants fluoxetine and paroxetine [36,37]. Nonetheless, the studies aimed at establishing a causal connection between brain serotonin and exercise-induced fatigue were inconclusive or contradictory and, at present, it is not clear whether moderately elevated levels of brain serotonin can actually cause fatigue or merely coincide with the onset of exercise-induced fatigue [29,34]. The original serotonin hypothesis of central fatigue has been later modified to account for the role of dopamine in the development of fatigue [38], as discussed in more detail in Section 3.e. The latest version of the theory proposes that central fatigue is associated with an increase of the ratio of extracellular serotonin to dopamine in the brain [29]. It should be mentioned that some researchers take issue with the separation of fatigue into "central" (related to the CNS) and "peripheral" (related to skeletal muscle), since the mechanisms of fatigue that can be arbitrarily labeled as central and peripheral are often interrelated and mutually dependent [29]. The definition of fatigue that seems to be widely accepted in the field of sports medicine is a reduction in the force output of skeletal muscle after exertion, which will result in an inability to continue exercise at the same intensity [39-42]. The reduced force output of skeletal muscle may be caused by reduced electrical drive delivered by motoneurons [43,44] and also by the depletion of energy stores in skeletal [45,46] muscle or from the combination of these two factors.

Precisely how physical exercise can lead to the elevated level of serotonin in the brain is not well understood but the theory that is mostly supported by experimental evidence explains this effect by increased availability of plasma tryptophan for transport through the blood-brain barrier [29,32]. It is thought that increased sympathetic nervous system activity during exercise, in particular the hormone epinephrine, leads to lipolysis and the release of free fatty acids into the circulation from adipose tissue. Free fatty acids are used by skeletal muscle as a source of energy and when the muscle tissue nears depletion of glycogen stores, the uptake of free fatty acids from circulation starts to lag behind their release from adipose tissue and their plasma level rises [29]. Free fatty acids can displace tryptophan from albumin (most tryptophan is normally bound to albumin) in the blood plasma, which leads to an elevated plasma level of "free available tryptophan". This free tryptophan can then cross the blood-brain barrier and is converted into serotonin in the brain (the first reaction is catalyzed by an enzyme called tryptophan hydroxylase) [29,32]. One additional factor that is believed to play a role in this chain of events is branched-chain amino acids (valine, leucine and isoleucine). The branched-chain amino acids in the blood plasma can be depleted during the course of physical exercise and because they share the same transporter-protein in the blood-brain barrier with tryptophan, the low level of plasma branched-chain amino acids can facilitate penetration of free tryptophan through the blood-brain barrier [34]. All these events would be expected to increase the level of serotonin in the brain.

With respect to exposure to cold, studies suggest that it reduces the level of serotonin in most regions of the brain [47,48] except the rostral brainstem [49], which would be consistent with diminished fatigue according to the above-mentioned serotonin hypothesis of central fatigue [29,34]. Two studies showed that the total concentration of serotonin (intracellular plus extracellular) in the brain of laboratory animals declines after exposure to cold [47,48]. Other studies have shown that body cooling results in the drop of plasma concentration of prolactin in human subjects [50-52] (contrary evidence [53]), which would also be consistent with reduced serotonin level or activity in the brain because plasma prolactin is believed to be an indicator of cerebral serotonergic activity [35]. Some investigators have pointed out that the plasma level of prolactin is not a very reliable marker of central serotonin activity because the release of prolactin from the pituitary into the bloodstream is controlled by several other neurotransmitter systems, most notably, by the dopamine system [29,54].

It is not known how body cooling can reduce the level of serotonin in the brain, but one possibility is the reduced level or total plasma tryptophan (both free and albumin-bound) as a result of activation of the liver enzyme tryptophan pyrrolase by exposure to cold [55,56]. Another possible explanation is inhibition of serotonergic pathways in the brain due to activation of noradrenergic neurons of locus ceruleus [57-59], which may be related to activation of the sympathetic nervous system in response to cold exposure [57]. Noradrenergic neurons often have an inhibitory effect on serotonergic neurons in the brain (and vice versa) [60,61] and this kind of inhibition may result in a reduced release of serotonin into the extracellular space, and therefore reduced serotonin turnover and synthesis. Interestingly, several studies have shown that exposure to cold activates some serotonergic neurons in the reticular activating system (in some raphe nuclei) [58,62-64] and also increases the level of serotonin in a small brain region called rostral brainstem [49]. However, the decline of the total brain serotonin level that was shown in experimental animals after exposure to cold [47,48] suggests that activity of the majority of serotonergic neurons in the brain is most likely inhibited by systemic cooling of the body.

Since serotonin is believed to play an important role in the regulation of mood and pharmacological agents that increase extracellular level of cerebral serotonin (SSRIs) are used for the treatment of clinical depression [65], a legitimate question may arise whether exposure to cold can worsen mood or exacerbate symptoms of depression, since cooling can temporarily reduce serotonin content of the brain. The answer appears to be "no" because the role of serotonin in depression is rather complicated [66] and, paradoxically, a pharmacological agent that has the opposite effect to that of SSRIs, the selective serotonin reuptake *enhancer* tianeptine (brand names "Coaxil" and "Stablon") can also serve as an effective antidepressant [67]. Additionally, several studies have shown that brief cooling of the body tends to improve rather than worsen mood in human subjects [5,14,15,68-73].

The effect of cooling on cerebral serotonin described in this subsection may be relevant to the pathophysiology of CFS because some studies have shown that this disorder is associated with excessive serotonergic activity in the brain [74-79]. Consequently, a temporary reduction of brain serotonin level could potentially be beneficial for CFS patients. It should be mentioned that some studies have failed to support this supposition [80,81], namely they could not establish an elevated cerebral serotonergic activity in CFS patients.

3.b. Stress-Response Pathways

Exposure to cold is known to activate the hypothalamic-pituitary-adrenal (HPA) axis [82,83] and many components of the sympathetic nervous system [82,84], the two stress response pathways that are believed to play a crucial role in the "fight-or-flight" response to external threats [85,86]. The sympathetic nervous system, in particular, is known to be responsible for priming the body for action by increasing the blood flow to skeletal muscle and causing vasoconstriction in most other organs and systems except brain parenchyma and heart [84,86-88]. These changes should theoretically favor improved physical performance compared to the baseline state of the body. Importantly, clinical studies have shown rather frequent occurrence of the sympathetic nervous system dysfunction in patients with CFS [89-91], but it is unclear at this point, whether this dysfunction is a primary factor in CFS or a symptom that is secondary to other factors associated with CFS, such as low physical activity and deconditioning. Therapeutic approaches aimed at correcting the sympathetic nervous system dysfunction have so far had limited success in CFS patients [92-94]. It should also be added that while moderate cooling stimulates many components of the sympathetic nervous system, it inhibits some of them, for example, the heart rate slows down (due to the baroreflex as a result of increased blood pressure) and activity of sweat glands is suppressed [95].

Dysfunction (insufficient function) of the HPA axis has also been found to correlate with fatigue [96], for example, a lowered plasma level of stress hormone cortisol (secreted by adrenal glands) is one of the few consistent endocrine changes found in CFS in numerous studies [93]. There is some evidence of another deficiency of the HPA axis in various disorders associated with fatigue: hypofunction of corticotropin-releasing hormone-producing neurons (located in hypothalamus) [96-98]. Nonetheless, the causal relationship between HPA hypofunction and fatigue has been difficult to establish so far [92,93]. For example, cortisol injections have shown a rather limited effect on CFS symptoms [92,93].

As mentioned above, body cooling is known to transiently activate the HPA axis [82,83] as evidenced by a brief increase in the plasma levels of adrenocorticotropic hormone [99,100] and beta-endorphin [101,102], as well as a modest elevation in the level of cortisol [103,104]. Some studies reported no significant change in cortisol levels following cold stress [105,106], which may be due to gender or diurnal variation of this effect [103,104]. Repeated cold stress has been shown to enhance HPA axis responsiveness to other stressors [107,108] and to enhance cortisol responses to combined heat-cold stress [109]. Therefore, repeated exposure to cold could potentially restore normal function of the HPA axis in CFS patients, but whether this improvement will result in reduced fatigue is not known. Similarly, repeated stimulation of the sympathetic nervous system by exposure to cold [82,84] may or may not restore its normal function in CFS patients and it is not clear if this will have any significant effect on fatigue.

3.c.The Analgesic Effect of Cooling

Cold hydrotherapy is known to produce a significant analgesic effect [110-112], and reduced muscle pain may to some extent be responsible for the reduction of fatigue that is observed following exposure to cold. There are several possible mechanisms of cold-induced analgesia. Numerous experiments show that laboratory animals subjected to a brief cold water swim experience substantial analgesia for 1-2 hours after the procedure in experiments involving tonic pain and for 5-10 minutes in experiments with phasic pain [110,113-116]. This effect may in part mediated by a many-fold increase in the plasma level of beta-endorphin after exposure to cold [101,102,117] (also reported in humans [103,118,119]), which is an opioid peptide and an endogenous painkiller [101]. The other component of this systemic analgesic effect is non-opioid in nature and appears to be mediated by noradrenergic pathways in the spinal cord and locus ceruleus in the brain [120-122]. While the non-opioid component of analgesia appears to be attenuated with repeated cold swimming [123,124], the opioid component was shown to be augmented [123,125]. An additional possible component of cold swim-induced analgesia is the gate control effect of local sensory stimulation [126]. The gate control theory of pain suggests that pain in the foot, for example, can be relieved by stimulating sensory receptors in the foot through vibration or immersion in cold or hot water, etc [127]. Some regions in the dorsal horn of the spinal cord, called laminae, transmit signals received from both nociceptors and tactile receptors [128]. Stimulation of tactile receptors can suppress transmission of impulses received from pain fibers, in a sense "blocking the gate" for nociception [128]. This gate control effect may explain the analgesic effect of local application of ice or cold water [129-131].

This analgesic effect could be beneficial in CFS, where pain symptoms are rather common [132,133]. In particular, muscle pain is believed to be one of the contributing factors of fatigue in many CFS patients, especially those with comorbid fibromyalgia [134].

3.d. The Reticular Activating System

There is evidence that exposure to cold can activate some components of the reticular activating system [49,58,135] also known as the diffuse modulatory system. It consists of a group of nuclei located mostly in the brainstem and responsible for regulation of the sleep/wake cycle [136,137]. In particular, body cooling appears to stimulate activity of serotonergic neurons of raphe nuclei [58,62-64] and noradrenergic neurons of locus ceruleus [57-59] the changes that can lead to activation of behavior and enhanced somatomotor function of the brain [136,138-142]. In particular, exposure to cold can increase locomotor activity of laboratory animals [143]. Some studies have also reported increased alertness as a result of exposure to cold [4,144,145] in addition to reduction of fatigue [4]. Both of these effects may be related to functionality of the reticular activation system because reduced electrical activity in this system appears to correlate with fatigue in laboratory animals [146-148]. In patients with multiple sclerosis and in polio survivors, the presence of minor lesions in the reticular activating system correlates with severe chronic fatigue [149,150]. This kind of lesions can also cause lethargy in laboratory animals [137,140,151]. Psychostimulant drugs are known to activate components of the reticular activating system, which is believed to be the likely mechanism of their wakefulness-promoting and fatigue-reducing effects [152-156].

Stimulation of the diffuse modulatory system by repeated exposure to cold would be expected to enhance somatomotor function of the brain and could potentially be beneficial in CFS because abnormally high fatigability of CFS patients appears to be mediated by a reduction in the ability of the CNS to generate motor neurotransmission [157-159]. Existing evidence suggests that CFS patients do not have lesions in the reticular activating system [140,160], although there are some data pointing to abnormalities of metabolism, blood flow, and electrical activity in the brainstem [161-164], the anatomical site of the reticular activating system [136,137].

3.e. Dopamine and Fatigue

The strong anti-fatigue and performance-enhancing effects of amphetamine (a psychostimulant drug) have led researchers to examine the role of dopamine in fatigue [165-168]. Amphetamine is a dopamine-norepinephrine reuptake inhibitor and also a dopamine-releasing agent; administration of amphetamine quickly elevates the extracellular level of dopamine in many areas of the brain [169]. Several studies on laboratory animals indeed showed that dopamine may be involved in the development of fatigue; in particular, the extracellular dopamine level in the brain tends to decline during prolonged exercise [38,170]. Additionally, inhibition of dopaminergic activity reduces exercise performance, which can be restored by means of dopamine agonists [171,172]. Administration of amphetamine has been shown to delay the onset of fatigue and to reduce pre-existing fatigue, thus improving exercise performance in both humans and laboratory animals [165-168]. These observations led to the modified version of the serotonin hypothesis of central fatigue, which holds that fatigue may be caused by the increased ratio of cerebral serotonin to dopamine; conversely, a low ratio of central serotonin to dopamine is believed to promote arousal and motivation, resulting in improved endurance performance [29,38].

Interestingly, body cooling can affect cerebral dopamine activity, and one experiment on rats has shown that exposure to cold increases the synthesis of dopamine in the striatum by about 50% [173], which could be one of the possible mechanisms of the anti-fatigue effect of cooling. The increase in the striatal dopamine synthesis is most likely the result of increased firing rate of dopaminergic neurons that project to this brain region from the substantia nigra or from the ventral tegmental area [174]. It can be hypothesized that the activation of dopaminergic neurons of the ventral tegmental area may be responsible for reduction of fatigue because these neurons are thought to control the level of arousal (active wakefulness vs. passive wakefulness) [175].

The dopamine system also controls prolactin release from the pituitary, namely, dopaminergic neurons cause tonic inhibition of the prolactin release [54]. As was mentioned in Section 3.a, serotonergic neurons have the opposite effect and stimulate the release of prolactin from the pituitary [54]. Serotonergic neurons often have inhibitory projections to dopaminergic neurons in the brain [61]. Both dopamine antagonists (such as neuroleptic drugs) and serotonin agonists (such as SSRIs) can cause hyperprolactinemia, i.e. elevated plasma level of prolactin [176,177]. Importantly, exposure to cold has been shown to reduce the plasma level of prolactin [50-52], which can be the result of reduced serotonergic activity or enhanced dopaminergic activity or both [54]. In any of these cases, the drop of plasma prolactin would be consistent with reduced fatigue according to the latest version of the serotonin hypothesis of central fatigue [29,38]. Interestingly, psychostimulant drugs, most of which are known to reduce fatigue [156], also reduce the plasma level of prolactin [178-180].

3.f. The Thyroid and Fatigue

Insufficient function of the thyroid gland (hypothyroidism) is typically associated with the symptom of fatigue [181], while chronically hyperactive state of the thyroid (hyperthyroidism) may be associated with higher prevalence of hypomania and mania [182]. Exposure to cold transiently activates the thyroid as evidenced by an increased plasma level of thyroid stimulating hormone, thyroxine and triiodothyronine [183-185]. This could be yet another possible mechanism of cold-induced reduction of fatigue. The thyroid hormones (mainly triiodothyronine) drive metabolism and are involved in thermogenesis (heat production) that is necessary to maintain normal core temperature of the body upon exposure to cold [186]. In particular, body cooling is known to increase metabolic rate: for instance, head-out immersion in cold water of 20°C almost doubles metabolic rate, while at 14°C it is more than quadrupled [187]. Theoretically, the high metabolic rate may accelerate [188,189] the process of recovery of muscle tissues from fatigue in CFS [190-193] and some studies indeed show accelerated muscle recovery following immersion in cold water [194,195]. In combination with cold-induced analgesia described above, the increased metabolic rate would be expected to reduce fatigue by both improving muscle recovery after exertion and by reducing muscle pain [134]. It should be pointed out that, currently, there is no evidence that CFS is associated with insufficient function of the thyroid or with low cerebral metabolic rate [196-198].

3.g. Fever and Fatigue

Fever as a symptom that can result from a number of medical conditions is almost always associated with fatigue [199,200] while hyperthermia is known to induce fatigue [201-206]. The precise mechanism of hyperthermia-induced fatigue is not clear, however heating of the body can increase the level of serotonin and tryptophan in blood plasma and in the brain [207-209] and is also known to increase the plasma level of prolactin [210], the observations that seem to be consistent with the serotonin hypothesis of central fatigue [29]. These effects of hyperthermia led some investigators to hypothesize that hyperthermia may play a significant role in exercise-induced fatigue, since prolonged exercise usually increases core body temperature [35]. Hyperthermia can also increase permeability of the blood-brain barrier [209] and cause accumulation of various metabolites in the CNS that may have negative effects on its functioning. Therefore, normalizing of elevated body temperature by itself may be expected to diminish fatigue.

One of the first scientific reports of cold water treatments of fever was written by Scottish botanist and military physician William Wright (1735-1819) at the end of the 18th century [211], which was a departure from the then prevailing paradigm according to which fever should be assisted and promoted in order to allow agents of disease to come out of the body with sweat [1]. This is what he wrote about one of his first experiments during a febrile illness that he caught on a boat near Jamaica in 1777:

"September 9th, having given the necessary directions, about three o'clock in the afternoon I stripped off all my cloaths, and threw a sea cloak loosely about me till I got upon deck, when the cloak also was laid aside: three buckets full of cold salt water were then thrown at once on me; the shock was great, but I felt immediate relief. The head-ach and other pains instantly abated, and a fine glow and diaphoresis succeeded. Towards evening, however, the febrile symptoms threatened a return, and I had recourse again to the same method, as before, with the same good effect. I now took food with an appetite, and, for the first time, had a sound night's rest" [211].

He continued the cold affusions twice a day for two additional days, to prevent a relapse [1,211]. The method was later promoted by another Scottish physician James Currie (1756-1805), who went on to test this approach on scarlet fever, smallpox, measles, influenza, as well as shipboard fevers and tropical fevers (malaria) [1]. Unfortunately, James Currie published most of his findings in his books rather than peer-reviewed journals [212].

Cold water treatments were met with initial enthusiasm, especially in Germany and were used rather widely in Central Europe and in the United States in the late 18th/early 19th century [212]. The interest gradually abated by the 1830s, and cold water treatments of fever were virtually abandoned afterwards [1]. The biographers of James Currie cite several reasons:

1. Cold affusions were too stressful and frightening for patients, and were often vehemently opposed by a patient's family [1]. Patients often preferred the less stressful tepid washings (the equivalent of modern sponging [213]) or tepid baths instead of cold water affusions [1].
2. Reports of success with febrile infections lead to indiscriminate use for other non-febrile conditions and resulted in patient discomfort and disappointing results when used in inappropriate circumstances [1]. This situation was aggravated by the fact that body temperature of patients was rarely measured at the time [1,212].
3. There were other, less stressful treatments of fever, which were often preferred by patients and doctors. Some of these other antipyretic treatments, such as James Currie's favorite bloodletting, could reduce the temperature of limbs but had no actual effect on core body temperature as we know today; these other modalities gradually replaced cold water treatments [1].

As described in Section 5, a cold water treatment may be designed such that it is effective, yet minimally stressful, for example, adapted cold showers at 20°C. This author's personal observations suggest that this method is effective in common febrile conditions such as upper respiratory tract infections [70], but, unfortunately, there is no statistically significant evidence that this procedure can serve as an effective antipyretic therapy. It is worth mentioning that physical cooling methods such as ice-water immersion and cold water spraying/evaporation are a quickest and most reliable way of lowering core body temperature known today [206,214]. Some reports show that a cooling speed of up to 0.3°C per minute can be achieved [215,216]. In modern clinical practice, cold baths are not normally used for reducing fever (antipyretic drugs are usually prescribed [217]), although sponging with tepid water is sometimes used instead of antipyretic drugs [213]. Sponging with tepid water (around 30°C) can reduce fever within 1.5 hours and was found to be less effective than acetaminophen in one study [213]. Cold water treatments on the other hand, are routinely used in the management of heatstroke and severe hyperthermia and can quickly reduce body temperature [206,214]. Despite the cooling effect in the case of elevated body temperature [1,215,216], immersion in 16-23°C water cannot normally cause hypothermia (core body temperature of 35°C or lower) in humans, even if the immersion lasts for several hours [218]. Therefore, it can be hypothesized that cold showers or cold baths at 20°C could be used to achieve rather quick elimination of fever with minimal risk of hypothermia. The procedure may have to be repeated several times per day in order to maintain near-normal temperature [1,211]. Interestingly, there is evidence that exposure to cold can abolish febrile responses to endogenous pyrogens [219], suggesting that the antipyretic effect of exposure to cold is mediated not only by physical cooling but also by neuroendocrine changes. Further studies would be necessary to establish the safety and effectiveness of cold water treatments in febrile conditions. Finally, although CFS patients often report experiencing low-grade fever, there is no evidence that the average body temperature of CFS patients is different from normal [196,220].

4. Potential Adverse Effects of Cold Hydrotherapy

As reported in several studies, moderate (and brief) cold hydrotherapy appears to be safe and does not seem to have either short-term or long-term adverse effects on health [84,221-225]. The effect of moderately cold hydrotherapy (16-23°C) on normal core body temperature is expected to be very small and therefore hypothermia is hardly a concern [218,226,227]. A near-life-time experiment on rats by Holloszy and Smith [222], where the animals had to stand in 23°C water for 4 hours 5 days a week, showed that repeated moderate cooling does not have observable adverse effects on health and actually extended average lifespan of the rats by a statistically insignificant 5% compared to control rats [222]. Two of the biggest studies on healthy human subjects, one lasting 5 weeks (daily 1-hour immersion in 20°C water) [221] and the other 6 weeks (1-hour immersion in 14°C water 3 times a week) [223] also did not report adverse effects on health. Further studies would be necessary to assess the safety of moderate cooling in healthy subjects and in patients.

Review of available literature suggests that the key factors determining safety and comfortable application of cold hydrotherapy are the following: (A) use of moderately cold water (around 20°C), rather than very cold water (12°C and lower [228-230]); (B) gradual adaptation to cold water instead of a stressful sudden whole-body exposure [231,232]; (C) monitoring of body temperature and avoiding cold hydrotherapy in rare cases of hypothermia. Some adverse effects of exposure to cold have been reported in literature and are outlined in detail below.

1. Raynaud's syndrome, which is characterized by abnormal sensitivity to cold, would be an obvious contraindication for cold hydrotherapy [233].

2. Prolonged exposure to acute cold can cause severe hypothermia, which has a number of negative effects on health such as hypovolemia, ataxia, atrial dysrhythmias, pulmonary edema, and mental confusion [227,234]. On the other hand, brief immersion (under 1 hour) in moderately cold water (16-23°C) appears to be safe and does not result in hypothermia in healthy human subjects. During this procedure, core body temperature stays almost unchanged during the first hour [218] due to unusual efficiency of the human thermoregulatory system [226]. However, in the elderly or people with certain metabolic disorders, there is a risk of hypothermia even in these moderate conditions, and therefore monitoring of body temperature is necessary and warming techniques such as a warm shower may be needed after cold hydrotherapy [227,234].

3. Water of 14°C and colder can cause pain in the skin [228,235] and may also cause transient slight reddening of the skin [236]. Immersion in water that is 14°C or colder will also cause hypothermia in human subjects [237].

4. As already mentioned above, exposure to acute cold such as swimming in ice-cold water can cause transient pulmonary edema in humans [238], especially after exercise [239,240]. Pulmonary edema in this case is most likely the result of severe hypothermia [227].

5. Sudden acute exposure to cold such as swimming in ice-cold water has been shown to increase permeability of the blood-brain barrier in laboratory animals [229,241]. In particular, this treatment repeated daily was shown to increase mortality of neurovirulent viral infections in mice [231,232], the effect that Ben-Nathan et al. attribute to the stressful nature of the sudden plunge into ice-cold water and to dramatic hypothermia induced by the cold swim [241]. Hypothermia is known to increase permeability of the blood brain barrier in normal test subjects (laboratory animals) [242].

6. Some stressful treatments such as isolation have been shown to increase permeability of the blood-brain barrier and increase mortality of neurovirulent viral infections in laboratory animals [231,241]. Therefore, it would be important to design a body cooling procedure that is not stressful, since winter swimming and sudden cold showers are known to be highly stressful [1,16].

7. Studies show that coldest months of the year are associated with higher incidence of stroke and acute heart failure and the difference is most pronounced among the elderly [243-245]. There is also evidence that immersion in cold water can cause transient arrhythmias in some patients with heart problems [246-248]. In the study by Holloszy and Smith [222], where rats were immersed in cold water repeatedly, starting from the age of 6 months to the age of 32 months, prevalence of heart disease as a possible cause of death was increased (while the prevalence of

malignancies was diminished and the average lifespan of the cold-exposed rats was slightly increased).

8. There is evidence that influenza epidemics occur predominantly during the winter season, however it is not known if this is due to the exposure to cold environment or to other factors, such as changes in nutrition and lifestyle [249,250]. One possible explanation is that inhalation of cold air can compromise immune defenses of the respiratory tract mucosa [251], and this may allow influenza virus to proliferate there freely, lysing epithelial cells and causing the corollary illness [252]. For this reason, a body cooling procedure that does not involve inhalation of cold air would not be expected to increase susceptibility to respiratory infections. For example, brief cooling of the body using 20°C water (such as a shower or immersion) in the atmosphere of room temperature air (20-25°C) is not expected to lower the temperature of the respiratory tract because core body temperature in humans will remain above 35°C [218]. Yet, this author's personal experience (unpublished) suggests that if cough is present, cold showers at 20°C may worsen this symptom.

Based on the literature cited above, the practice of winter swimming may carry some risks to health because of the psychological stress and the possibility of hypothermia. Nevertheless, it should be mentioned that the 4-month-long study of winter swimming (performed 4 times a week) did not report adverse effects on health among participants [5].

5. Conclusion

As discussed in the section about possible mechanisms of cold-induced reduction of fatigue, some of these mechanisms may be relevant to the pathophysiology of CFS. These relevant mechanisms include inhibition of cerebral serotonergic activity, activation of the HPA axis, the analgesic effect, and possibly also stimulation of the reticular activating system. The evidence for some of these effects is statistically insignificant and/or comes from animal models only and further studies would be needed for confirmation. Nonetheless, the totality of the currently available mechanistic evidence combined with the evidence of the anti-fatigue effect in healthy subjects and some groups of patients suggests that repeated moderate cooling could have some therapeutic or possibly prophylactic value for CFS patients.

A possible procedure that could test this hypothesis has been proposed by this author in a recent theoretical paper [16] and is briefly outlined below. It was designed to be minimally stressful and to carry little or no risk of hypothermia. The intervention consists of adapted cold showers, 20°C, at a constant flow rate selected from the range 16 to 24 L/min, lasting 3 minutes, and preceded by a 5-minute gradual adaptation phase (expansion of the area of contact with cold water from the feet up, to make the cold shower less shocking), the whole procedure being repeated 2 times per day (morning and afternoon, no later than 7 p.m.). Sample size estimates for the possible clinical study can be found in that same article [16]. At present, it is not known if repeated moderate cooling is beneficial for CFS patients, and this author is not aware of any ongoing studies.

Interestingly, some (but not all) of the physiological effects of body cooling resemble those of psychostimulant agents. In particular, body cooling can enhance dopaminergic activity in the striatum and can reduce the plasma level of prolactin; it stimulates components of the reticular activating system and of the sympathetic nervous system; it can increase locomotor activity of laboratory animals [143,153,253], as described in more detail above. Unfortunately, several studies have shown that psychostimulants are either not effective or only marginally beneficial for CFS patients [254-257], despite the fact that these medications can be effective at reducing fatigue associated with such medical conditions as major depressive disorder [258-262], idiopathic Parkinson disease [263], primary biliary cirrhosis [264], Charcot-Marie-Tooth disease [265], amyotrophic lateral sclerosis [266], acquired immune deficiency syndrome [267,268], narcolepsy [269], multiple sclerosis [270-273], and occupational sleep deprivation [156,274,275]. Similarly, body cooling may or may not be effective in CFS. Further clinical studies would be needed to determine whether repeated moderate cooling has a significant clinical benefit for CFS patients. Further research would also be needed to assess the safety of this approach in healthy subjects and in patients.

References

[1] Pratusevich, IM; Shustruiskaia, LN. Change in the cortical and subcortical reactions in children during mental fatigue and its elimination by means of cold and muscular work. *Gig Sanit*, 1962, vol. 27, 103-109.

[2] Roundy, ES; Cooney, LD. Effectiveness of rest, abdominal cold packs, and cold showers in relievng fatigue. *Res Q*, 1968, vol. 39, 690-695.

[3] Flensner, G; Lindencrona, C. The cooling-suit: case studies of its influence on fatigue among eight individuals with multiple sclerosis. *J Adv Nurs*, 2002, vol. 37, 541-550.

[4] Huttunen, P; Kokko, L; Ylijukuri, V. Winter swimming improves general well-being. *Int J Circumpolar Health*, 2004, vol. 63, 140-144.

[5] Vaile, J; Halson, S; Gill, N; Dawson, B. Effect of hydrotherapy on recovery from fatigue. *Int J Sports Med*, 2008, vol. 29, 539-544.

[6] Clarke, DH; Royce, J. Rate of muscle tension development and release under extreme temperatures. *Int Z Angew Physiol*, 1962, vol. 19, 330-336.

[7] Clarke, RS; Hellon, RF; Lind, AR. The duration of sustained contractions of the human forearm at different muscle temperatures. *J Physiol*, 1958, vol. 143, 454-473.

[8] Edwards, RH; Harris, RC; Hultman, E; Kaijser, L; Koh, D; Nordesjo, LO. Effect of temperature on muscle energy metabolism and endurance during successive isometric contractions, sustained to fatigue, of the quadriceps muscle in man. *J Physiol*, 1972, vol. 220, 335-352.

[9] Lind, AR. Muscle fatigue and recovery from fatigue induced by sustained contractions. *J Physiol*, 1959, vol. 147, 162-171.

[10] McGown, HL. Effects of cold application on maximal isometric contraction. *Phys Ther*, 1967, vol. 47, 185-192.

[11] Freal, JE; Kraft, GH; Coryell, JK. Symptomatic fatigue in multiple sclerosis. *Arch Phys Med Rehabil*, 1984, vol. 65, 135-138.

[12] Flensner, G; Lindencrona, C. The cooling-suit: a study of ten multiple sclerosis patients' experiences in daily life. *J Adv Nurs,* 1999, vol. 29, 1444-1453.

[13] Hirvonen, J; Lindeman, S; Matti, J; Huttunen, P. Plasma catecholamines, serotonin and their metabolites and beta-endorphin of winter swimmers during one winter. Possible correlations to psychological traits. *Int J Circumpolar Health,* 2002, vol. 61, 363-372.

[14] Lindeman, S; Hirvonen, J; Joukamaa, M. Neurotic psychopathology and alexithymia among winter swimmers and controls--a prospective study. *Int J Circumpolar Health,* 2002, vol. 61, 123-130.

[15] Shevchuk, NA. Possible use of repeated cold stress for reducing fatigue in chronic fatigue syndrome: a hypothesis. *Behav Brain Funct,* 2007, vol. 3, 55.

[16] Gray, JB; Martinovic, AM. Eicosanoids and essential fatty acid modulation in chronic disease and the chronic fatigue syndrome. *Med Hypotheses,* 1994, vol. 43, 31-42.

[17] Verducci, FM. Interval cryotherapy and fatigue in university baseball pitchers. *Res Q Exerc Sport,* 2001, vol. 72, 280-287.

[18] Verducci, FM. Interval Cryotherapy Decreases Fatigue During Repeated Weight Lifting. *J Athl Train,* 2000, vol. 35, 422-426.

[19] Bergh, U; Ekblom, B. Influence of muscle temperature on maximal muscle strength and power output in human skeletal muscles. *Acta Physiol Scand,* 1979, vol. 107, 33-37.

[20] Oksa, J; Rintamaki, H; Rissanen, S. Muscle performance and electromyogram activity of the lower leg muscles with different levels of cold exposure. *Eur J Appl Physiol Occup Physiol,* 1997, vol. 75, 484-490.

[21] Cornwall, MW. Effect of temperature on muscle force and rate of muscle force production in men and women. *J Orthop Sports Phys Ther,* 1994, vol. 20, 74-80.

[22] Galloway, SD; Maughan, RJ. Effects of ambient temperature on the capacity to perform prolonged cycle exercise in man. *Med Sci Sports Exerc,* 1997, vol. 29, 1240-1249.

[23] Olschewski, H; Bruck, K. Thermoregulatory, cardiovascular, and muscular factors related to exercise after precooling. *J Appl Physiol,* 1988, vol. 64, 803-811.

[24] Davies, CT; Mecrow, IK; White, MJ. Contractile properties of the human triceps surae with some observations on the effects of temperature and exercise. *Eur J Appl Physiol Occup Physiol,* 1982, vol. 49, 255-269.

[25] Davies, CT; Young, K. Effect of temperature on the contractile properties and muscle power of triceps surae in humans. *J Appl Physiol,* 1983, vol. 55, 191-195.

[26] Sargeant, AJ. Effect of muscle temperature on leg extension force and short-term power output in humans. *Eur J Appl Physiol Occup Physiol,* 1987, vol. 56, 693-698.

[27] Bruck, K; Olschewski, H. Body temperature related factors diminishing the drive to exercise. *Can J Physiol Pharmacol,* 1987, vol. 65, 1274-1280.

[28] Meeusen, R; Watson, P; Hasegawa, H; Roelands, B; Piacentini, MF. Central fatigue: the serotonin hypothesis and beyond. *Sports Med,* 2006, vol. 36, 881-909.

[29] Romanowski, W; Grabiec, S. The role of serotonin in the mechanism of central fatigue. *Acta Physiol Pol,* 1974, vol. 25, 127-134.

[30] Soares, DD; Coimbra, CC; Marubayashi, U. Tryptophan-induced central fatigue in exercising rats is related to serotonin content in preoptic area. *Neurosci Lett,* 2007, vol. 415, 274-278.

[31] Fernstrom, JD; Fernstrom, MH. Exercise, serum free tryptophan, and central fatigue. *J Nutr,* 2006, vol. 136, 553S-559S.

[32] Davis, JM. Carbohydrates, branched-chain amino acids, and endurance: the central fatigue hypothesis. *Int J Sport Nutr,* 1995, vol. 5 Suppl, S29-38.

[33] Blomstrand, E. A role for branched-chain amino acids in reducing central fatigue. *J Nutr,* 2006, vol. 136, 544S-547S.

[34] Low, D; Cable, T; Purvis, A. Exercise thermoregulation and hyperprolactinaemia. *Ergonomics,* 2005, vol. 48, 1547-1557.

[35] Aman, MG; Kern, RA; Osborne, P; Tumuluru, R; Rojahn, J; del Medico, V. Fenfluramine and methylphenidate in children with mental retardation and borderline IQ: clinical effects. *Am J Ment Retard,* 1997, vol. 101, 521-534.

[36] Hu, XH; Bull, SA; Hunkeler, EM; Ming, E; Lee, JY; Fireman, B; Markson, LE. Incidence and duration of side effects and those rated as bothersome with selective serotonin reuptake inhibitor treatment for depression: patient report versus physician estimate. *J Clin Psychiatry,* 2004, vol. 65, 959-965.

[37] Davis, JM; Bailey, SP. Possible mechanisms of central nervous system fatigue during exercise. *Med Sci Sports Exerc,* 1997, vol. 29, 45-57.

[38] Weir, JP; Beck, TW; Cramer, JT; Housh, TJ. Is fatigue all in your head? A critical review of the central governor model. *Br J Sports Med,* 2006, vol. 40, 573-586.

[39] Gandevia, SC. Some central and peripheral factors affecting human motoneuronal output in neuromuscular fatigue. *Sports Med,* 1992, vol. 13, 93-98.

[40] Guessous, I; Favrat, B; Cornuz, J; Verdon, F. Fatigue: review and systematic approach to potential causes. *Rev Med Suisse,* 2006, vol. 2, 2725-2731.

[41] Evans, WJ; Lambert, CP. Physiological basis of fatigue. *Am J Phys Med Rehabil,* 2007, vol. 86, S29-46.

[42] Dalsgaard, MK; Secher, NH. The brain at work: a cerebral metabolic manifestation of central fatigue? *J Neurosci Res,* 2007, vol. 85, 3334-3339.

[43] Gandevia, SC. Spinal and supraspinal factors in human muscle fatigue. *Physiol Rev,* 2001, vol. 81, 1725-1789.

[44] Schillings, ML; Kalkman, JS; Janssen, HM; van Engelen, BG; Bleijenberg, G; Zwarts, MJ. Experienced and physiological fatigue in neuromuscular disorders. *Clin Neurophysiol,* 2007, vol. 118, 292-300.

[45] Shulman, RG; Rothman, DL. The "glycogen shunt" in exercising muscle: A role for glycogen in muscle energetics and fatigue. *Proc Natl Acad Sci U S A,* 2001, vol. 98, 457-461.

[46] Aly, MS; Mohamed, MI; Rahman, TA; Moustafa, S. Studies of contents of norepinephrine and 5-hydroxytryptamine in brain--I. Normal and cold exposure. *Comp Biochem Physiol C,* 1985, vol. 82, 155-158.

[47] Toh, CC. Effects of temperature on the 5-hydroxytryptamine (serotonin) content of tissues. *J Physiol,* 1960, vol. 151, 410-415.

[48] Passerin, AM; Bellush, LL; Henley, WN. Activation of bulbospinal serotonergic neurons during cold exposure. *Can J Physiol Pharmacol,* 1999, vol. 77, 250-258.

[49] Hermanussen, M; Jensen, F; Hirsch, N; Friedel, K; Kroger, B; Lang, R; Just, S; Ulmer, J; Schaff, M; Ahnert, P; et al. Acute and chronic effects of winter swimming on LH,

FSH, prolactin, growth hormone, TSH, cortisol, serum glucose and insulin. *Arctic Med Res,* 1995, vol. 54, 45-51.

[50] O'Malley, BP; Cook, N; Richardson, A; Barnett, DB; Rosenthal, FD. Circulating catecholamine, thyrotrophin, thyroid hormone and prolactin responses of normal subjects to acute cold exposure. *Clin Endocrinol (Oxf),* 1984, vol. 21, 285-291.

[51] Rauhala, P; Idanpaan-Heikkila, JJ; Lang, A; Tuominen, RK; Mannisto, PT. Cold exposure attenuates effects of secretagogues on serum prolactin and growth hormone levels in male rats. *Am J Physiol,* 1995, vol. 268, E758-765.

[52] Jobin, M; Ferland, L; Cote, J; Labrie, F. Effect of exposure to cold on hypothalamic TRH activity and plasma levels of TSH and prolactin in the rat. *Neuroendocrinology,* 1975, vol. 18, 204-212.

[53] Freeman, ME; Kanyicska, B; Lerant, A; Nagy, G. Prolactin: structure, function, and regulation of secretion. *Physiol Rev,* 2000, vol. 80, 1523-1631.

[54] Francesconi, RP; Boyd, AE, 3rd; Mager, M. Human tryptophan and tyrosine metabolism: effects of acute exposure to cold stress. *J Appl Physiol,* 1972, vol. 33, 165-169.

[55] Sitaramam, V; Ramasarma, T. Nature of induction of tryptophan pyrrolase in cold exposure. *J Appl Physiol,* 1975, vol. 38, 245-249.

[56] Jiang, XH; Guo, SY; Xu, S; Yin, QZ; Ohshita, Y; Naitoh, M; Horibe, Y; Hisamitsu, T. Sympathetic nervous system mediates cold stress-induced suppression of natural killer cytotoxicity in rats. *Neurosci Lett,* 2004, vol. 358, 1-4.

[57] Yuan, L; Brewer, C; Pfaff, D. Immediate-early Fos protein levels in brainstem neurons of male and female gonadectomized mice subjected to cold exposure. *Stress,* 2002, vol. 5, 285-294.

[58] Beley, A; Beley, P; Rochette, L; Bralet, J. Time-dependent changes in the rate of noradrenaline synthesis in various rat brain areas during cold exposure. *Pflugers Arch,* 1977, vol. 368, 225-229.

[59] Plaznik, A; Danysz, W; Kostowski, W; Bidzinski, A; Hauptmann, M. Interaction between noradrenergic and serotonergic brain systems as evidenced by behavioral and biochemical effects of microinjections of adrenergic agonists and antagonists into the median raphe nucleus. *Pharmacol Biochem Behav,* 1983, vol. 19, 27-32.

[60] Guiard, BP; El Mansari, M; Merali, Z; Blier, P. Functional interactions between dopamine, serotonin and norepinephrine neurons: an in-vivo electrophysiological study in rats with monoaminergic lesions. *Int J Neuropsychopharmacol,* 2008, vol. 11, 625-639.

[61] Dickenson, AH. Specific responses of rat raphe neurones to skin temperature. *J Physiol,* 1977, vol. 273, 277-293.

[62] McAllen, RM; Farrell, M; Johnson, JM; Trevaks, D; Cole, L; McKinley, MJ; Jackson, G; Denton, DA; Egan, GF. Human medullary responses to cooling and rewarming the skin: a functional MRI study. *Proc Natl Acad Sci U S A,* 2006, vol. 103, 809-813.

[63] Ootsuka, Y; Blessing, WW. Inhibition of medullary raphe/parapyramidal neurons prevents cutaneous vasoconstriction elicited by alerting stimuli and by cold exposure in conscious rabbits. *Brain Res,* 2005, vol. 1051, 189-193.

[64] Deshauer, D; Moher, D; Fergusson, D; Moher, E; Sampson, M; Grimshaw, J. Selective serotonin reuptake inhibitors for unipolar depression: a systematic review of classic long-term randomized controlled trials. *CMAJ,* 2008, vol. 178, 1293-1301.

[65] Lacasse, JR; Leo, J. Serotonin and depression: a disconnect between the advertisements and the scientific literature. *PLoS Med,* 2005, vol. 2, e392.

[66] Olie, JP; Bayle, F; Kasper, S. A meta-analysis of randomized controlled trials of tianeptine versus SSRI in the short-term treatment of depression. *Encephale,* 2003, vol. 29, 322-328.

[67] Berger, BG; Owen, DR. Mood alteration with swimming--swimmers really do "feel better". *Psychosom Med,* 1983, vol. 45, 425-433.

[68] Forrester, JM. The origins and fate of James Currie's cold water treatment for fever. *Med Hist,* 2000, vol. 44, see page 61.

[69] Shevchuk, NA. Adapted cold shower as a potential treatment for depression. *Med Hypotheses,* 2008, vol. 70, 995-1001.

[70] Rymaszewska, J; Bialy, D; Zagrobelny, Z; Kiejna, A. The influence of whole body cryotherapy on mental health. *Psychiatr Pol,* 2000, vol. 34, 649-653.

[71] Rymaszewska, J; Ramsey, D; Chladzinska-Kiejna, S. Whole-body cryotherapy as adjunct treatment of depressive and anxiety disorders. *Arch Immunol Ther Exp (Warsz),* 2008, vol. 56, 63-68.

[72] Wehr, TA; Sack, DA; Rosenthal, NE. Seasonal affective disorder with summer depression and winter hypomania. *Am J Psychiatry,* 1987, vol. 144, 1602-1603.

[73] Cleare, AJ; Bearn, J; Allain, T; McGregor, A; Wessely, S; Murray, RM; O'Keane, V. Contrasting neuroendocrine responses in depression and chronic fatigue syndrome. *J Affect Disord,* 1995, vol. 34, 283-289.

[74] Bakheit, AM; Behan, PO; Dinan, TG; Gray, CE; O'Keane, V. Possible upregulation of hypothalamic 5-hydroxytryptamine receptors in patients with postviral fatigue syndrome. *BMJ,* 1992, vol. 304, 1010-1012.

[75] Sharpe, M; Hawton, K; Clements, A; Cowen, PJ. Increased brain serotonin function in men with chronic fatigue syndrome. *BMJ,* 1997, vol. 315, 164-165.

[76] Spath, M; Welzel, D; Farber, L. Treatment of chronic fatigue syndrome with 5-HT3 receptor antagonists--preliminary results. *Scand J Rheumatol Suppl,* 2000, vol. 113, 72-77.

[77] Badawy, AA; Morgan, CJ; Llewelyn, MB; Albuquerque, SR; Farmer, A. Heterogeneity of serum tryptophan concentration and availability to the brain in patients with the chronic fatigue syndrome. *J Psychopharmacol,* 2005, vol. 19, 385-391.

[78] Georgiades, E; Behan, WM; Kilduff, LP; Hadjicharalambous, M; Mackie, EE; Wilson, J; Ward, SA; Pitsiladis, YP. Chronic fatigue syndrome: new evidence for a central fatigue disorder. *Clin Sci (Lond),* 2003, vol. 105, 213-218.

[79] Yatham, LN; Morehouse, RL; Chisholm, BT; Haase, DA; MacDonald, DD; Marrie, TJ. Neuroendocrine assessment of serotonin (5-HT) function in chronic fatigue syndrome. *Can J Psychiatry,* 1995, vol. 40, 93-96.

[80] Vassallo, CM; Feldman, E; Peto, T; Castell, L; Sharpley, AL; Cowen, PJ. Decreased tryptophan availability but normal post-synaptic 5-HT2c receptor sensitivity in chronic fatigue syndrome. *Psychol Med,* 2001, vol. 31, 585-591.

[81] Nakamoto, M. Responses of sympathetic nervous system to cold exposure in vibration syndrome subjects and age-matched healthy controls. *Int Arch Occup Environ Health,* 1990, vol. 62, 177-181.

[82] Nakane, T; Audhya, T; Kanie, N; Hollander, CS. Evidence for a role of endogenous corticotropin-releasing factor in cold, ether, immobilization, and traumatic stress. *Proc Natl Acad Sci U S A,* 1985, vol. 82, 1247-1251.

[83] Jansky, L; Sramek, P; Savlikova, J; Ulicny, B; Janakova, H; Horky, K. Change in sympathetic activity, cardiovascular functions and plasma hormone concentrations due to cold water immersion in men. *Eur J Appl Physiol Occup Physiol,* 1996, vol. 74, 148-152.

[84] Hellstrom, PM; Olerup, O; Tatemoto, K. Neuropeptide Y may mediate effects of sympathetic nerve stimulations on colonic motility and blood flow in the cat. *Acta Physiol Scand,* 1985, vol. 124, 613-624.

[85] Jansen, AS; Nguyen, XV; Karpitskiy, V; Mettenleiter, TC; Loewy, AD. Central command neurons of the sympathetic nervous system: basis of the fight-or-flight response. *Science,* 1995, vol. 270, 644-646.

[86] Handa, Y; Caner, H; Hayashi, M; Tamamaki, N; Nojyo, Y. The distribution pattern of the sympathetic nerve fibers to the cerebral arterial system in rat as revealed by anterograde labeling with WGA-HRP. *Exp Brain Res,* 1990, vol. 82, 493-498.

[87] Sinski, M; Lewandowski, J; Abramczyk, P; Narkiewicz, K; Gaciong, Z. Why study sympathetic nervous system? *J Physiol Pharmacol,* 2006, vol. 57 Suppl 11, 79-92.

[88] Freeman, R; Komaroff, AL. Does the chronic fatigue syndrome involve the autonomic nervous system? *Am J Med,* 1997, vol. 102, 357-364.

[89] Wyller, VB; Godang, K; Morkrid, L; Saul, JP; Thaulow, E; Walloe, L. Abnormal thermoregulatory responses in adolescents with chronic fatigue syndrome: relation to clinical symptoms. *Pediatrics,* 2007, vol. 120, e129-137.

[90] Centers for Disease Control and Prevention, Atlanta, GA, USA. Chronic fatigue syndrome: possible causes [online].2007 [cited 2008 September 30]. Available from: URL: http://www.cdc.gov/cfs/cfscauses.htm

[91] Centers for Disease Control and Prevention, Atlanta, GA, USA. Chronic fatigue syndrome: Treatment options [online].2007 [cited 2008 September 30]. Available from: URL: http://www.cdc.gov/cfs/cfstreatmentHCP.htm

[92] Cleare, AJ. The neuroendocrinology of chronic fatigue syndrome. *Endocr Rev,* 2003, vol. 24, 236-252.

[93] Peterson, PK; Pheley, A; Schroeppel, J; Schenck, C; Marshall, P; Kind, A; Haugland, JM; Lambrecht, LJ; Swan, S; Goldsmith, S. A preliminary placebo-controlled crossover trial of fludrocortisone for chronic fatigue syndrome. *Arch Intern Med,* 1998, vol. 158, 908-914.

[94] Korhonen, I. Blood pressure and heart rate responses in men exposed to arm and leg cold pressor tests and whole-body cold exposure. *Int J Circumpolar Health,* 2006, vol. 65, 178-184.

[95] Swain, MG. Fatigue in chronic disease. *Clin Sci (Lond),* 2000, vol. 99, 1-8.

[96] Gold, PW; Licinio, J; Wong, ML; Chrousos, GP. Corticotropin releasing hormone in the pathophysiology of melancholic and atypical depression and in the mechanism of action of antidepressant drugs. *Ann N Y Acad Sci,* 1995, vol. 771, 716-729.

[97] Neeck, G; Crofford, LJ. Neuroendocrine perturbations in fibromyalgia and chronic fatigue syndrome. *Rheum Dis Clin North Am,* 2000, vol. 26, 989-1002.

[98] Ohno, H; Yahata, T; Yamashita, K; Kuroshima, A. Effect of acute cold exposure on ACTH and zinc concentrations in human plasma. *Jpn J Physiol,* 1987, vol. 37, 749-755.

[99] Goundasheva, D; Andonova, M; Ivanov, V. Changes in some parameters of the immune response in rats after cold stress. *Zentralbl Veterinarmed B,* 1994, vol. 41, 670-674.

[100] Vaswani, KK; Richard, CW, 3rd; Tejwani, GA. Cold swim stress-induced changes in the levels of opioid peptides in the rat CNS and peripheral tissues. *Pharmacol Biochem Behav,* 1988, vol. 29, 163-168.

[101] Giagnoni, G; Santagostino, A; Senini, R; Fumagalli, P; Gori, E. Cold stress in the rat induces parallel changes in plasma and pituitary levels of endorphin and ACTH. *Pharmacol Res Commun,* 1983, vol. 15, 15-21.

[102] Gerra, G;, volpi, R; Delsignore, R; Maninetti, L; Caccavari, R; Vourna, S; Maestri, D; Chiodera, P; Ugolotti, G; Coiro, V. Sex-related responses of beta-endorphin, ACTH, GH and PRL to cold exposure in humans. *Acta Endocrinol (Copenh),* 1992, vol. 126, 24-28.

[103] Smith, DJ; Deuster, PA; Ryan, CJ; Doubt, TJ. Prolonged whole body immersion in cold water: hormonal and metabolic changes. *Undersea Biomed Res,* 1990, vol. 17, 139-147.

[104] Koska, J; Ksinantova, L; Sebokova, E; Kvetnansky, R; Klimes, I; Chrousos, G; Pacak, K. Endocrine regulation of subcutaneous fat metabolism during cold exposure in humans. *Ann N Y Acad Sci,* 2002, vol. 967, 500-505.

[105] Marino, F; Sockler, JM; Fry, JM. Thermoregulatory, metabolic and sympathoadrenal responses to repeated brief exposure to cold. *Scand J Clin Lab Invest,* 1998, vol. 58, 537-545.

[106] Pardon, MC; Ma, S; Morilak, DA. Chronic cold stress sensitizes brain noradrenergic reactivity and noradrenergic facilitation of the HPA stress response in Wistar Kyoto rats. *Brain Res,* 2003, vol. 971, 55-65.

[107] Ma, S; Morilak, DA. Chronic intermittent cold stress sensitises the hypothalamic-pituitary-adrenal response to a novel acute stress by enhancing noradrenergic influence in the rat paraventricular nucleus. *J Neuroendocrinol,* 2005, vol. 17, 761-769.

[108] Dugue, B; Leppanen, E. Adaptation related to cytokines in man: effects of regular swimming in ice-cold water. *Clin Physiol,* 2000, vol. 20, 114-121.

[109] Truesdell, LS; Bodnar, RJ. Reduction in cold-water swim analgesia following hypothalamic paraventricular nucleus lesions. *Physiol Behav,* 1987, vol. 39, 727-731.

[110] Kenunen, OG; Prakh'e, IV; Kozlovskii, BL. A change in the alarm level entails a change in behavioural strategy of mice in stress and a change in analgesia induced by it. *Ross Fiziol Zh Im I M Sechenova,* 2004, vol. 90, 1555-1562.

[111] LaFoy, J; Geden, EA. Postepisiotomy pain: warm versus cold sitz bath. *J Obstet Gynecol Neonatal Nurs,* 1989, vol. 18, 399-403.

[112] Hua, S; Hermanussen, S; Tang, L; Monteith, GR; Cabot, PJ. The neural cell adhesion molecule antibody blocks cold water swim stress-induced analgesia and cell adhesion between lymphocytes and cultured dorsal root ganglion neurons. *Anesth Analg,* 2006, vol. 103, 1558-1564.

[113] Parsons, CG; Herz, A. Peripheral opioid receptors mediating antinociception in inflammation. Evidence for activation by enkephalin-like opioid peptides after cold water swim stress. *J Pharmacol Exp Ther,* 1990, vol. 255, 795-802.

[114] Bodnar, RJ; Komisaruk, BR. Reduction in cervical probing analgesia by repeated prior exposure to cold-water swims. *Physiol Behav,* 1984, vol. 32, 653-655.

[115] Metzger, D; Zwingmann, C; Protz, W; Jackel, WH. Whole-body cryotherapy in rehabilitation of patients with rheumatoid diseases--pilot study. *Rehabilitation (Stuttg),* 2000, vol. 39, 93-100.

[116] Sasaki, F; Wu, P; Rougeau, D; Unabia, G; Childs, GV. Cytochemical studies of responses of corticotropes and thyrotropes to cold and novel environment stress. *Endocrinology,* 1990, vol. 127, 285-297.

[117] Glickman-Weiss, EL; Nelson, AG; Hearon, CM; Goss, FL; Robertson, RJ. Are beta-endorphins and thermoregulation during cold-water immersion related? *Undersea Hyperb Med,* 1993, vol. 20, 205-213.

[118] Suzuki, K; Maekawa, K; Minakuchi, H; Yatani, H; Clark, GT; Matsuka, Y; Kuboki, T. Responses of the hypothalamic-pituitary-adrenal axis and pain threshold changes in the orofacial region upon cold pressor stimulation in normal, volunteers. *Arch Oral Biol,* 2007, vol. 52, 797-802.

[119] Bodnar, RJ; Kelly, DD; Spiaggia, A; Ehrenberg, C; Glusman, M. Dose-dependent reductions by naloxone of analgesia induced by cold-water stress. *Pharmacol Biochem Behav,* 1978, vol. 8, 667-672.

[120] Kepler, KL; Bodnar, RJ. Yohimbine potentiates cold-water swim analgesia: re-evaluation of a noradrenergic role. *Pharmacol Biochem Behav,* 1988, vol. 29, 83-88.

[121] Rochford, J; Henry, JL. Analgesia induced by continuous versus intermittent cold water swim in the rat: differential effects of intrathecal administration of phentolamine and methysergide. *Pharmacol Biochem Behav,* 1988, vol. 31, 27-31.

[122] Lapo, IB; Konarzewski, M; Sadowski, B. Effect of cold acclimation and repeated swimming on opioid and nonopioid swim stress-induced analgesia in selectively bred mice. *Physiol Behav,* 2003, vol. 78, 345-350.

[123] Hamm, RJ; Knisely, JS; Lyons, CM. Adaptation of body temperature and nociception to cold stress in preweanling rats. *Physiol Behav,* 1990, vol. 47, 895-897.

[124] Bragin, EO; Popkova, EV; Vasilenko, GF. Changes in pain reactions and 3H-naloxone binding to opiate receptors of the hypothalamus and midbrain in rats after repeated swimming in cold water. *Biull Eksp Biol Med,* 1989, vol. 108, 292-294.

[125] Nadler, SF; Weingand, K; Kruse, RJ. The physiologic basis and clinical applications of cryotherapy and thermotherapy for the pain practitioner. *Pain Physician,* 2004, vol. 7, 395-399.

[126] DeLeo, JA. Basic science of pain. *J Bone Joint Surg Am,* 2006, vol. 88 Suppl 2, 58-62.

[127] Kandel, ER; Schwartz, JH; Jessell, TM. Principles of Neural Science. 4th edn. New York: McGraw-Hill; 2000.

[128] Diamond, S; Freitag, FG. Cold as an adjunctive therapy for headache. *Postgrad Med,* 1986, vol. 79, 305-309.

[129] Robbins, LD. Cryotherapy for headache. *Headache,* 1989, vol. 29, 598-600.

[130] Singh, RK; Martinez, A; Baxter, P. Head cooling for exercise-induced headache. *J Child Neurol,* 2006, vol. 21, 1067-1068.

[131] Fukuda, K; Straus, SE; Hickie, I; Sharpe, MC; Dobbins, JG; Komaroff, A. The chronic fatigue syndrome: a comprehensive approach to its definition and study. International Chronic Fatigue Syndrome Study Group. *Ann Intern Med,* 1994, vol. 121, 953-959.

[132] Meeus, M; Nijs, J. Central sensitization: a biopsychosocial explanation for chronic widespread pain in patients with fibromyalgia and chronic fatigue syndrome. *Clin Rheumatol,* 2007, vol. 26, 465-473.

[133] Cook, DB; Nagelkirk, PR; Poluri, A; Mores, J; Natelson, BH. The influence of aerobic fitness and fibromyalgia on cardiorespiratory and perceptual responses to exercise in patients with chronic fatigue syndrome. *Arthritis Rheum,* 2006, vol. 54, 3351-3362.

[134] Baffi, JS; Palkovits, M. Fine topography of brain areas activated by cold stress. A fos immunohistochemical study in rats. *Neuroendocrinology,* 2000, vol. 72, 102-113.

[135] Kayama, Y; Ito, S; Koyama, Y; Jodo, E. Tonic and phasic components of the ascending reticular activating system. *Fukushima J Med Sci,* 1991, vol. 37, 59-74.

[136] Siegel, J. Brain mechanisms that control sleep and waking. *Naturwissenschaften,* 2004, vol. 91, 355-365.

[137] Stone, EA; Lin, Y; Ahsan, R; Quartermain, D. Role of locus coeruleus alpha1-adrenoceptors in motor activity in rats. *Synapse,* 2004, vol. 54, 164-172.

[138] Lovick, TA. The medullary raphe nuclei: a system for integration and gain control in autonomic and somatomotor responsiveness? *Exp Physiol,* 1997, vol. 82, 31-41.

[139] Dickinson, CJ. Chronic fatigue syndrome--aetiological aspects. *Eur J Clin Invest,* 1997, vol. 27, 257-267.

[140] Kiyashchenko, LI; Mileykovskiy, BY; Lai, YY; Siegel, JM. Increased and decreased muscle tone with orexin (hypocretin) microinjections in the locus coeruleus and pontine inhibitory area. *J Neurophysiol,* 2001, vol. 85, 2008-2016.

[141] Hornung, JP. The human raphe nuclei and the serotonergic system. *J Chem Neuroanat,* 2003, vol. 26, 331-343.

[142] Chambers, JB; Williams, TD; Nakamura, A; Henderson, RP; Overton, JM; Rashotte, ME. Cardiovascular and metabolic responses of hypertensive and normotensive rats to one week of cold exposure. *Am J Physiol Regul Integr Comp Physiol,* 2000, vol. 279, R1486-1494.

[143] Mahapatra, AP; Mallick, HN; Kumar, VM. Changes in sleep on chronic exposure to warm and cold ambient temperatures. *Physiol Behav,* 2005, vol. 84, 287-294.

[144] Giesbrecht, GG; Arnett, JL; Vela, E; Bristow, GK. Effect of task complexity on mental performance during immersion hypothermia. *Aviat Space Environ Med,* 1993, vol. 64, 206-211.

[145] Derevenco, P; Stoica, N; Sovrea, I; Imreh, S. Central and peripheral effects of 6-hydroxydopamine on exercise performance in rats. *Psychoneuroendocrinology,* 1986, vol. 11, 141-153.

[146] Boev, VM; Krauz, VA. Functional state of the hippocampo-reticular complex during submaximal physical loading and fatigue. *Zh Vyssh Nerv Deiat Im I P Pavlova,* 1981, vol. 31, 1029-1037.

[147] Fornal, CA; Martin-Cora, FJ; Jacobs, BL. "Fatigue" of medullary but not mesencephalic raphe serotonergic neurons during locomotion in cats. *Brain Res,* 2006, vol. 1072, 55-61.

[148] Staub, F; Bogousslavsky, J. Fatigue after stroke: a major but neglected issue. *Cerebrovasc Dis,* 2001, vol. 12, 75-81.

[149] Bruno, RL; Cohen, JM; Galski, T; Frick, NM. The neuroanatomy of post-polio fatigue. *Arch Phys Med Rehabil,* 1994, vol. 75, 498-504.

[150] Szymusiak, R; Iriye, T; McGinty, D. Sleep-waking discharge of neurons in the posterior lateral hypothalamic area of cats. *Brain Res Bull,* 1989, vol. 23, 111-120.

[151] Hou, RH; Freeman, C; Langley, RW; Szabadi, E; Bradshaw, CM. Does modafinil activate the locus coeruleus in man? Comparison of modafinil and clonidine on arousal and autonomic functions in human, volunteers. *Psychopharmacology (Berl),* 2005, vol. 181, 537-549.

[152] Alttoa, A; Eller, M; Herm, L; Rinken, A; Harro, J. Amphetamine-induced locomotion, behavioral sensitization to amphetamine, and striatal D2 receptor function in rats with high or low spontaneous exploratory activity: differences in the role of locus coeruleus. *Brain Res,* 2007, vol. 1131, 138-148.

[153] Colussi-Mas, J; Geisler, S; Zimmer, L; Zahm, DS; Berod, A. Activation of afferents to the ventral tegmental area in response to acute amphetamine: a double-labelling study. *Eur J Neurosci,* 2007, vol. 26, 1011-1025.

[154] Nikolaou, A; Schiza, SE; Giakoumaki, SG; Roussos, P; Siafakas, N; Bitsios, P. The 5-min pupillary alertness test is sensitive to modafinil: a placebo controlled study in patients with sleep apnea. *Psychopharmacology (Berl),* 2008, vol. 196, 167-175.

[155] Pigeau, R; Naitoh, P; Buguet, A; McCann, C; Baranski, J; Taylor, M; Thompson, M; Mac, KII. Modafinil, d-amphetamine and placebo during 64 hours of sustained mental work. I. Effects on mood, fatigue, cognitive performance and body temperature. *J Sleep Res,* 1995, vol. 4, 212-228.

[156] Schillings, ML; Kalkman, JS; van der Werf, SP; van Engelen, BG; Bleijenberg, G; Zwarts, MJ. Diminished central activation during maximal, voluntary contraction in chronic fatigue syndrome. *Clin Neurophysiol,* 2004, vol. 115, 2518-2524.

[157] Siemionow, V; Fang, Y; Calabrese, L; Sahgal, V; Yue, GH. Altered central nervous system signal during motor performance in chronic fatigue syndrome. *Clin Neurophysiol,* 2004, vol. 115, 2372-2381.

[158] Kent-Braun, JA; Sharma, KR; Weiner, MW; Massie, B; Miller, RG. Central basis of muscle fatigue in chronic fatigue syndrome. *Neurology,* 1993, vol. 43, 125-131.

[159] Lewis, DH; Mayberg, HS; Fischer, ME; Goldberg, J; Ashton, S; Graham, MM; Buchwald, D. Monozygotic twins discordant for chronic fatigue syndrome: regional cerebral blood flow SPECT. *Radiology,* 2001, vol. 219, 766-773.

[160] Tirelli, U; Chierichetti, F; Tavio, M; Simonelli, C; Bianchin, G; Zanco, P; Ferlin, G. Brain positron emission tomography (PET) in chronic fatigue syndrome: preliminary data. *Am J Med,* 1998, vol. 105, 54S-58S.

[161] Neri, G; Bianchedi, M; Croce, A; Moretti, A. "Prolonged" decay test and auditory brainstem responses in the clinical diagnosis of the chronic fatigue syndrome. *Acta Otorhinolaryngol Ital,* 1996, vol. 16, 317-323.

[162] Bianchedi, M; Croce, A; Moretti, A; Neri, G; Barberio, A; Iezzi, A; Pizzigallo, E. Auditory brain stem evoked potentials in the evaluation of chronic fatigue syndrome. *Acta Otorhinolaryngol Ital,* 1995, vol. 15, 403-410.

[163] Costa, DC; Tannock, C; Brostoff, J. Brainstem perfusion is impaired in chronic fatigue syndrome. *QJM,* 1995, vol. 88, 767-773.

[164] Borg, G; Edstrom, CG; Linderholm, H; Marklund, G. Changes in physical performance induced by amphetamine and amobarbital. *Psychopharmacologia,* 1972, vol. 26, 10-18.

[165] Chandler, JV; Blair, SN. The effect of amphetamines on selected physiological components related to athletic success. *Med Sci Sports Exerc,* 1980, vol. 12, 65-69.

[166] Gerald, MC. Effects of (+)-amphetamine on the treadmill endurance performance of rats. *Neuropharmacology,* 1978, vol. 17, 703-704.

[167] Oliverio, A. Analysis of the "anti-fatigue" activity of amphetamine. Role of central adrenergic mechanisms. *Farmaco [Sci],* 1967, vol. 22, 441-449.

[168] Atianjoh, FE; Ladenheim, B; Krasnova, IN; Cadet, JL. Amphetamine causes dopamine depletion and cell death in the mouse olfactory bulb. *Eur J Pharmacol,* 2008, vol. 589, 94-97.

[169] Bailey, SP; Davis, JM; Ahlborn, EN. Effect of increased brain serotonergic activity on endurance performance in the rat. *Acta Physiol Scand,* 1992, vol. 145, 75-76.

[170] Heyes, MP; Garnett, ES; Coates, G. Central dopaminergic activity influences rats ability to exercise. *Life Sci,* 1985, vol. 36, 671-677.

[171] Kalinski, MI; Dluzen, DE; Stadulis, R. Methamphetamine produces subsequent reductions in running time to exhaustion in mice. *Brain Res,* 2001, vol. 921, 160-164.

[172] Beley, A; Beley, P; Rochette, L; Bralet, J. Effect of cold exposure on synthesis of cerebral dopamine (author's transl). *J Physiol (Paris),* 1976, vol. 72, 1029-1034.

[173] Sagvolden, T; Johansen, EB; Aase, H; Russell, VA. A dynamic developmental theory of attention-deficit/hyperactivity disorder (ADHD) predominantly hyperactive/impulsive and combined subtypes. *Behav Brain Sci,* 2005, vol. 28, 397-419; discussion 419-368.

[174] Lee, RS; Steffensen, SC; Henriksen, SJ. Discharge profiles of ventral tegmental area GABA neurons during movement, anesthesia, and the sleep-wake cycle. *J Neurosci,* 2001, vol. 21, 1757-1766.

[175] Damsa, C; Bumb, A; Bianchi-Demicheli, F; Vidailhet, P; Sterck, R; Andreoli, A; Beyenburg, S. "Dopamine-dependent" side effects of selective serotonin reuptake inhibitors: a clinical review. *J Clin Psychiatry,* 2004, vol. 65, 1064-1068.

[176] Dickson, RA; Glazer, WM. Neuroleptic-induced hyperprolactinemia. *Schizophr Res,* 1999, vol. 35 Suppl, S75-86.

[177] Klenerova, V; Sida, P; Hynie, S; Jurcovicova, J. Rat strain differences in responses of plasma prolactin and PRL mRNA expression after acute amphetamine treatment or restraint stress. *Cell Mol Neurobiol,* 2001, vol. 21, 91-100.

[178] Samuels, ER; Hou, RH; Langley, RW; Szabadi, E; Bradshaw, CM. Comparison of pramipexole and modafinil on arousal, autonomic, and endocrine functions in healthy, volunteers. *J Psychopharmacol,* 2006, vol. 20, 756-770.

[179] Shaywitz, BA; Shaywitz, SE; Sebrechts, MM; Anderson, GM; Cohen, DJ; Jatlow, P; Young, JG. Growth hormone and prolactin response to methylphenidate in children with attention deficit disorder. *Life Sci,* 1990, vol. 46, 625-633.

[180] Kumar, N; Allen, KA; Riccardi, D; Bercu, BB; Cantor, A; Minton, S; Balducci, L; Jacobsen, PB. Fatigue, weight gain, lethargy and amenorrhea in breast cancer patients on chemotherapy: is subclinical hypothyroidism the culprit? *Breast Cancer Res Treat,* 2004, vol. 83, 149-159.

[181] Bunevicius, R; Velickiene, D; Prange, AJ, Jr. Mood and anxiety disorders in women with treated hyperthyroidism and ophthalmopathy caused by Graves' disease. *Gen Hosp Psychiatry,* 2005, vol. 27, 133-139.

[182] Savourey, G; Caravel, JP; Barnavol, B; Bittel, JH. Thyroid hormone changes in a cold air environment after local cold acclimation. *J Appl Physiol,* 1994, vol. 76, 1963-1967.

[183] Quintanar-Stephano, JL; Quintanar-Stephano, A; Castillo-Hernandez, L. Effect of the exposure to chronic-intermittent cold on the thyrotropin and thyroid hormones in the rat. *Cryobiology,* 1991, vol. 28, 400-403.

[184] Reed, HL; Quesada, M; Hesslink, RL, Jr.; D'Alesandro, MM; Hays, MT; Christopherson, RJ; Turner, BV; Young, BA. Changes in serum triiodothyronine kinetics and hepatic type I 5'-deiodinase activity of cold-exposed swine. *Am J Physiol,* 1994, vol. 266, E786-795.

[185] Silvestri, E; Schiavo, L; Lombardi, A; Goglia, F. Thyroid hormones as molecular determinants of thermogenesis. *Acta Physiol Scand,* 2005, vol. 184, 265-283.

[186] Sramek, P; Simeckova, M; Jansky, L; Savlikova, J; Vybiral, S. Human physiological responses to immersion into water of different temperatures. *Eur J Appl Physiol,* 2000, vol. 81, 436-442.

[187] St Rose, JE; Murray, GW; Howe, SA. Effect of alterations in metabolic rate on the duration of tolerance in neonatally injected animals. *Int Arch Allergy Appl Immunol,* 1976, vol. 52, 183-187.

[188] Vallerand, AL; Zamecnik, J; Jacobs, I. Plasma glucose turnover during cold stress in humans. *J Appl Physiol,* 1995, vol. 78, 1296-1302.

[189] Wong, R; Lopaschuk, G; Zhu, G; Walker, D; Catellier, D; Burton, D; Teo, K; Collins-Nakai, R; Montague, T. Skeletal muscle metabolism in the chronic fatigue syndrome. *In vivo* assessment by ^{31}P nuclear magnetic resonance spectroscopy. *Chest,* 1992, vol. 102, 1716-1722.

[190] Jammes, Y; Steinberg, JG; Mambrini, O; Bregeon, F; Delliaux, S. Chronic fatigue syndrome: assessment of increased oxidative stress and altered muscle excitability in response to incremental exercise. *J Intern Med,* 2005, vol. 257, 299-310.

[191] McCully, KK; Natelson, BH. Impaired oxygen delivery to muscle in chronic fatigue syndrome. *Clin Sci (Lond),* 1999, vol. 97, 603-608; discussion 611-603.

[192] Fulle, S; Mecocci, P; Fano, G; Vecchiet, I; Vecchini, A; Racciotti, D; Cherubini, A; Pizzigallo, E; Vecchiet, L; Senin, U; Beal, MF. Specific oxidative alterations in vastus

lateralis muscle of patients with the diagnosis of chronic fatigue syndrome. *Free Radic Biol Med,* 2000, vol. 29, 1252-1259.

[193] Nomura, T; Kawano, F; Kang, MS; Lee, JH; Han, EY; Kim, CK; Sato, Y; Ohira, Y. Effects of long-term cold exposure on contractile muscles of rats. *Jpn J Physiol,* 2002, vol. 52, 85-93.

[194] Yanagisawa, O; Niitsu, M; Yoshioka, H; Goto, K; Kudo, H; Itai, Y. The use of magnetic resonance imaging to evaluate the effects of cooling on skeletal muscle after strenuous exercise. *Eur J Appl Physiol,* 2003, vol. 89, 53-62.

[195] Hamilos, DL; Nutter, D; Gershtenson, J; Ikle, D; Hamilos, SS; Redmond, DP; Di Clementi, JD; Schmaling, KB; Jones, JF. Circadian rhythm of core body temperature in subjects with chronic fatigue syndrome. *Clin Physiol,* 2001, vol. 21, 184-195.

[196] Abu-Judeh, HH; Levine, S; Kumar, M; el-Zeftawy, H; Naddaf, S; Lou, JQ; Abdel-Dayem, HM. Comparison of SPET brain perfusion and ^{18}F-FDG brain metabolism in patients with chronic fatigue syndrome. *Nucl Med Commun,* 1998, vol. 19, 1065-1071.

[197] Siessmeier, T; Nix, WA; Hardt, J; Schreckenberger, M; Egle, UT; Bartenstein, P. Observer independent analysis of cerebral glucose metabolism in patients with chronic fatigue syndrome. *J Neurol Neurosurg Psychiatry,* 2003, vol. 74, 922-928.

[198] Anand, AC; Kumar, R; Rao, MK; Dham, SK. Low grade pyrexia: is it chronic fatigue syndrome? *J Assoc Physicians India,* 1994, vol. 42, 606-608.

[199] Camus, F; Henzel, D; Janowski, M; Raguin, G; Leport, C; Vilde, JL. Unexplained fever and chronic fatigue: abnormal circadian temperature pattern. *Eur J Med,* 1992, vol. 1, 30-36.

[200] Koltyn, KF; Robins, HI; Schmitt, CL; Cohen, JD; Morgan, WP. Changes in mood state following whole-body hyperthermia. *Int J Hyperthermia,* 1992, vol. 8, 305-307.

[201] Yamamoto, S; Iwamoto, M; Inoue, M; Harada, N. Evaluation of the effect of heat exposure on the autonomic nervous system by heart rate variability and urinary catecholamines. *J Occup Health,* 2007, vol. 49, 199-204.

[202] McMorris, T; Swain, J; Smith, M; Corbett, J; Delves, S; Sale, C; Harris, RC; Potter, J. Heat stress, plasma concentrations of adrenaline, noradrenaline, 5-hydroxytryptamine and cortisol, mood state and cognitive performance. *Int J Psychophysiol,* 2006, vol. 61, 204-215.

[203] Chad, KE; Brown, JM. Climatic stress in the workplace: its effect on thermoregulatory responses and muscle fatigue in female workers. *Appl Ergon,* 1995, vol. 26, 29-34.

[204] Gonzalez-Alonso, J; Teller, C; Andersen, SL; Jensen, FB; Hyldig, T; Nielsen, B. Influence of body temperature on the development of fatigue during prolonged exercise in the heat. *J Appl Physiol,* 1999, vol. 86, 1032-1039.

[205] Glazer, JL. Management of heatstroke and heat exhaustion. *Am Fam Physician,* 2005, vol. 71, 2133-2140.

[206] Wu, TC; He, HZ; Tanguay, RM; Wu, Y; Xu, DG; Currie, RW; Qu, S; Feng, JD; Zhang, GG. The combined effects of high temperature and carbon monoxide on heat stress response. *J Tongji Med Univ,* 1995, vol. 15, 178-183.

[207] Dey, S; Dey, PK; Sharma, HS. Regional metabolism of 5-hydroxytryptamine in brain under acute and chronic heat stress. *Indian J Physiol Pharmacol,* 1993, vol. 37, 8-12.

[208] Sharma, HS; Dey, PK. Influence of long-term acute heat exposure on regional blood-brain barrier permeability, cerebral blood flow and 5-HT level in conscious normotensive young rats. *Brain Res,* 1987, vol. 424, 153-162.

[209] Koska, J; Rovensky, J; Zimanova, T; Vigas, M. Growth hormone and prolactin responses during partial and whole body warm-water immersions. *Acta Physiol Scand,* 2003, vol. 178, 19-23.

[210] Wright, W. Remarks on malignant fevers; and their cure by cold water and fresh air. *Lond Med J,* 1796, vol. 7, 109-115.

[211] Cosby, CB. James Currie and hydrotherapy. *J Hist Med Allied Sci,* 1950, vol. 5, 280-288.

[212] Agbolosu, NB; Cuevas, LE; Milligan, P; Broadhead, RL; Brewster, D; Graham, SM. Efficacy of tepid sponging versus paracetamol in reducing temperature in febrile children. *Ann Trop Paediatr,* 1997, vol. 17, 283-288.

[213] Wexler, RK. Evaluation and treatment of heat-related illnesses. *Am Fam Physician,* 2002, vol. 65, 2307-2314.

[214] Hadad, E; Rav-Acha, M; Heled, Y; Epstein, Y; Moran, DS. Heat stroke : a review of cooling methods. *Sports Med,* 2004, vol. 34, 501-511.

[215] Harker, J; Gibson, P. Heat-stroke: a review of rapid cooling techniques. *Intensive Crit Care Nurs,* 1995, vol. 11, 198-202.

[216] Botting, R. Antipyretic therapy. *Front Biosci,* 2004, vol. 9, 956-966.

[217] Tikuisis, P. Heat balance precedes stabilization of body temperatures during cold water immersion. *J Appl Physiol,* 2003, vol. 95, 89-96.

[218] Stitt, JT; Shimada, SG. The effect of low ambient temperature on the febrile responses of rats to semi-purified human endogenous pyrogen. *Yale J Biol Med,* 1985, vol. 58, 189-194.

[219] Hamilos, DL; Nutter, D; Gershtenson, J; Redmond, DP; Clementi, JD; Schmaling, KB; Make, BJ; Jones, JF. Core body temperature is normal in chronic fatigue syndrome. *Biol Psychiatry,* 1998, vol. 43, 293-302.

[220] O'Brien, C; Young, AJ; Lee, DT; Shitzer, A; Sawka, MN; Pandolf, KB. Role of core temperature as a stimulus for cold acclimation during repeated immersion in 20 degrees C water. *J Appl Physiol,* 2000, vol. 89, 242-250.

[221] Holloszy, JO; Smith, EK. Longevity of cold-exposed rats: a reevaluation of the "rate-of-living theory". *J Appl Physiol,* 1986, vol. 61, 1656-1660.

[222] Jansky, L; Pospisilova, D; Honzova, S; Ulicny, B; Sramek, P; Zeman, V; Kaminkova, J. Immune system of cold-exposed and cold-adapted humans. *Eur J Appl Physiol Occup Physiol,* 1996, vol. 72, 445-450.

[223] Castellani, JW; IK, MB; Rhind, SG. Cold exposure: human immune responses and intracellular cytokine expression. *Med Sci Sports Exerc,* 2002, vol. 34, 2013-2020.

[224] Banerjee, SK; Aviles, H; Fox, MT; Monroy, FP. Cold stress-induced modulation of cell immunity during acute *Toxoplasma gondii* infection in mice. *J Parasitol,* 1999, vol. 85, 442-447.

[225] Doufas, AG; Sessler, DI. Physiology and clinical relevance of induced hypothermia. *Neurocrit Care,* 2004, vol. 1, 489-498.

[226] McCullough, L; Arora, S. Diagnosis and treatment of hypothermia. *Am Fam Physician*, 2004, vol. 70, 2325-2332.

[227] Julien, N; Marchand, S. Endogenous pain inhibitory systems activated by spatial summation are opioid-mediated. *Neurosci Lett*, 2006, vol. 401, 256-260.

[228] Arican, N; Kaya, M; Kalayci, R; Kucuk, M; Cimen, V; Elmas, I. Effects of acute cold exposure on blood-brain barrier permeability in acute and chronic hyperglycemic rats. *Forensic Sci Int*, 2002, vol. 125, 137-141.

[229] Casey, KL; Minoshima, S; Morrow, TJ; Koeppe, RA. Comparison of human cerebral activation pattern during cutaneous warmth, heat pain, and deep cold pain. *J Neurophysiol*, 1996, vol. 76, 571-581.

[230] Ben-Nathan, D; Lustig, S; Feuerstein, G. The influence of cold or isolation stress on neuroinvasiveness and virulence of an attenuated variant of West Nile virus. *Arch Virol*, 1989, vol. 109, 1-10.

[231] Ben-Nathan, D; Lustig, S; Kobiler, D; Danenberg, HD; Lupu, E; Feuerstein, G. Dehydroepiandrosterone protects mice inoculated with West Nile virus and exposed to cold stress. *J Med Virol*, 1992, vol. 38, 159-166.

[232] Bakst, R; Merola, JF; Franks, AG, Jr.; Sanchez, M. Raynaud's phenomenon: pathogenesis and management. *J Am Acad Dermatol*, 2008, vol. 59, 633-653.

[233] Day, MP. Hypothermia: a hazard for all seasons. *Nursing*, 2006, vol. 36, 44-47.

[234] Misasi, S; Morin, G; Kemler, D; Olmstead, PS; Pryzgocki, K. The effect of a toe cap and bias on perceived pain during cold water immersion. *J Athl Train*, 1995, vol. 30, 49-52.

[235] Wingfield, DL; Fraunfelder, FT. Possible complications secondary to cryotherapy. *Ophthalmic Surg*, 1979, vol. 10, 47-55.

[236] Jansky, L; Janakova, H; Ulicny, B; Sramek, P; Hosek, V; Heller, J; Parizkova, J. Changes in thermal homeostasis in humans due to repeated cold water immersions. *Pflugers Arch*, 1996, vol. 432, 368-372.

[237] Roeggla, M; Roeggla, G; Seidler, D; Muellner, M; Laggner, AN. Self-limiting pulmonary edema with alveolar hemorrhage during diving in cold water. *Am J Emerg Med*, 1996, vol. 14, 333.

[238] Wilmshurst, PT. Pulmonary oedema induced by emotional stress, by sexual intercourse, and by exertion in a cold environment in people without evidence of heart disease. *Heart*, 2004, vol. 90, 806-807.

[239] Biswas, R; Shibu, PK; James, CM. Pulmonary oedema precipitated by cold water swimming. *Br J Sports Med*, 2004, vol. 38, e36.

[240] Ben-Nathan, D; Lustig, S; Danenberg, HD. Stress-induced neuroinvasiveness of a neurovirulent noninvasive Sindbis virus in cold or isolation subjected mice. *Life Sci*, 1991, vol. 48, 1493-1500.

[241] Elmas, I; Kucuk, M; Kalayci, RB; Cevik, A; Kaya, M. Effects of profound hypothermia on the blood-brain barrier permeability in acute and chronically ethanol treated rats. *Forensic Sci Int*, 2001, vol. 119, 212-216.

[242] Myint, PK; Vowler, SL; Woodhouse, PR; Redmayne, O; Fulcher, RA. Winter excess in hospital admissions, in-patient mortality and length of acute hospital stay in stroke: a

hospital database study over six seasonal years in Norfolk, UK. *Neuroepidemiology,* 2007, vol. 28, 79-85.

[243] Milo-Cotter, O; Setter, I; Uriel, N; Kaluski, E; Vered, Z; Golik, A; Cotter, G. The daily incidence of acute heart failure is correlated with low minimal night temperature: cold immersion pulmonary edema revisited? *J Card Fail,* 2006, vol. 12, 114-119.

[244] Sheth, T; Nair, C; Muller, J; Yusuf, S. Increased winter mortality from acute myocardial infarction and stroke: the effect of age. *J Am Coll Cardiol,* 1999, vol. 33, 1916-1919.

[245] Lader, EW; Kronzon, I. Ice-water-induced arrhythmias in a patient with ischemic heart disease. *Ann Intern Med,* 1982, vol. 96, 614-615.

[246] Doubt, TJ; Mayers, DL; Flynn, ET. Transient cardiac sinus dysrhythmia occurring after cold water immersion. *Am J Cardiol,* 1987, vol. 59, 1421-1422.

[247] Houdas, Y; Deklunder, G; Lecroart, JL. Cold exposure and ischemic heart disease. *Int J Sports Med,* 1992, vol. 13 Suppl 1, S179-181.

[248] Fiore, AE; Shay, DK; Haber, P; Iskander, JK; Uyeki, TM; Mootrey, G; Bresee, JS; Cox, NJ. Prevention and control of influenza. Recommendations of the Advisory Committee on Immunization Practices (ACIP), 2007. *MMWR Recomm Rep,* 2007, vol. 56, 1-54.

[249] Reichert, TA; Simonsen, L; Sharma, A; Pardo, SA; Fedson, DS; Miller, MA. Influenza and the winter increase in mortality in the United States, 1959-1999. *Am J Epidemiol,* 2004, vol. 160, 492-502.

[250] Davis, MS; Williams, CC; Meinkoth, JH; Malayer, JR; Royer, CM; Williamson, KK; McKenzie, EC. Influx of neutrophils and persistence of cytokine expression in airways of horses after performing exercise while breathing cold air. *Am J Vet Res,* 2007, vol. 68, 185-189.

[251] Herold, S; von Wulffen, W; Steinmueller, M; Pleschka, S; Kuziel, WA; Mack, M; Srivastava, M; Seeger, W; Maus, UA; Lohmeyer, J. Alveolar epithelial cells direct monocyte transepithelial migration upon influenza virus infection: impact of chemokines and adhesion molecules. *J Immunol,* 2006, vol. 177, 1817-1824.

[252] Dietz, DM; Dietz, KC; Moore, S; Ouimet, CC; Kabbaj, M. Repeated social defeat stress-induced sensitization to the locomotor activating effects of d-amphetamine: role of individual differences. *Psychopharmacology (Berl),* 2008, vol. 198, 51-62.

[253] Wyller, VB. The chronic fatigue syndrome--an update. *Acta Neurol Scand Suppl,* 2007, vol. 187, 7-14.

[254] Valdizan Uson, JR; Idiazabal Alecha, MA. Diagnostic and treatment challenges of chronic fatigue syndrome: role of immediate-release methylphenidate. *Expert Rev Neurother,* 2008, vol. 8, 917-927.

[255] Blockmans, D; Persoons, P; Van Houdenhove, B; Bobbaers, H. Does methylphenidate reduce the symptoms of chronic fatigue syndrome? *Am J Med,* 2006, vol. 119, 167 e123-130.

[256] Randall, DC; Cafferty, FH; Shneerson, JM; Smith, IE; Llewelyn, MB; File, SE. Chronic treatment with modafinil may not be beneficial in patients with chronic fatigue syndrome. *J Psychopharmacol,* 2005, vol. 19, 647-660.

[257] Fava, M; Thase, ME; DeBattista, C; Doghramji, K; Arora, S; Hughes, RJ. Modafinil augmentation of selective serotonin reuptake inhibitor therapy in MDD partial responders with persistent fatigue and sleepiness. *Ann Clin Psychiatry,* 2007, vol. 19, 153-159.

[258] Konuk, N; Atasoy, N; Atik, L; Akay, O. Open-label study of adjunct modafinil for the treatment of patients with fatigue, sleepiness, and major depression treated with selective serotonin reuptake inhibitors. *Adv Ther,* 2006, vol. 23, 646-654.

[259] Thase, ME; Fava, M; DeBattista, C; Arora, S; Hughes, RJ. Modafinil augmentation of SSRI therapy in patients with major depressive disorder and excessive sleepiness and fatigue: a 12-week, open-label, extension study. *CNS Spectr,* 2006, vol. 11, 93-102.

[260] Ninan, PT; Hassman, HA; Glass, SJ; McManus, FC. Adjunctive modafinil at initiation of treatment with a selective serotonin reuptake inhibitor enhances the degree and onset of therapeutic effects in patients with major depressive disorder and fatigue. *J Clin Psychiatry,* 2004, vol. 65, 414-420.

[261] DeBattista, C; Doghramji, K; Menza, MA; Rosenthal, MH; Fieve, RR. Adjunct modafinil for the short-term treatment of fatigue and sleepiness in patients with major depressive disorder: a preliminary double-blind, placebo-controlled study. *J Clin Psychiatry,* 2003, vol. 64, 1057-1064.

[262] Mendonca, DA; Menezes, K; Jog, MS. Methylphenidate improves fatigue scores in Parkinson disease: a randomized controlled trial. *Mov Disord,* 2007, vol. 22, 2070-2076.

[263] Jones, DE; Newton, JL. An open study of modafinil for the treatment of daytime somnolence and fatigue in primary biliary cirrhosis. *Aliment Pharmacol Ther,* 2007, vol. 25, 471-476.

[264] Carter, GT; Han, JJ; Mayadev, A; Weiss, MD. Modafinil reduces fatigue in Charcot-Marie-Tooth disease type 1A: a case series. *Am J Hosp Palliat Care,* 2006, vol. 23, 412-416.

[265] Carter, GT; Weiss, MD; Lou, JS; Jensen, MP; Abresch, RT; Martin, TK; Hecht, TW; Han, JJ; Weydt, P; Kraft, GH. Modafinil to treat fatigue in amyotrophic lateral sclerosis: an open label pilot study. *Am J Hosp Palliat Care,* 2005, vol. 22, 55-59.

[266] Rabkin, JG; McElhiney, MC; Rabkin, R; Ferrando, SJ. Modafinil treatment for fatigue in HIV+ patients: a pilot study. *J Clin Psychiatry,* 2004, vol. 65, 1688-1695.

[267] Breitbart, W; Rosenfeld, B; Kaim, M; Funesti-Esch, J. A randomized, double-blind, placebo-controlled trial of psychostimulants for the treatment of fatigue in ambulatory patients with human immunodeficiency virus disease. *Arch Intern Med,* 2001, vol. 161, 411-420.

[268] Becker, PM; Schwartz, JR; Feldman, NT; Hughes, RJ. Effect of modafinil on fatigue, mood, and health-related quality of life in patients with narcolepsy. *Psychopharmacology (Berl),* 2004, vol. 171, 133-139.

[269] Nagels, G; D'Hooghe M, B; Vleugels, L; Kos, D; Despontin, M; De Deyn, PP. P300 and treatment effect of modafinil on fatigue in multiple sclerosis. *J Clin Neurosci,* 2007, vol. 14, 33-40.

[270] Zifko, UA; Rupp, M; Schwarz, S; Zipko, HT; Maida, EM. Modafinil in treatment of fatigue in multiple sclerosis. Results of an open-label study. *J Neurol,* 2002, vol. 249, 983-987.

[271] Rammohan, KW; Rosenberg, JH; Lynn, DJ; Blumenfeld, AM; Pollak, CP; Nagaraja, HN. Efficacy and safety of modafinil (Provigil) for the treatment of fatigue in multiple sclerosis: a two centre phase 2 study. *J Neurol Neurosurg Psychiatry,* 2002, vol. 72, 179-183.

[272] Weinshenker, BG; Penman, M; Bass, B; Ebers, GC; Rice, GP. A double-blind, randomized, crossover trial of pemoline in fatigue associated with multiple sclerosis. *Neurology,* 1992, vol. 42, 1468-1471.

[273] Wesensten, NJ; Belenky, G; Thorne, DR; Kautz, MA; Balkin, TJ. Modafinil vs. caffeine: effects on fatigue during sleep deprivation. *Aviat Space Environ Med,* 2004, vol. 75, 520-525.

[274] Li, YF; Zhan, H; Xin, YM; Tang, GX; Wei, SH; Li, T. Effects of modafinil on visual and auditory reaction abilities and subjective fatigue level during 48 h sleep deprivation. *Space Med Med Eng (Beijing),* 2003, vol. 16, 277-280.

In: Chronic Fatigue Syndrome: Symptoms, Causes & Prevention   ISBN: 978-1-60741-493-3
Editor: E. Svoboda and K. Zelenjcik, pp. 89-101   © 2010 Nova Science Publishers, Inc.

Chapter 4

Chronic Fatigue Syndrome: Metabolic and Electrophysiological Muscle Responses to Exercise

Yves Jammes, Stéphane Delliaux,
Jean Guillaume Steinberg and Fabienne Brégeon
UMR MD2 P2COE, IFR Jean Roche, Faculty of Medicine, University of Mediterranée
and Lung Function Laboratory, North Hospital, Assistance Publique – Hôpitaux de
Marseille, Marseille, France.

Abstract

Because chronic fatigue syndrome (CFS) is often diagnosed in later life of subjects who exercise frequently, exercise-induced causes of CFS are highly suspected. Muscle metabolism at rest, during, and after muscle contraction was explored in CFS patients using physiological (oxygen uptake (VO_2), arterio-venous oxygen difference) and biochemical assessment (^{31}P resonance magnetic spectroscopy, lactic acid, blood markers of oxidative stress, cytokines, and heat shock proteins, Hsp). In the majority of CFS patients, 1) muscle glycolysis is unaltered, 2) the aerobic capacity is often enhanced and about one-fourth of patients have an increased proportion of type 1 oxidative muscle fibre, 3) exercise-induced production of reactive oxygen species (ROS) is accentuated with reduction of antioxidant defences, 4) the immune response to exercise is rarely modified, 5) recent observations indicate a marked reduction of heat shock proteins (Hsp) expression in response to exercise. Because, in healthy individuals, Hsp protect the cells against the deleterious effects of ROS, it is tempting to speculate that the elevated oxidative stress in CFS patients might result from reduced Hsp expression. CFS patients have also reduced muscle excitability in response to direct stimulation (M wave) and a deregulation of the Na^+/K^+ and Ca^{2+}-ATPase pumps. M wave alterations are correlated with both the magnitude of reduced K^+ outflow from contracting muscles and accentuated oxidative stress. Thus, CFS is characterized by an altered muscle response to exercise which might result from an accentuated oxidative stress, possibly due to reduced Hsp expression.

Introduction

The term chronic fatigue syndrome (CFS) was recommended by the US Center for Disease Control and Prevention. This syndrome is characterized by persistent, relapsing fatigue, often associated with pain in muscles and several joints, post-exertional malaise, and unrefreshing sleep, for which there exists no clear etiology. Primary analyses of negative biological observations, including the absence of changes in light and electron microscopy of muscles biopsies [15] and contractile muscle properties [23], have led to the former conclusion that CFS is not a myopathy but that psychological/psychiatric factors appear to be of greater importance [17]. However, CFS is sometimes diagnosed in elite ultra-endurance cyclists [61] and in later life of subjects who exercised frequently [24]. CFS patients also often complain of delayed recovery after exercise, confirmed by lengthened recovery of maximal voluntary contraction after fatiguing efforts [51]. Thus, exercise-induced causes of CFS pathology are now highly suspected [56].

Biochemical Events

Muscle metabolism and cell signalling pathways were explored at rest, during and after muscle contraction in CFS patients. A large panel of histological, physiological and biochemical tools were used such as studies on muscle mitochondria, measurements of oxygen uptake (VO_2) and arteriovenous oxygen difference, ^{31}P magnetic resonance spectroscopy (MRS), and blood dosages of lactic acid, markers of oxidative stress, cytokines, and heat shock proteins (Hsp).

Metabolism

Glycolysis appears inconstantly abnormal

Concerning the glycolytic metabolic pathway, most of observations are in favour of an absence of increased lactic acid production in the majority of CFS patients [4,27,28,37]. Thus, Barnes et al. [4] did not report any significant abnormalities of intramuscular pH regulation in the majority of CFS patients explored using ^{31}P MRS spectroscopy, an increased acidification relative to PCr depletion occurring in only 6/46 subjects. In the Lane's studies [36,37], only a limited subgroup of CFS patients (8%) was characterized by an increased blood lactate response to subanaerobic threshold exercise with relative increase in type 2 glycolytic fibres in muscle biopsies. In the ^{31}P MRS study by Wong et al. [75] the changes in PCr and intramuscular pH occurred more rapidly in the *gastrocnemius* muscle of all CFS patients than in control subjects, indicating an acceleration of glycolysis. The aforementioned data suggest the existence of subgroups of CFS patients concerning their metabolic profiles. The absence of significant increase in post-exercise lactate level in the majority of CFS patients opposes the marked blood lactate accumulation after exercise always reported in patients with mitochondrial myopathy [39,42].

Aerobiosis and oxidative stress are often accentuated

There are no differences in the ultrastructural characteristics of muscle mitochondria in CFS patients [54] but, in the absence of data on mitochondrial respiration, including the cytochrome chain reactions, an altered mitochondrial functional capacity remains unknown. The histological study by Lane and co-workers [37] reports a predominance of type 1 oxidative muscle fibres in one fourth of CFS patients, favouring the elevation of aerobic pathways. From several reports [25,27,28,48,63], measurement of the oxygen uptake (VO_2) in exercising CFS patients indicated normal aerobic function, especially the relationship between VO_2 and work rate increases was similar to that expected in healthy subjects. Moreover, when CFS patients were compared to patients with a major depressive disorder but no muscle fatigue, Fulcher and White [18] found that CFS patients had significantly higher submaximal VO_2 during exercise despite their perceiving greater fatigue. The venous oxygen level (PvO_2) during exercise can also be used as an index of the oxidative metabolism, a reduced PvO_2 fall during exercise correlating closely with the severity of oxidative impairment [30,69]. In CFS patients, we measured a greater fall in oxygen content in venous blood for the same VO_2 level, suggesting the existence of accentuated aerobic pathways [27]. On the other hand, other observations, based on measurements of a reduced maximal oxygen uptake (VO_2max) [11,60] or ^{31}P MRS evaluation of muscle metabolism [46,75] concluded that the aerobic capacity was reduced in CFS patients. It must be pointed out that measurement of PCr recovery from static or dynamic contraction is not commonly accepted to explore the oxidative capacities. Indeed, Kemp et al. [32] have shown that the rate of PCr resynthesis after exercise may be normal despite an impaired oxygen supply to working muscles. Anyway, differences in muscle metabolism seem to really exist between subgroups of CFS patients—the study by Vanness et al. [71] in 189 CFS patients showing a large scattering to produce maximal aerobic capacity in response to cardiopulmonary exercise test. Finally, it seems accurate to consider that a majority of CSF patients have an accentuated aerobic muscle metabolism.

An elevated oxygen uptake during exercise is a major source of production of reactive oxygen species (ROS) by the mitochondrial activity [58]. The cellular redox status primarily is regulated by the balance between cellular oxidant and reductant levels and numerous cellular and blood antioxidants play key roles in this regulation. A moderate ROS production is necessary to optimize normal cell functioning, modulating membrane potassium and calcium channels [45,47], to facilitate the excitation-contraction coupling [55], and to regulate the contractile proteins [35]. Besides, an excessive ROS production, such as occurring during and after muscle contraction at a high strength, exerts well-known deleterious effects, including the inhibition of Na^+-K^+ pump activity [31] and also activation of local and systemic inflammatory responses with enhanced cytokines production [52]. Acute interrelationships exist between the redox status and the expression of heat shock proteins (Hsp). Indeed, both ROS and antioxidants regulate Hsp expression and, in turn, the reduction of Hsp expression increases the ROS generation [74]. The ROS production is regulated by another negative feed-back loop. ROS potentiate the action of uncoupling proteins (UCP) [14], namely the UCP3 which seems to protect mitochondria against lipid-induced oxidative stress in muscles [49]. UCP3 has been proposed to export fatty acid anions or fatty acid peroxides away from the matrix-side of the mitochondrial inner membrane to prevent their deleterious accumulation [64]. Figure 1 gives a schematic representation of interrelationships between ROS production—inflammation—Hsp expression. In healthy subjects, an enhanced ROS production in response to cycling or running exercise is well documented [1,26,65]. It is based on measurements of blood indices of lipid peroxidation (thiobarbituric acid reactive substances or TBARS, and isoprostanes) and the consumption of endogenous blood antioxidants (plasma reduced ascorbic acid, RAA, and erythrocyte reduced glutathione, GSH). The oxidative stress develops within the first minutes of the post-exercise recovery period and it is completed at the 20th min [26]. Recent general reviews on CFS genesis suggest a possible role of excessive ROS production following exertion [5,21]. Indeed, in CFS patients, an altered oxidant-antioxidant status of blood occurs early in response to maximal exercise and are prolonged compared to healthy sedentary subjects [27,28], both the TBARS increase and RAA decrease being respectively already significant at measurements of ventilatory threshold and VO_2max and persisting until the 30th min of recovery. An animal model of CFS, in which mice were forced to swim everyday for 7 days [66], also revealed that chronic swim test increased brain lipid peroxidation and intracellular antioxidant levels (catalase, superoxide dismutase). All the other studies in CFS patients were limited to the changes in resting blood oxidant-antioxidant status, reporting lower Vitamin E concentration, higher levels of oxidized LDL, TBARS and malondialdehyde (MAL) [59,72], and increased susceptibility of LDL and VLDL to copper-induced peroxidation [41]. Vecchiet et al. [72] also reported inverse proportionality between muscle symptoms of fatigue and blood levels of TBARS and Vit E. In biopsies of vastus lateralis muscle of CFS patients, Fule et al. [20] have detected oxidative damage to DNA and lipids as well as an increased activity of intracellular antioxidants (catalase, glutathione peroxidise, and transferase). Several authors also found in CFS patients a correlation between musculoskeletal symptoms and an accentuated lipid peroxidation at rest [33,43,72]. In fact, oxidative damage seems to be the common pathway of muscle cell death in most of muscular dystrophies [57,70].

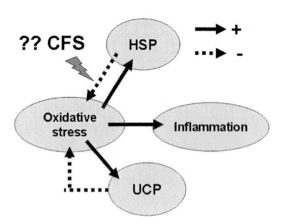

Figure 1. Relationships between oxidative stress, inflammation, and signalling proteins (Heat shock proteins, Hsp, and uncoupling proteins, UCP) and the possible role of a lowered Hsp expression in CFS pathophysiology.

Cell Signalling Pathways on Biochemical Changes

Innate immunity and inflammatory response to exercise

It has been hypothesized that cytokines may mediate some of the symptoms and immunological disturbances in CFS patients. Indeed, CFS patients present an immune imbalance, characterized by a depressed function of natural killer cells, reduced T cell responses to mitogens and specific antigens, IgG subclass deficiencies (IgG1, IgG3) and decreased complement levels [17]. On the other hand, several studies failed to demonstrate abnormal plasma cytokine levels in CFS patients at rest compared to healthy subjects [2,73] while others reported an elevation of plasma level of transforming growthfactor-beta level [6,53] and IL-6 and Il-1α [8-10,22,38]. Moreover, no clear evidence of a link between abnormal immunity and CFS was established [5]. At exertion, a 30-min walking at 1 mph provoked an increased blood level of TGFβ in CFSs [53] whereas other studies [8,41] did not report any elevation of plasma IL-6 and IL-1β in response to exercise. Recent observations by our team [27] confirm the absence of significant differences in the IL-6 response to maximal cycling exercise between CFSs and healthy sedentary subjects (Figure 2). At this time, it seems difficult to conclude that marked disorders in immune balance exist in CFS patients.

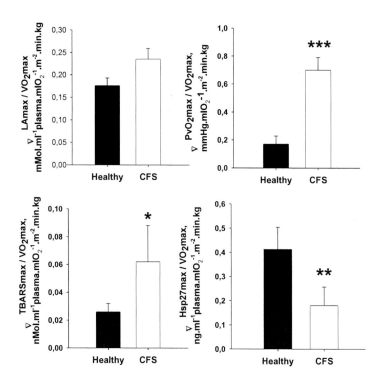

Figure 2. Comparison between maximal variations of plasma lactic acid level (LA), oxygen partial pressure in venous blood (PvO2), blood marker of lipid peroxidation (TBARS), and heat shock protein 27 (Hsp 27) measured in healthy sedentary subjects and CFS patients in response to maximal

incremental cycling exercise. Data are related to corresponding values of maximal oxygen uptake (VO2max). From data by Jammes et al. [27,28].

Expression of heat shock proteins

In healthy individuals, formation of Hsp20, Hsp27, and Hsp 70 occurs in contracting muscles and their plasmatic changes are detectable [50]. In CFS patients, we found no published data on the changes in plasma Hsp level at rest and after exercise. Our recent unpublished observations in 10 CFS patients reveal that the post-exercise increase in plasma Hsp27 was delayed and shortened and the peak Hsp 27 increase lowered compared to controls. These preliminary data suggest that the reduced expression of chaperone proteins (Hsp) in exercising CFS patients might explain the accentuation of exercise-induced oxidative stress.

Figure 2 summarizes our data on the differences between metabolic response to maximal cycling exercise in healthy subjects and CFS patients. Are shown the absence of differences in maximal post-exercise increase in plasma lactic acid, the significant increases in oxygen uptake by exercising muscle (accentuated fall in PvO_2) and lipid peroxidation (increased TBARS level), and the significant reduction of Hsp27 variation after exertion.

Electrophysiological Muscle Events

Electrophysiological muscle events are closely linked with biochemical changes in contracting muscles including the ionic fluxes through the membranes. Muscle fatigue primarily results from the incapacity of muscle fibres to contract and this muscle failure is called "peripheral fatigue". This may result from failure of metabolic processes due to the imbalance between oxygen demand and supply, reduced excitation-contraction coupling involving altered intracellular calcium release and mobilization, and also impaired muscle membrane excitability due to altered ionic fluxes through the sarcolemma. "Peripheral fatigue" is generally preceded by changes in recruitment of motoneurones, leading to the preferential firing of slow motoneurones which drive fatigue-resistant motor units. This phenomenon, called "central fatigue", results in reduced force production and tends to delay the occurrence of "peripheral fatigue" ("muscle wisdom" phenomenon) [16]. In humans, non invasive tools are used to explore "peripheral" and "central" fatigues. They are respectively, the contractile muscle response to direct electrical stimulation (twitch) with recording of the compound muscle action potential (M-wave), electromyographic recordings maximal or submaximal voluntary contractions with sometimes interpolation of twitches, and analysis of post-exercise recovery of maximal contraction [16].

Absence of "Central Fatigue"

Supporting the hypothesis of a "central fatigue" in CFS patients, some physiological studies using twitch interpolation technique and analyses of maximal voluntary contraction have concluded to the absence of any failure of the force production in response to the motor command [34,40,68]. On the other hand, data by Samii et al. [62] suggested that "post-exercise cortical excitability seems to be significantly reduced in CFS patients". Indeed, these authors measured a marked decrease in post-exercise facilitation of muscle action potentials evoked by transcranial magnetic stimulation. However, the existence of altered muscle membrane excitability in response to exercise in CFSs (see below) may simply explain Samii's observations [62], confirming the absence of "central fatigue" in these patients.

Altered Muscle Membrane Excitability

Recording the compound evoked muscle action potentials (M-wave) with surface electrodes (SEMG) is a non-invasive mean to explore peripheral muscle fatigue in exercising humans. An impaired excitation of the muscle fibres is suspected when the M-wave declines and becomes broader [7]. In healthy sedentary subjects, the M-wave duration modestly increases after a maximal incremental cycling exercise, indicating a post-exercise facilitation of membrane excitability [3,29]. On the other hand, after a maximal exercise bout, CFS patients present a significant reduction of muscle excitability in response to direct muscle stimulation [27,28] and impaired recovery of the maximal isometric torque [51]. Our studies in CFS patients [27,28] showed no change in the neuromuscular transmission (conduction time) whereas the M-wave amplitude decreased and its duration was lengthened, indicating a reduced muscle membrane excitability. M-wave alterations early began after the exercise had stopped and culminated at the end of the 30-min recovery period. Kent-Braun and coworkers [34] also recorded the M-wave and analysed its changes in amplitude in CFS patients executing intermitent submaximal contractions of the *tibialis anterior* muscle. These authors did not measure any significant differences in the M-wave variations between CFS and control subjects. However, their protocol was limited to a small muscle group and thus cannot be compared to an incremental cycling exercise until VO_2max which involves the participation of large muscle groups.

Altered Ionic Fluxes Through the Muscle Membrane

In healthy subjects, muscle biopsies have demonstrated a contraction-induced loss in myoplasmic potassium (K^+) concentration [66]. This potassium outflow is detectable in plasma and the kinetics of plasma K^+ increase during an incremental exercise is well known [44]. Increased ROS production with exercise exerts inhibitory action on the Na^+-K^+ pump activity [30], reducing the potassium outflow and also probably the muscle membrane excitability.

Collecting some of our published data [27,28], we noted that the magnitude of post-exercise altered muscle membrane excitability (reduced M-wave amplitude) was proportional to the decrease in potassium outflow and to the oxidative stress (increased TBARS level) (Figure 3.). Thus, in CFS patients, the accentuated and prolonged post-exercise oxidative stress may be responsible for muscle membrane alterations due to lipid hydroperoxides formation. The study by Fulle et al. [19] has confirmed in CFS patients a deregulation of the

Na^+/K^+ and Ca^{2+}-ATPase pumps and the alterations in ryanodine channels in the sarcoplasmic reticulum membranes. To explain their data of altered excitation-contraction coupling in skeletal muscle of CFS patients, Fulle et al. [19] suggested that the deregulation of pump activities could result from an increased fluidity of sarcoplasmic reticulum membrane. It must be pointed out that the association of an enhanced exercise-induced oxidative stress with reduced muscle membrane excitability seems rather specific of CFS. Indeed, in patients receiving a long-term treatment with statins and presenting chronic muscle weakness, the exercise-induced oxidative stress was markedly depressed or even suppressed and no post-exercise M-wave alteration was reported [12,13].

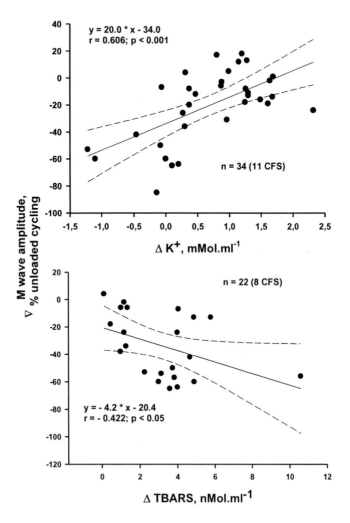

Figure 3. Correlations between maximal post-exercise changes in amplitude of compound muscle action potential (M-wave) and the corresponding changes in plasma potassium level (K^+) or peak increase in a blood marker of lipid peroxidation (TBARS) in CFS patients and healthy sedentary subjects. (Data from references 27 and 28). Linear regression with 95% confidence intervals are drawn and corresponding equations are reported.

Conclusion

Fatigue of CFS patients might result from altered muscle membrane excitability due to the accumulation of reactive oxygen species. The depressed Hsp response to exercise might explain the accentuated oxidative stress in these patients. Future studies should focus on the origin of such a reduced Hsp expression and also on the functional benefits of antioxidant supplementation to balance the accentuated exercise-induced oxidative stress in CFSs.

References

[1]   Alessio, HM. (1993). Exercise-induced oxidative stress. *Med Sci Sports Exerc* 1993, 25, 218-224.

[2]   Amel Kashipaz, MR; Swinden, D; Todd, I; Powell, RJ. (2003). Normal production of inflammatory cytokines in chronic fatigue and fibromyalgia syndromes determined by intracellular cytokine staining in short-term cultured blood mononuclear cells. *Clin Exp Immunol*, 2003, 132, 360-365.

[3]   Arnaud, S; Zattara-Hartmann, MC; Tomei, C; Jammes, Y. (1997). Correlation between muscle metabolism and changes in M-wave and surface electromyogram: dynamic constant load leg exercise in untrained subjects. *Muscle Nerve* 1997, 20, 1197-1199.

[4]   Barnes, PR; Taylor, DJ; Kemp, GJ; Radda, GK. (1993). Skeletal muscle bioenergetics in chronic fatigue syndrome. *J Neurol Neurosurg Psychiatry* 1993, 56, 679-683.

[5]   Bassi, N; Amital, D; Amital, H; Doria, A; Shoenfeld, Y. (2008). Chronic fatigue syndrome: characteristics and possible causes for its pathogenesis. *Isr Med Assoc J* 2008, 10, 79-82.

[6]   Bennett AL, Chao CC, Hu S, Buchwald D, Fagioli LR, Schur PH, Peterson PK, Komaroff AL. (1997). Elevation of bioactive transforming growth factor-beta in serum from patients with chronic fatigue syndrome. *J Clin Immunol.* 1997, 17, 160-166.

[7]   Bigland-Ritchie, B; Kukulka, CJ; Lippold, OCJ; Woods, JJ. (1982). The absence of neuromuscular transmission failure in sustained maximal voluntary contractions. *J Physiol* 1982, 330, 265-278

[8]   Cannon, JG; Angel, JB; Ball, RW; Abad, LW; Fagioli, L; Komaroff, AL. (1999). Acute phase responses and cytokine secretion in chronic fatigue syndrome. *J Clin Immunol* 1999, 19, 414-421.

[9]   Chao, CC; Gallagher, M; Phair, J; Peterson, PK. (1990). Serum neopterin and interleukin-6 levels in chronic fatigue syndrome. *J Infect Dis* 1990, 162,1412-1413.

[10] Chao, CC; Janoff, EN; Hu, SX; Thomas, K; Gallagher, M; Tsang, M; Peterson, PK. (1991). Altered cytokine release in peripheral blood mononuclear cell cultures from patients with the chronic fatigue syndrome. *Cytokine* 1991, 3, 292-298.

[11] De Becker, P; Roeykens, J; Reynders, M; McGregor, N; De Meirleir, K. (2000). Exercise capacity in chronic fatigue syndrome. *Arch Intern Med* 2000, 27, 3270-3277.

[12] Delliaux, S; Steinberg, JG; Lesavre, N; Paganelli, F; Oliver, C; Jammes, Y (2006). Effect of long-term atorvastatin treatment on the electrophysiological and mechanical functions of muscle. *Int J Pharmacol Ther*, 2006, 44, 251-261.

[13] Delliaux, S; Steinberg, JG; Bechis, G; Paganelli, F; Oliver, C; Lesavre, N; Jammes, Y (2007). Statins alter oxidant-antioxidant status and lower exercise-induced oxidative stress. *Int J Clin Pharmacol Ther*, 2007, 45, 244-252.

[14] Echtay, KS ; Roussel, D ; St-Pierre, J; Jekabsons, MB; Cadenas, S; Stuart, JA; Harper, JA; Roebuck, SJ; Morrison, A; Pickering, S; Clapham, JC; Brand, MD. (2002). Superoxide activates mitochondrial uncoupling proteins. *Nature* 2002, 415, 96-99.

[15] Edwards, RH; Gibson, H; Clague, JE; Helliwell, T. (1993). Muscle histopathology and physiology in chronic fatigue syndrome. *Ciba Found Symp* 1993,173, 102-117.

[16] Enoka, RM; Stuart, DG. (1992). Neurobiology of muscle fatigue. *J Appl Physiol* 72, 1631-1648.

[17] Evengard, B; Schacterle, RS; Komaroff, AL. (1999). Chronic fatigue syndrome: new insights and old ignorance. *J Intern Med* 1999, 246, 455-469.

[18] Fulcher, KY; White, PD. (2000). Strength and physiological response to exercise in patients with chronic fatigue syndrome. *J Neurol Neurosurg Psychiatry* 69, 302-307.

[19] Fulle, S; Belia, S; Vecchiet, J; Morabito, C; Vecchiet, L; Fano, G. (2003). Modification of the functional capacity of sarcoplasmic reticulum membranes in patients suffering from chronic fatigue syndrome. *Neuromusc Disorders* 2003, 13, 479-484.

[20] Fulle, S; Mecocci, P; Fanó, G; Vecchiet, I; Vecchini, A; Racciotti, D; Cherubini, A; Pizzigallo, E; Vecchiet, L; Senin, U; Beal, MF. (2000). Specific oxidative alterations in vastus lateralis muscle of patients with the diagnosis of chronic fatigue syndrome. *Free Radic Biol Med* 2000, 29, 1252-1259.

[21] Fulle, S; Pietrangelo, T; Mancinelli, R; Saggini, R; Fano, G. (2007). Specific correlations between muscle oxidative stress and chronic fatigue syndrome: a working hypothesis. *J Muscle Res Cell Motil* 2007, 28, 355-362.

[22] Gaab, J; Rohleder, N; Heitz, V; Engert, V; Schad, T; Schürmeyer, TH; Ehlert, U. (2005). Stress-induced changes in LPS-induced pro-inflammatory cytokine production in chronic fatigue syndrome. *Pychoneuroendocrinology* 2005, 30, 188-198.

[23] Gibson, H; Carroll, N; Clague, JE; Edwards, RH. (1993). Exercise performance and fatiguability in patients with chronic fatigue syndrome. *J Neurol Neurosurg Psychiatry* 1993, 56, 993-998.

[24] Harvey, SB; Wadsworth, M; Wessely, S; Hotopf, M. (2008). Etiology of chronic fatigue syndrome: testing popular hypotheses using a national birth cohort study. *Psychosom Med* 2008, 70, 488-495.

[25] Imbar, O; Dlin, R; Rotstein, A; Whipp BJ. (2201). Physiological responses to incremental exercise in patients with chronic fatigue syndrome. *Med Sci Sports Exerc* 2001, 33, 1463-1470.

[26] Jammes, Y; Steinberg, JG; Bregeon, F; Delliaux, S. (2004). The oxidative stress in response to routine incremental cycling exercise in healthy sedentary subjects. *Respir Physiol Neurobiol* 2004, 144, 81-90.

[27] Jammes, Y ; Steinberg, JG ; Delliaux, S : Brégeon F (2009). Chronic fatigue syndrome combines increased exercise-induced oxidative stress and reduced cytokine and Hsp responses. *J Intern Med* 2009, 266, 196-206.

[28] Jammes, Y; Steinberg, JG; Mambrini, O; Bregeon, F; Delliaux, S. (2005). Chronic fatigue syndrome: assessment of increased oxidative stress and altered muscle excitability in response to incremental exercise. *J Int Med* 2005, 257, 299-231.

[29] Jammes, Y; Zattara-Hartmann, MC; Caquelard, F; Arnaud, S; Tomei, C. (1997). Electromyographic changes in vastus lateralis during dynamic exercise. *Muscle Nerve* 1997, 20, 247-249.

[30] Jensen, TD; Kazemi-Esfarjani, P; Skomorowska, E; Vissing, J. (2002). A forearm exercise screening test for mitochondrial myopathy. *Neurology* 2002, 58, 1533-1538.

[31] Juel, C (2006). Muscle fatigue and reactive oxygen species. *J Physiol* 576, 279-288.

[32] Kemp, GJ; DJ, Taylor; CH, Thompson; LJ, Hands; B, Rajagopalan; P, Styles; GK, Radda.(1993). Quantitative analysis by 31P magnetic resonance spectroscopy of abnormal mitochondrial oxidation in skeletal muscle during recovery from exercise. *NMR Biomed* 1993, 6, 302-310.

[33] Kennedy, G; Spence, VA; McLaren, M; Hill, A; Underwood, C; Belch, JJ. (2005). Oxidative stress levels are raised in chronic fatigue syndrome and are associated with clinical symptoms. *Free Radic Biol Med* 2005, 39, 584-589.

[34] Kent-Braun, JA; Sharma, KR; Weiner, MW; Massie, B; Miller, RG. (1993). Central basis of muscle fatigue in chronic fatigue syndrome. *Neurology* 1993, 43, 124-131.

[35] Könczöl, F; Lorinczy, D; Belagyi, J. (1998). Effect of oxygen free radicals on myosin in muscle fibres. *FEBS Lett* 1998, 427, 341-344.

[36] Lane, RJ; Barrett, MC; Taylor, DJ; Kemp, GJ; Lodi, R. (1998). Heterogeneity in chronic fatigue syndrome: evidence from magnetic resonance spectroscopy of muscle. *Neuromuscul Disord* 1998, 8, 204-209.

[37] Lane, RJ; Barrett, MC; Woodrow, D; Moss, J; Fletcher, R; Archard, LC. (1998). Muscle fibre characteristics and lactate responses to exercise in chronic fatigue syndrome. *J Neurol Neurosurg Psychiatry* 1998, 64, 362-367.

[38] Linde, A; Andersson, B; Svenson, SB; Ahrne, H; Carlsson, M; Forsberg, P; Hugo, H; Karstorp, A; Lenkei, R; Lindwall, A.; et al. (1992). Serum levels of lymphokines and soluble cellular receptors in primary Epstein-Barr virus infection and in patients with chronic fatigue syndrome. *J Infect Dis* 1992, 165, 994-1000.

[39] Lindholm, H; Lofberg, M; Somer, H; Naveri, H; Sovijarji, A. (2004). Abnormal blood lactate accumulation after exercise in patients with multiple mitochondrial DNA deletions and minor muscular symptoms. *Clin Physiol Funct Imaging* 2004, 24, 109-115.

[40] Lloyd, AR; Gandevia, SC; Hales, JP. (1991). Muscle performance, voluntary activation, twitch properties and perceived efforts in normal subjects and patients with the chronic fatigue syndrome. *Brain* 1991, 114, 85-98.

[41] Lloyd, A; Gandevia, SC; Brockman, A; Hales, J; Wakefield, D. (1994). Cytokine production and fatigue in patients with chronic fatigue syndrome and healthy control subjects in response to exercise. *Clin Infect Dis* 1994, 18 Suppl 1:S142-146.

[42] Lofberg, M; Lindholm, H; Naveri, H; Majander, A; Suomalainen, A; Paetau, A; Sovijarvi, A; Harkonen, M; Somer, H. (2001). ATP, phosphocreatine and lactate in exercising muscle in mitochondrial disease and McArdle's disease. *Neuromuscul Disord* 2001, 11, 370-375.

[43] Manuel y Keenoy, B; Moorkens, G; Vertommen, J; De Leeuw, I. (2001). Antioxidant status and lipoprotein peroxidation in chronic fatigue syndrome. *Life Sci* 2001, 68, 2037-2049.

[44] Marcos, E; Ribas, J. (1995). Kinetics of plasma potassium concentrations during exhausting exercise in trained and untrained men. *Eur J Appl Physiol* 1995, 71, 207-214.

[45] Matalon, S; Hardiman, KM; Jain, L; Eaton, DC; Kotlikoff, M; Eu, JP; Sun, J; Meissner, G; Stamler, JS. (2003). Regulation of ion channel structure and function by reactive oxygen-nitrogen species. *Am J Physiol Lung Cell Mol Physiol* 2003, 285, L1184-1189.

[46] McCully, KK; Natelson, BH; Iotti, S; Sisto, S; Leigh, JS Jr. (1996). Reduced oxidative muscle metabolism in chronic fatigue syndrome. *Muscle Nerve* 1996, 19, 621-625.

[47] McKenna, MJ; Medved, I; Goodman, CA; Brown, MJ; Bjorksten, AR; Murphy, KT; Petersen, AC; Sostaric, S; Gong, X. (2006). N-acetylcysteine attenuates the decline in muscle Na^+,K^+-pump activity and delays fatigue during prolonged exercise in humans. *J Physiol* 2006, 576, 279-288.

[48] Mullis, R; Campbell, IT; Wearden, AJ; Morriss, RK; Pearson, DJ.(1999). Prediction of peak oxygen uptake in chronic fatigue syndrome. *Br J Sports Med* 1999, 33, 352-356.

[49] Nabben, M; Hoeks, J. (2008). Mitochondrial uncoupling protein 3 and its role in cardiac- and skeletal muscle metabolism. *Physiol Behav* 2008, 94: 259-269.

[50] Noble, EG. Heat shock proteins and their induction with exercise. In: Locke, M; Noble, M, editors. *Exercise and Stress Response*, Boca Raton, London, New York, Washington DC: CRC Press, 2002, pp. 43-78.

[51] Paul, L; Wood, L; Behan, WM; Maclaren, WM. (1999). Demonstration of delayed recovery of fatiguing exercise in chronic fatigue syndrome. *Eur J Neurol* 1999, 6, 63-69.

[52] Pedersen, BK;   Hoffman-Goetz, L. (2000). Exercise and the immune system: regulation, integration, and adaptation. *Physiol Rev* 2000, 80, 1055-1081.

[53] Peterson, PK; Sirr, SA; Grammith, FC; Schenck, CH; Pheley, AM; Hu, S; Chao, CC. (1994). Effects of mild exercise on cytokines and cerebral blood flow in chronic fatigue syndrome. *Clin Diagn Lab Immunol* 1994, 1, 222-226.

[54] Plioplys, AV; Plioplys, S. (1995). Electron-microscopic investigation of muscle mitochondria in chronic fatigue syndrome. *Neuropsychobiology* 1995, 32, 175-181.

[55] Posterino, GS; Cellini, MA; Lamb, GD. (2003). Effects of oxidation and cytosolic redox conditions on excitation-contraction coupling in rat skeletal muscle. *J Physiol* 2003, 547, 807-823.

[56] Prins, JB; Van der Meer, JWM; Bleijenberg, G. (2006). Chronic fatigue syndrome. *Lancet* 2006, 367, 346-355.

[57] Rando, TA. (2002). Oxidative stress and the pathogenesis of muscular dystrophies. *Am J Phys Med Rehabil* 2002, 81(11 Suppl), S175-186.

[58] Reid, MB. (2001). Invited Review: redox modulation of skeletal muscle contraction: what we know and what we don't. *J Appl Physiol* 2001, 90, 724-731.

[59] Richards, RS; Roberts, TK; McGregor, NR; Dunstan, RH; Butt, HL. (2000). Blood parameters indicative of oxidative stress are associated with symptom expression in chronic fatigue syndrome. *Redox Rep* 2000, 5, 35-41.

[60] Riley, MS; O'Brien, CJ; McCluskey, DR; Bell, NP; Nicholls, DP. (1990). Aerobic work capacity in patients with chronic fatigue syndrome. *Brit Med J* 1990, 27, 953-956.

[61] Rowbottom, DG; Keast, D; Green, S; Kakulas, B; Morton, AR. (1998). The case history of an elite ultra-endurance cyclist who developed chronic fatigue syndrome. *Med Sci Sports Exerc* 1998, 30, 1345-1348.

[62] Samii, A; Wassermann, EM; Ikoma, K; Mercuri, B; George, MS; O'Fallon, A; Dale, JK; Straus, SE; Hallett, M. (1996). Decreased postexercise facilitation of motor evoked potentials in patients with chronic fatigue syndrome or depression. *Neurology* 1996, 47, 1410-1414.

[63] Sargent, C; Scroop, GC; Nemeth, PM; Burnet, RB; Buckley, JD. (2002). Maximal oxygen uptake and lactate metabolism are normal in chronic fatigue syndrome. *Med Sci Sports Med* 2002, 34, 51-56.

[64] Schrauwen, P; Hoeks, J; Hesselink, MK. (2006). Putative function and physiological relevance of the mitochondrial uncoupling protein-3: involvement in fatty acid metabolism? *Prog Lipid Res*.2006, 45, 17-41.

[65] Sen, C.K. (1995). Oxidants, antioxidants in exercise. *J Appl Physiol* 1995, 79, 675-686.

[66] Singh, A; Garg, V; Gupta, S; Kulkarni, SK. (2002). Role of antioxidants in chronic fatigue syndrome. *Indian J Exp Biol* 2002, 40, 1240-1244.

[67] Sjøgaard, G. (1990). Exercise-induced muscle fatigue: the significance of potassium. *Acta Physiol Scand Suppl* 1990, 593, 1-63.

[68] Stokes, MJ; Cooper, RG; Edwards, RH. (1988). Normal muscle strength and fatigability in patients with effort syndromes. *Brit Med J* 1988, 297, 1014-1017.

[69] Taivassalo, T; Abbott, A; Wyrick, P; Haller, G. (2002). Venous oxygen levels during aerobic forearm exercise: an index of impaired oxidative metabolism in mitochondrial myopathy. *Ann Neurol* 2002, 51, 38-44.

[70] Trenell, MI; CM, Sue; GJ, Kemp; T, Sachinwalla; CH, Thompson. (2006). Aerobic exercise and muscle metabolism in patients with mitochondrial myopathy. *Muscle Nerve* 2006, 33, 524-531.

[71] Vanness, JM; Snell, CR; Strayer, DR; Dempsey, L 4th; Stevens, SR. (2003). Subclassifying chronic fatigue syndrome through exercise testing. *Med Sci Sports Exerc* 2003, 35, 908-913.

[72] Vecchiet, J ; Cipollone, F ; Falasca, K ; Mezzetti, A ; Pizzigallo, E ; Bucciarelli, T ; De Laurentis, S ; Affaitati, G ; De Cesare, D ; Giamberardino, MA. (2003). Relationship between musculoskeletal symptoms and blood markers of oxidative stress in patients with chronic fatigue syndrome. *Neurosci Lett* 2003, 335, 151-154.

[73] Vollmer-Conna, U; Cameron, B; Hadzi-Pavlovic, D; Singletary, K; Davenport, T; Vernon, S; Reeves, WC; Hickie, I; Wakefield, D; Llyod, AR. (2007). Dubbo Infective Outcomes Study Group. Postinfective fatigue syndrome is not associated with altered cytokine production. *Clin Infect Dis* 2007, 45, 732-735.

[74] Whitam, M; Fortes, MB. (2008). Heat shock protein 72: release and biological significance during exercise. *Frontiers in Biosci* 2008, 13, 1328-1339.

[75] Wong, R; Lopaschuk, G; Zhu, G; Walker, D; Catellier, D; Burton, D; Teo, K; Collins-Nakai, R; Montague, T. (1992). Skeletal muscle metabolism in the chronic fatigue syndrome. In vivo assessment by [31] P nuclear magnetic resonance spectroscopy. *Chest* 1992, 102, 1716-1722.

In: Chronic Fatigue Syndrome: Symptoms, Causes and Prevention ISBN: 978-1-60741-493-3
Editor: E. Svoboda and K. Zelenjcik, pp. 103-124   © 2010 Nova Science Publishers, Inc.

Chapter 5

Characteristic Features of Dysautonomia Distinguishing Chronic Fatigue Syndrome from Fibromyalgia – One Clinic's Experience

Jochanan E. Naschitz* and Itzhak Rosner **
Departments of Internal Medicine A* and Rheumatology**,
The Bnai-Zion Medical Center and Bruce and Ruth Rappaport Faculty of Medicine,
Technion-Israel Institute of Technology, Haifa, Israel.

Abstract

Substantial clinical overlap may exist amongst functional somatic syndromes, in general, and chronic fatigue syndrome (CFS) and fibromyalgia (FM), in particular. The underlying pathophysiology of these disorders is unclear. In this article we review studies performed at our institution, exploring similarities and dissimilarities between CFS and FM based on autonomic nervous functioning and electrocardiographic QT. Two methods were recently developed to assess autonomic nervous functioning via cardiovascular reactivity in response to a standardized postural challenge. The 'hemodynamic instability score' (HIS) computes blood pressure and heart rate changes along the tilt test and the resulting measurements are processed by image analysis techniques. Three studies assessed the HIS in CFS patients. Group averages of HIS were CFS = +3.72 (SD 5.02) vs. healthy = -4.62 (SD 2.26) and FM -3.25 (SD 2.63) (p <0.0001). An other technique is based on beat-to-beat heart rate and pulse transit time recordings during the tilt test, data processing by fractal and recurrence plot analysis and computing a 'Fractal & Recurrence Analysis-based Score' (FRAS). FRAS values >0.22 were specific for CFS vs. healthy subjects and FM (2 studies). A different approach, measurement of the QT interval on the surface electrocardiogram found that the corrected QT in CFS patients is relatively shortened and thereby differs from QT in FM (p <0.0001). Jointly, these records show characteristic features to the CFS dysautonomia phenotype, supporting the distinction between CFS and FM. This data may be relevant in providing objective criteria for CFS diagnosis and distinction from other functional somatic syndromes.

Key words: chronic fatigue syndrome, fibromyalgia, tilt test, fractal analysis, dysautonomia, QT interval

Running head: Chronic fatigue syndrome

Chronic fatigue is reported in more than 20% of people seen in primary care. Chronic fatigue can be a manifestation of a medical disease, psychiatric or neurologic disturbances, or a side effect of drugs prescribed for previous disorders [2]. Clinically evaluated, medically unexplained fatigue of at least six months duration, that is of new onset, is not a result of ongoing exertion, not substantially alleviated by rest, and substantially reducing previous levels of activity is called chronic fatigue syndrome (CFS) [29]. Two US community-based CFS studies found prevalences among adults of 0·23% and 0·42%; the rates were higher in women, members of minority groups, and people with lower educational attainment and occupational status [38,77]. Though chronic fatigue syndrome (CFS) has received considerable attention, it remains a controversial disorder. Heterogeneity within patient groups labeled as having CFS makes it likely that there are multiple factors contributing to this disorder [43.

Clinical practice guidelines for diagnosis and treatment of CFS have been recently published by independent working groups [43,54,71,76,106]. Accordingly, the diagnosis of CFS is based on patient history and exclusion of other diagnosable medical or psychiatric illness. The most widely supported scientific case definition is the 1994 definition from the US Centers for Disease Control and Prevention, which is now considered the standard [29]. However, the CFS definition was shown to lack specificity by comparison of groups of patients who met the case definition but had different symptom severities [55]. Also, heterogeneity has been found within samples of patients with chronic fatigue [107]. Between 2000 and 2002, international experts joined forces and identified ambiguities in the case definition for CFS. Guidelines for systematic and uniform case ascertainment and specific instruments for classification were developed to resolve ambiguities [75]. In 2003, another case definition was proposed in an attempt to exclude psychiatric cases [11]. Although they differ, all case definitions select severely fatigued groups of patients.

The main problem is the descriptive character of the definition of CFS. In all CFS case definitions, the illness is identified by means of symptoms, disability, and exclusion of explanatory illnesses, and not by means of physical signs or abnormalities in laboratory test results. As such, CFS belongs to the spectrum of functional somatic syndromes. These include, besides CFS, irritable bowel syndrome, chronic pelvic pain, fibromyalgia, non-cardiac chest pain, tension headache, hyperventilation syndrome and the Gulf war syndrome [1,48,101].

Wessely et al. suggested in 1999 that there was substantial overlap between these conditions and challenged the acceptance of distinct syndromes as defined in the medical literature [101]. The dispute between 'splitters' and 'lumpers' of functional somatic syndrome is still pertinent. Indeed, community studies find lower rates of overlap of functional somatic syndromes than do secondary care studies; there is little overlap in the main symptoms of the two most common functional somatic syndromes - irritable bowel syndrome and fibromyalgia [39,105]; the risk factor of childhood sexual abuse varies six-fold across different functional somatic syndromes [79]; antidepressant efficacy ranges widely in different functional somatic syndromes [3]; and the concept of a general functional somatic syndrome does not predict prognosis, which varies by specific syndromes [101].

A recent review article by Prins et al. [71] recapitulates the difficulties with the definition and understanding the pathophysiology of CFS. The authors suggest a framework for future studies by following two strategies: the aims at distinguishing CFS from other disorders; the other explores similarities and dissimilarities in functional somatic syndromes based on neurosciences. This is exactly the kind of studies we were conducting over the last decade.

Pathophysiology

Predisposition to CFS may originate in personality and lifestyle. Thus, neuroticism and introversion have been reported as risk factors for the disorder [35]. Inactivity in childhood and inactivity after infectious mononucleosis have been found to increase the risk of CFS in adults [99,104]. Studies on twins [8,34,42,65,82] and an association with HLA-DR4 [51] indicate a possible genetic predisposition to the disease. However, some studies have failed to find an association between HLA class II alleles and CFS [41,95]. Smith's study [88],not in twins, found that CFS might be associated with HLA DQA1*01, but this finding must be confirmed in a large independent cohort. *Precipitating factors* of CFS are: acute physical or psychological stress [32,83,92], infections such as a cold, flu-like illness, or infectious mononucleosis [9,19,44,83,103], Q fever and Lyme disease [92]. Once CFS has developed, several *maintaining factors* can impede recovery. Psychological processes seem to be involved in the perpetuation of complaints in patients with CFS [33,40,97].

The nature of the underlying pathophysiology of CFS is unclear. Many mechanisms have been hypothesised. Neuroendocrine dysregulations are supported by challenge tests showing lower than normal cortisol response to increased corticotropin concentrations and upregulation of the serotonergic system [13,30]. Studies of immunological functions have not consistently shown immunological abnormalities [45,82]. Also, cerebral abnormalities have not been constantly observed [50] on magnetic resonance imaging [68] and single photon emission tomography [16,20]. Two studies have also found a reduction in the volume of grey matter in patients with CFS [21,70]. CFS have reduced absolute cortical blood flow when compared with from healthy controls [110]. A recent study assessed cerebrospinal fluid proteins that were differentially expressed in this CFS-spectrum of illnesses compared to control subjects [4]. The authors suggested that a proteomic "biosignature" may provide an insight to the pathophsyilogy of CFS and may become diagnostically import, provided sensitivity, and specificity of the proteomic pattern is proven in prospective studies.

A close connection between impairment of autonomic nervous functions, i.e. dysautonomia, and CFS has been demonstrated. Evidence for this comes from overlapping symptoms between autonomic disorders and CFS, the common occurrence of neurally mediated hypotension during head-up tilt (HUTT) in patients with CFS [6,53,80], and the improvement of symptoms of CFS following therapy directed at neurally mediated hypotension [56]. The postural tachycardia syndrome, which has been attributed to a partial dysautonomia involving the vasculature of the legs, has also been described in CFS [28,56,85].

Our studies of the past decade began with attempts to clarify the dysautonomia of CFS. We proceeded thereafter by focusing on cardiovascular reactivity as a reflection of autonomic nervous activity in CFS. These studies lead to the description of a characteristic pattern of cardiovascular reactivity in CFS, which is specific to CFS [60,62,64,66,67].

The Hemodynamic Instability Score (HIS)

The HIS involves computing BP- and HR- changes during the course of a head-up tilt test, followed by processing the data curves generated by utilizing image analysis techniques [58].

In a first study [67], patients with CFS (n = 25) and their age and sex-matched healthy controls (n = 37) as well as patients with fibromyalgia (n= 30), generalized anxiety disorder (n = 15) and essential hypertension (n = 20) were evaluated with the aid of a head-up tilt test (HUTT). The protocol of the HUTT was based on the 10-minute supine/30 minute head-up tilt test as previously described [65]. Testing was conducted from 8:00 to 11:00 a.m., in a quiet environment, and at constant room temperature of 22-25° C. The patients maintained a regular meal schedule, but were restricted from smoking and caffeine ingestion for 6 hours prior to the examination. Intake of food products and medications with sympathomimetic activity prior to the study was prohibited. Manual BP readings were taken by a physician certified in the BP measurement technique according to American Heart Association recommendations [94]. We favored the mercury column sphygmomanometer (Baumanometer, standby model 0661-0250), since this is the standard non-invasive method for BP measurement, and is the most accurate for evaluation of BP at rest [69,87] and during HUTT [58,59]. The HR measurements were recorded on an electrocardiographic monitor. The patient lay in a supine position on the tilt table, secured to the table at the chest, hips and knees with adhesive girdles. The cuff of the BP recording device was attached to the left arm, which was supported at heart level at all times during the study. Three measurements in the supine position were recorded at 5-minute intervals. The table was then gently tilted head-up to an angle of 70°. The duration of the tilt was 30 minutes. During the initial 5 minutes of tilt, measurements were obtained at one-minute intervals, followed by readings every 5 minutes. When dizziness or faintness occurred, repeated measurements were taken at 30-second intervals. In the event of a loss of consciousness the test was discontinued.

Parameters. The 'BP-change' and 'HR-change' were computed.

a) Systolic and diastolic BP-changes were defined as the differences between individual BP values measured during HUTT and the last recumbent BP value, and divided by the last recumbent BP value. The result is BP change, expressed as a relative value by comparison to the last supine measurement, and calculated according to the following equation:

Equation 1: BP change = $BP_{(n1....n13)} - BP_{n3}/BP_{n3})$.

The averages and SD of the current values of the systolic and diastolic BP changes was calculated for each subject and labeled SYST-AVG.cur, DIAST-AVG.cur, SYST-SD.cur and DIAST SD.cur, respectively (Figure 1).

FD = log (number of self-similar pieces) / log (magnification factor)

	syst	diast	HR	syst.difs.cur	syst.difs.abs	HR.difs.cur
supine 1	122	70	52	0.109	0.109	0.106
supine 5	116	72	42	0.055	0.055	-0.106
supine10	110	70	47	0.000	0.002	0.000
tilt 1	94	76	82	-0.145	0.145	0.745
tilt 2	100	76	84	-0.091	0.091	0.787
tilt 3	102	74	84	-0.073	0.073	0.787
tilt 4	102	78	84	-0.073	0.073	0.787
tilt 5	102	76	82	-0.073	0.073	0.745
tilt 10	106	76	87	-0.036	0.036	0.851
tilt 15	106	78	88	-0.036	0.036	0.872
tilt 20	104	78	90	-0.055	0.055	0.915
tilt 25	100	76	89	-0.091	0.091	0.894
tilt 30	106	76	86	-0.036	0.036	0.830

B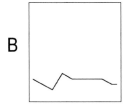

SYST-SD.cur	0.062
HR-SD.cur	0.366
SYST-FD.cur	1.132
HIS	16.48

C

Figure 1. Processing the HIS. Systolic, diastolic BP, and HR values of a CFS patient, taken throughout the HUTT are represented in Figure 1A. From the measured values, the relative changes of BP and HR were calculated, according to the equation: BP difference = $BP_{(n1...n13)}$ - BP_{n3} /BP_{n3}. Absolute values were then obtained by converting all results to positive numbers. Shown in the table are systolic BP differences as current (c) and absolute (a) values, as well as HR differences in current values (c). The BP and HR changes were utilized to calculate the SYS-DIF-c-SD and HR-DIF-c-SD (Figure 1C), which are independent predictors of the HIS. The third independent predictor of HIS is the SYS-DIF-a-FD, and it was processed from the time-curve of the systolic BP differences (Figure 1B) by a fractal analysis program. Finally, the three independent predictors were applied to compute the HIS (Figure 1C). In this specific case, HIS +5.137 is typical for a CFS patient.

The BP changes were also represented graphically in time-curves (Figure 2). These figures were constructed in a fixed template on Microsoft Excel graphics. The frame measured 2 standard rectangles on the horizontal axis (72 pixels width each) and 12 rectangles on the vertical axis (21 pixels height each). The X-axis was calibrated from 1 to 13 representing the sequentially fixed measurements. The Y-axis was calibrated from 0 to 0.6 representing the amplitude of the BP change. The default of the time-curves was set such as to modify BP changes < 0.02 to be represented = 0.02, and BP changes > 0.6 to be represented = 0.6. The time-curves were depicted as continuous, thin, black lines on white background. Subsequently, the time-curves were loaded on the MS Windows Paintbrush program. The field size was 320 x 320 pixels. The original colors were inverted to white line on black background. The images were saved as 24-bit Bitmap image format. The images were loaded in the computerized image analyzer Benoit Version 1.3 (Trusoft Int'l, Inc, 1999, St. Petersburg, Florida). The time-curve's fractal dimension (FD) was automatically assessed by using the box counting method. FD represents a 'self-similarity' in dynamic behavior over multiple scales of time. FD is calculated

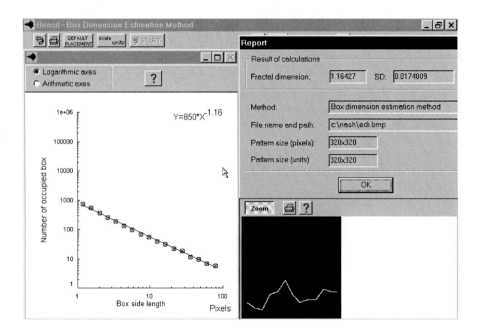

Figure 2. Computation of the fractal dimension of the heart rate by the box method method.

The side length of the largest box of the grid was 80 pixels. The coefficient of box size decrease was 1.3. The number of box sizes used was 17. The increment of grid rotation was 15 degrees. The length of the time-curve outlines was automatically measured. The outline ratio (OR) was calculated by dividing the length of the outline curve by the length of a straight line on the horizontal axis from intervals 1 to 13.

b) 'Absolute systolic and diastolic BP changes' were computed by transforming positive and negative BP changes into positive values. The relative values of BP changes were calculated as above. Subsequently, the average, SD, OR and FD of the absolute BP changes were calculated and labeled SYST-AVG.abs, SYST-SD.abs, SYST-OR.abs, SYST-FD.abs, DIAST-AVG.abs, DIAST-SD.abs, DIAST-OR.abs and DIAST-FD.abs.

c). 'Heart rate change' was defined as the difference between successive HR values and the last recumbent HR value, and divided by the last recumbent HR value:

$$\text{Equation 2: HR change} = HR_{(n1....n13)} - HR_{n3} / HR_{n3}$$

The HR changes average, SD, OR and FD were calculated and labeled HR-AVG.cur, HR-SD.cur, HR-OR.cur, and HR-FD.cur.

d) Absolute HR changes were derived from the transformation of positive and negative HR change values into positive numbers. The absolute HR changes average, SD, OR and FD were calculated: HR-AVG.abs, HR-SD.abs, HR-OR.abs, HR-FD.abs.

Overall, 24 variables were defined and collectively called 'cardiovascular instability indices'. A multivariate analysis of all 24 parameters was conducted, evaluating independent predictors of CFS versus healthies. Results of multivariate analysis identified the best predictors for the assessment of CFS versus healthy to be SYST-FD.abs, SYST-SD.cur and HR-SD.cur. Based on the regression coefficients (slopes and intercept) of these predictors, a linear discriminant score was computed for each subject. This discriminant score was called 'hemodynamic instability score' (HIS).

Equation 3: HIS = 64.3303 + (SYST-FD.abs x -68.0135) + (SYST-SD.cur x 111.3726) + HR-SD.cur x 60.4164)

In this equation, SYST-FD.abs = the fractal dimension of absolute values of the systolic BP changes, SYST-SD.cur = the standard deviation of the current values of the systolic BP changes, and HR-SD.cur = the standard deviation of the current values of the heart rate changes. Group averages (SD) of HIS were: CFS = +3.72 (SD 5.02) and healthy = -4.62 (SD 2.26). The best cut-off differentiating CFS from healthy was HIS –0.98. HIS values >-0.98 was associated with CFS (sensitivity 97% specificity 96.6%).

With the aid of Equation 3, HIS values were calculated in the other groups (Table 1 and Figure 3). Comparison of HIS values showed significant differences ($p < 0.0001$) between CFS and healthy, hypertensives and FM groups, but not versus generalized anxiety disorder.

Table 1. HIS values in CFS compared with other groups of subjects

Group (No Cases)	HIS avg (SD), 95% CI	P value
CFS (n = 25)	+3.72 (5.02), +1.65 to +5.8	
Generalized anxiety disorder (n = 15)	+1.08 (5.2), -1.81 to +3.97	NS
Fibromyalgia (n = 25)	-3.27 (2.63), -4.14 to –2.41	<0.0001
Healthy (n = 37)	-4.62 (2.26), -5.37 to –3.86	<0.0001
Hypertension (n = 20)	-5.53 (2.24), -6.58 to –4.48	<0.0001

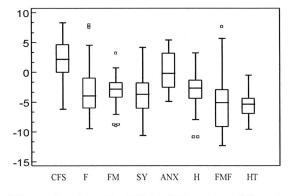

Figure 3. HIS values in different disorders. The HIS in CFS patients differs significantly from other patients groups, except for patients with anxiety disorder. CFS = chronic fatigue syndrome, F = non-CFS fatigue, FM = fibromyalgia, SY = neuraly mediated syncope, ANX = generalized anxiety disorder, H = healthy, FMF = familial Mediterranean fever, HT = essential hypertension.

In a second study, the specificity of the proposed HIS threshold of -0.98 for CFS was evaluated comparing patients with CFS and non-CFS chronic fatigue and patients with recurrent syncope [62]. These groups were chosen for their clinical similarity to CFS and possible dysautonomic background. In this second study, the HIS threshold -0.98 differentiated between CFS patients (HIS = +2.02 (SD 4.07)) and healthy subjects (HIS = -2.48 (SD 4.07)) as well other groups. Subsequent studies confirmed these observations [61,64]. The overall specificity of the HIS for the diagnosis of CFS was 85.1% .

Thus, in the appropriate clinical context, a HIS value greater than −0.98 is consistent with a diagnosis of CFS, providing certain confounding conditions are excluded. As a general rule, patients with any other medical or psychiatric illness should not be diagnosed with CFS [29]. In particular, patients with generalized anxiety disorder were found to have comparable HIS values to CFS patients. Pathologically elevated HIS may be expected to occur in cardiovascular deconditioning following prolonged bed rest or under zero-gravity [78], in autonomic dysfunction associated with neurological or chronic inflammatory disorders [17,93], or as result of drug effects on the autonomic nervous system, though no systematical studies have appraised the effects of any of these conditions on the HIS. From the clinician's point of view, differentiation of these disorders from CFS is usually simple. Overall, the potential utility of the HIS for diagnostic purposes can be assumed from the data presented in this study. The HIS can reinforce the clinician's diagnosis by providing objective criteria to the assessment of CFS, which until now, could only be subjectively inferred.

Distinguishing CFS from fibromyalgia may be difficult on clinical grounds since fibromyalgia shares many features with CFS. Fibromyalgia is a clinical syndrome characterized by widespread pain and abnormal sensitivity on palpation of specific tender points [109]. The pathogenesis of FM has been elusive, made difficult by the absence of distinctive biochemical or histological abnormalities. There is much debate and controversy about this condition. On the one side are those who deny the existence of fibromyalgia as a nosologic entity and consider it an artificial summation of unrelated symptoms [31,72]. On the other side are clinicians and researchers who define fibromyalgia as a distinct clinico-pathologic disorder and suggest that it is a genetically based disease with autosomal-dominant transmission [10]. A point of obfuscation in classifying patients with fibromyalgia lies in the overlap of this syndrome with other functional somatic and pain syndromes [14,47]. By applying the HIS methodology, dissimilar cardiovascular responses to postural challenge were observed in CFS (HIS = +3.72 (SD 5.02) and FM (HIS = -3.25 (SD 2.63)) (p <0.0001) [67]. This was again demonstrated in another study: in CFS, HIS = +2.14(SD 4.67) and in FM, HIS = -2.81(SD 2.62) [62]. The unique features to the CFS dysautonomia phenotype were not observed in FM patients, supporting the separation of FM from CFS in terms of autonomic nervous activity.

The 'Fractal & Recurrence Analysis-Based Score' (FRAS)

To further support the prospect of defining a characteristic dysautonomia in CFS patients, an additional technique was proposed to assess the cardiovascular reactivity during the HUTT.

The protocol of the tilt test and PTT (pulse transit time) recordings were also based on the 10-minute supine - 30 minute head-up tilt test as previously described [65]. In a first study [66], patients with CFS (n=23), familial Mediterranean fever (n=15), psoriatic arthritis (n=10), generalized anxiety disorder (n=12), neurally mediated syncope (n=20), and healthy subjects (n=20) were evaluated. The patient lay in a supine position on the tilt table, secured to the table at the chest, hips and knees with adhesive girdles. The cuff of the BP recording device was attached to the left arm, which was supported at heart level at all times during the study. The right forearm and hand were supported by a cast, and suspended with a sling to the patient's neck. The fingers pointed to the mid-axillary line at the level of the fourth intercostal space. The photoelectric sensor of the photoplethysmograph (PPG) was placed on the distal phalanx of the second or third finger. The hand was held in a relaxed semi-open position, with the palm turned downward and fixed with adhesive strips, taking care not to apply pressure to the PPG transducer. The electrocardiogram (ECG) and PPG were recorded on a Datex-Engstrom Cardiocap^{TM} II instrument (Datex Instrumentation Corporation, Helsinki, Finland), connected to the Biopac MP 100 data acquisition system (Biopac,Santa Barbara, California). The PTT was automatically computed on the AcqKnowledge software, and the tracings were continuously displayed on the computer screen. The computer program identified the PTT as the time interval between the peak of the electrocardiographic R wave and the peak of the pressure wave at the finger, as measured by the pulse plethysmograph. A sample rate of 500 samples per second provided 1/500 Hz resolution for the HR and PTT measurements. Measurements were acquisitioned in the supine position over a 10-minute period. The table was then gently tilted head-up to an angle of 70° and the acquisition continued for a total of 600 cardiac cycles (usually 5 to 10 minutes).

Data processing The RR intervals on ECG recordings and the corresponding PTT values were automatically computed with the AcqKnowledge software. Four sets of values were obtained each comprising approximately 600 measurements – the HR supine, PTT supine, HR tilt, and PTT tilt. Later the measurements were reviewed and edited. For this purpose, the computer program signaled HR values less than 45 bpm or in excess of 110 bpm, and PTT values less than 0.2 sec or longer than 0.4 sec. For each of the aberrant measurements the investigator decided whether or not it was likely in the context of 30-40 contiguous measurements. PTT measurements less than 0.2 sec were considered to be artifacts, based on our experience that such values occurred only upon movement of the transducer. PTT values greater than 0.4 seconds were considered artifacts when occurring alone or as couples, but when clustering in series of 3 or more spikes the occurrence was considered to be authentic. Suspicious HR values were deleted together with the concomitant PTT measurements, and suspicious PTT values were deleted together with the concomitant HR measurements. After editing, the data were advanced to mathematical analysis.

Mathematical processing of data Three mathematical methods were applied: general statistics, recurrence plot analysis, and fractal analysis.

Fractal analysis For fractal analysis, time series of 500-600 consecutive edited measurements, either HR or PTT, were loaded into the Benoit Version 1.3 analyzer (Trusoft Int'l, Inc, 1999, St. Petersburg, Florida). Time curves were constructed. The fractal dimension of the time curve (FD) was calculated with the aid of four different methods: R/S, roughness-length, variogram, and wavelets analysis. Typical tracings are shown in **Figure 4**. *Recurrence Quantitative Analysis (RQA):* In our study, we utilized the Visual Recurrence Analysis computer program version 4.2 developed by Eugene Kononov, 1999. Recurrence plot analysis is a relatively new technique for the qualitative assessment of time series [25,46]. Technically, this method expands a one-dimensional time series into a higher dimensional space. This is done by using a "delayed coordinate embedding", which creates a phase space portrait (recurrence plot) of the system. To start RQA calculations, 500-600 consecutive edited HR or PTT measurements were loaded in the computer program. The embedding dimension, time delay and false nearest neighbor were determined. On this basis, the RQA variables were computed: recurrence, determinism, ratio, entropy, maxline, trend, and spatio-temporal entropy. **Figure 5** illustrates the recurrence plot of the HR in a patient with CFS. A 'structured pattern' is seen on gross. Besides the global impression given by the appearance of the recurrent plot, quantitative descriptors were developed and are included in the recurrence quantification analysis method (RQA). These are: recurrence, determinism, ratio, entropy, maxline, trend, and spatio-temporal entropy [25,46]. Recurrence quantifies the percentage of the plot occupied by recurrent points. Determinism is the percentage of recurrent points that appear in sequence, forming diagonal line structures in the distance matrix. Entropy, measures the richness of deterministic structuring of the series. Trend is the regression coefficient of the relation between time and the amount of recurrence.

On collecting all computed variables derived by analysis of time series measurements, thirteen variables were obtained. By summarizing the four data sets in each patient, including HR and PTT in supine and tilt positions, a total of 52 variables of cardiovascular reactivity were obtained.

Study phases I and II Phase I of the study ('training phase') compared the data of CFS patients with data of a heterogenous control population. This data was tailored to differentiate the phenotype of cardiovascular reactivity in CFS patients versus a spectrum of other clinical entities, some with an exaggerated reactivity and others with a normal cardiovascular reactivity. For this purpose, in the control group patients with syncope and patients with FMF were included. Patients with recurrent syncope often have increased cardiovascular reactivity and may show overlapping features with CFS patients, while FMF patients usually have normal reactivity (Naschitz et al, personal communication). In study phase I, means and SDs of all 52 cardiovascular reactivity variables were calculated and comparisons between the data of CFS patients and controls were performed. A multivariate analysis was conducted, evaluating independent predictors of CFS. Based on the regression coefficients (slopes and intercept) of these predictors, a linear discriminant score was computed for each subject. This discriminant score was called 'Fractal & Recurrence Analysis-based Score' (FRAS). The best cut-off between the FRAS of patients and controls was established. In CFS patients and the mixed control group including patients with neurally mediated syncope and patients with FMF, the average and SD of the 52 variables of cardiovascular reactivity were calculated and group comparisons were performed. On univariate analysis, 13 variables showed significant differences between CFS and controls. These included 6 fractal parameters, 5 RQA parameters and 2 parameters derived from summary statistic analysis.

The multivariate model identified the best predictors for the assessment of CFS versus mixed control patients to be: 1. HR on tilt - fractal dimension by roughness-length analysis (HR-tilt-R/L) (p = 0.0063), 2. PTT on tilt - fractal dimension by roughness-length analysis (PTT-tilt-R/L) (p = 0.0035), 3. HR supine – determinism on recurrence quantification analysis (HR-supine-DET) (p = 0.0009), 4. PTT on tilt - fractal dimension by wavelets analysis (PTT-tilt-WAVE) (p = 0.0003), and 5. HR on tilt standard deviation (HR-tilt-SD) (p = 0.0001). Based on the regression coefficients (slopes and intercept) of these predictors, a linear discriminant score was computed for each subject, called FRAS.

Equation 1: FRAS = 76.2 + 0.04*HR-supine-DET – 12.9*HR-tilt-R/L – 0.31*HR-tilt-SD - 19.27*PTT-tilt-R/L – 9.42* PTT-tilt-WAVE

The best cut-off differentiating CFS from the control population was FRAS = +0.22.

With the aid of Equation 1, FRAS values were calculated in study phase II in the other patient groups. Comparison of FRAS values in CFS patients and in the other groups showed significant differences compared to healthy subjects (p <0.0001), FMF patients (p <0.0001), psoriatic arthritis (0.03), syncope (p <0.0001), but not between CFS and generalized anxiety disorder. FRAS >0.22 was associated with CFS (sensitivity 70% and specificity 88%). A subsequent study [60] confirmed these observations.

Fractal dimension of the HR by different methods

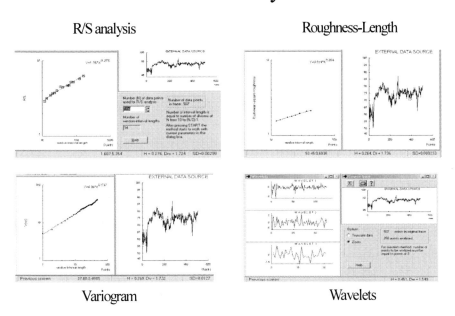

Figure 4. Computation of the heart rate fractal dimension based on a time series of 500 continuous cardiac cycles. Four different methods are implemented.

Recurrence Quantitative Analysis of the HR

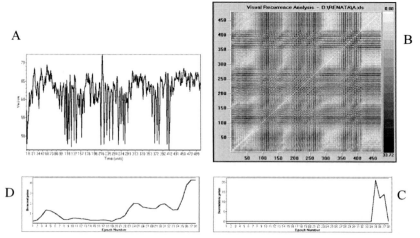

Figure 5. Steps in processing the heart rate recurrence plot. Time series of the HR are displayed in A. The visual recurrence plot in shown in B, recurrence points in C, and deterministic points in D.

Based on the method of the FRAS we conducted a study to evaluate cardiovascular reactivity in fibromyalgia [63]. The study group included 30 women with FM, average age of 46.7 years (SD 7.03). An age matched group of 30 women with other rheumatic disorders or having a dysautonomic background - chronic fatigue syndrome (CFS), non-CFS fatigue, neurally mediated syncope and psoriatic arthritis – served as controls. Variables acting as independent predictors of the cardiovascular reactivity in FM patients versus the comparison group were identified. By univariate analysis comparing variables of the cardiovascular reactivity in FM patients against control patients, no statistically significant differences were found between the groups.

Thus, study of the cardiovascular reactivity utilizing a head-up tilt test and processing the data with the method of the 'Fractal and Recurrence Analysis Score' did not reveal a specific, FM-associated abnormality. These data confirmed prior studies that utilized a variety of other methodologies and reached similar conclusions. FM patients represent a heterogenic group with respect to their pattern of cardiovascular reactivity. These findings appear consistent with the concept that fibromyalgia is a common symptomatic framework, rather than a separate disease entity [31,73], and therefore patients' cardiovascular reactivity patterns are accordingly, heterogenic. Thus, a distinctive cardiovascular reactivity was identified in CFS patients but not in FM.

Mechanisms Involved in Disease-Related Cardiovascular Reactivity Patterns

Cardiovascular reactivity is relatively reproducible within individuals [37].The conventional understanding that cardiovascular reactivity is merely the result of arterial baroreflexes is simplistic and no longer tenable. Indeed, numerous factors modulate the response to baroreflex activation apart from strength of the activating stimulus. These include the set point of the reflex, neuronal input from hypothalamus, cortical centers, brainstem centers, the responsiveness of cardiovascular receptors and structures, interactions of aortocarotid with chemoreflex arcs, as well as modulatory influences of neuro-humoral and vasoactive substances [5,18,23,49,86,89]. Serotonin, adenosine and opioids are additional triggers of the Betzold-Jarisch reflex; peripheral sympathetic afferents are directly activated by circulating mediators; and higher nervous centers modulate the cardiovascular reflexes. Disease-specific cardiovascular reactivity patterns may be explained by the existence of unique permutations in the cardiovascular, neuro-endocrine and paracrine changes present in certain disorders.

In applying the FRAS to the study of cardiovascular reactivity in healthy subjects, no specific reactivity pattern was observed [60]. We speculate that CVR in healthy individuals is heterogenic, not modulated by a specific pathologic mechanism into uniformity. The present study conducted in patients with FM did not disclose a specific CVR pattern. These findings appear consistent with the concept that fibromyalgia is a common symptomatic framework, rather than a separate disease entity [31,36,63], and therefore patients' cardiovascular reactivity patterns are, accordingly, heterogenic.

Shortened Electrocardiographic QT Interval

It is known that QT interval on the electrocardiogram is influenced among others by autonomic nervous function. Since a specificity of cardiovascular reactivity, as an expression of autonomic dysfunction, had been noted in CFS, it was elected to examine the QT interval in this disorder as well.

The QT interval on the surface electrocardiogram (ECG) reflects depolarization and repolarization of myocardial cells. A variety of factors may influence the QT interval, including heart rate, genetic abnormalities of the potassium channel, electrolyte disturbances, myocardial ischemia, drugs, and sympathetic and parasympathetic tone [7,26,52,74,100]. Changes in autonomic tone may condition the QT interval directly by altering repolarization kinetics of myocardial cells through influences on ion currents or indirectly by modulating the heart rate [7]. The effects of the autonomic nervous system on the QT interval have been studied in patients with combined sympathetic and parasympathetic failure, such are patients with idiopathic pure autonomic failure, familial dysautonomia, multiple system atrophy and Parkinson's disease as well as patients with diabetic autonomic neuropathy and chronic liver disease [7,12,22]. The above conditions often are associated with abnormally prolonged QT intervals. In contrast, patients with isolated sympathetic failure, such as subjects with congenital deficiency of dopamine-beta-hydroxylase, have a normal duration of the QT interval [7].

We examined whether the corrected QT interval (QTc) in CFS differs from QTc in other populations [57]. On search of the literature no previous publications on QT interval in patients with CFS were found. The QTc was calculated at the end of 10 minutes of recumbence and the end of 10 minutes of head-up tilt. In a pilot study, groups of 15 subjects, CFS and controls matched for age and gender, were investigated. In a second phase of the study, the QTc was measured in larger groups of CFS (n=30) and control patients (n=96), not matched for demographic features. In the pilot study, the average supine QTc in CFS was 0.371 ± 0.02 sec and QTc on tilt 0.385 ± 0.02 sec, significantly shorter than in controls (p = 0.0002 and 0.0003, respectively). Results of phase II confirmed this data (**Figure 6**). Thus, relative short QTc intervals are features of the CFS-related dysautonomia.

In a follow-up study, we evaluated whether fibromyalgia and CFS can be distinguished by QTc (Naschitz et al, personal communication).The study groups were comprised of women with fibromyalgia (n = 30) and with CFS (n = 28). The patients were evaluated with a 10 minute supine-30 minute head-up tilt test. The electrocardiographic QT interval was corrected for heart rate (HR) according to Fridericia's equation (QTc). In addition, cardiovascular reactivity was assessed based on blood pressure and HR changes and was expressed as the 'hemodynamic instability score' (HIS). The average supine QTc in fibromyalgia was 0.417 ± 0.025 sec versus 0.372 ± 0.022 sec in CFS (p <0.0001); the supine QTc cut-off <0.385.7 sec was 79% sensitive and 87% specific for CFS vs. fibromyalgia. The average QTc at the 10th minute of tilt was 0.409 ± 0.018 sec in fibromyalgia versus 0.367 ± 0.021 in CFS (p <0.0001); the tilt QTc cut-off <383.3 msec was 71% sensitive and 91% specific for CFS vs. fibromyalgia. In this study, the average HIS in fibromyalgia patients was -3.52 ± 1.96 vs. +3.21 ± 2.43 in CFS (p <0.0001). Thus, the QTc and HIS were within the normal range in the large majority of fibromyalgia patients. In contrast, a short QTc interval and increased HIS characterized CFS patients.

The mechanisms underlying the relatively short QTc in CFS have not been investigated. Prior studies in CFS, based on spectral analysis of HR and BP, showed that the vagal tone is reduced in these patients [15,91]. Decreased vagal tone may provide the mechanism for QTc shortening in CFS; however, it should be noted that not all studies have confirmed that vagal tone is diminished in CFS [24]. Both HIS and QTc are influenced by autonomic nervous activity. Thus, an alteration in autonomic function which is operative in CFS but not in fibromyalgia may explain the differences in QTc and HIS.

There are important limitations to these studies, which were limited to CFS patients in one city, presenting mild-to-moderate degrees of severity of fatigue. CFS is, however, a heterogeneous disorder. Subgroups of patients according to features such as chronicity, immunology, activity, and neurobiology were not addressed in our studies.

Future Studies

A first step in understanding the pathophysiology of CFS is to separate it from other similar and overlapping functional somatic syndromes [71]. To this end, we proceded by evaluating dysautonomia in CFS especially in terms of cardiovascular reactivity. A specific cardiovascular reactivity pattern was defined in CFS utilizing both the HIS and FRAS methodologies. Thereafter, a unique finding of the electrocardiographic QTc interval in CFS was established. Subsequently, the above described methodologies were applied to fibromyalgia in direct comparison to CFS. Our findings of a relatively short QTc interval and positive HIS as features of CFS-related dysautonomia were not present in the large majority of fibromyalgia patients. These data support the contention that FM and CFS are distinct disorders. Thus, evidence has accumulated demonstrating characteristic features to the CFS dysautonomia phenotype. This enables the separation of CFS from FM in terms of cardiovascular reactivity patterns and electrocardiographic parameters. These observations may be clinically relevant: provide objective criteria for CFS diagnosis, suggest therapeutic targets [61,64] and aid in monitoring response to therapy.

The upcoming challenge is to find out what is disturbed in the molecular interplay at the level of the central nervous system [71]. Successful molecular profiling of CFS will require the integration of genetic, genomic and proteomic data with environmental and behavioral data to define the heterogeneity in order to optimize intervention [27,98,102]. Innovative analytical methodologies needs to be developed to investigate the complex interacting influences operative in functional somatic syndromes [96,98].

QTc in CFS versus other groups

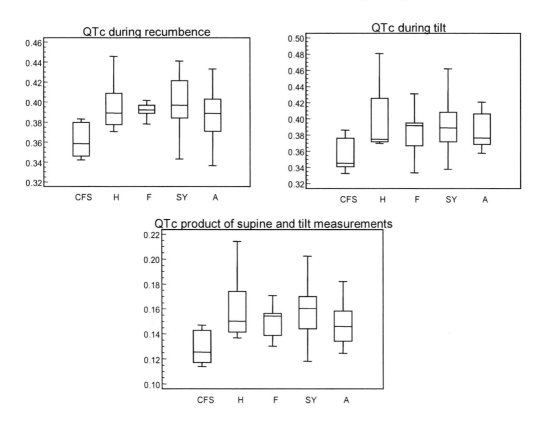

Figure 6. QTc values in five groups matched for age and gender. QTc in CFS differs significantly from QTc in each control group. CFS = chronic fatigue syndrome, H = healthy subjects, F = non-CFS fatigue, SY = neurally mediated syncope, A = psoriatic arthritis. The boxes contain the 50% of values falling between the 25th and 75th percentiles, the horizontal line within the box represents the median value, and the "whiskers" are the lines that extend from the box to the highest and lowest values, excluding the outliers.

References

[1] Aaron, LA; Burke, MM; Buchwald, D. Overlapping conditions among patients with chronic fatigue syndrome, fibromyalgia and temporomandibular disorder. Arch Intern Med, 2000, 160, 221-227.

[2] Adams, RD; Victor, AH. Fatigue, asthenia, anxiety and depressive reactions. In : Adams, RD; Victor, A; Topper, AH; eds. Principles of neurology, 6th edn. New York: McGraw-Hill, 1997, 497-507.

[3] Allen, LA; Escobar, JI; Lehrer, PM; Gara, MA; Woolfolk, RL. Psychosocial treatmentsfor multiple unexplained physical symptoms: a review of the literature. Psychosomatic Medicine, 2002, 64, 939 -950.

[4] Baraniuk, JN; Casado, B; Maibach, H; Clauw, DJ; Pannell, LK; Hess, SS. A Chronic Fatigue Syndrome - related proteome in human cerebrospinal fluid. BMC Neurol., 2005, 5, 22.

[5] Barraco, RA; Janusz, CJ; Polasek, PM; Parizon, M; Roberts, PA. Cardiovascular effectsof microinjection of adenosine into the nucleus tractus solitarius. Brain Res Bull, 1988, 20, 129-132.

[6] Bou-Holaigah, I; Rowe, PC; Kan, J; Calkins, H. The relationship between neurally mediated hypotension and the chronic fatigue syndrome. JAMA, 1995, 274, 961-967.

[7] Browne, KF; Zipes, DP; Heger, JJ; Prystowsky, EN. Influence of the autonomous nervous system on the QT interval in man. Am J Cardiol, 1982, 50, 1099-1103.

[8] Buchwald, D; Herell, R; Ashton, Sl. A twin study of chronic fatigue. Psychosom Med, 2001, 63, 936–943.

[9] Buchwald, DS; Rea, TD; Katon, WJ; Russo, JE; Ashley, RL. Acute infectious mononucleosis: characteristics of patients who report failure to recover. Am J Med, 2000, 109, 531–537.

[10] Buskila, D; Neumann, L. Fibromyalgia syndrome (FM) and nonarticular tendernessin relatives of patients with FM. J Rheumatol, 1997, 24, 941–944.

[11] Carruthers, BM; Jain, AK; De Meirleir, KL. Myalgic encephalomyelitis/ chronic fatigue syndrome: clinical working case definition, diagnostic and treatment protocols, J Chronic Fatigue Syndr, 2003, 11, 7–115.

[12] Choy, AMJ; Lang, CJ; Roden, DM; Robertson, D; Wood, AJJ; Robertson RM; Biaggioni I. Abnormalities of the QT in primary disorders of autonomic failure. Am Heart J, 1998, 136, 664-671.

[13] Cleare, AJ. The neuroendocrinology of chronic fatigue syndrome, Endocr Rev, 2003, 24, 236–252.

[14] Cohen, H; Neumann, L; Shore, M; Amir, M; Cassuto, Y; Buskila, D. Autonomic dysfunction in patients with fibromyalgia: application of power spectral analysisof heart rate variability. Semin Arthritis Rheum, 2000, 29, 217–227.

[15] Cordero, DL; Sisto, SA; Tapp, WN; LaManca, JJ; Pareja, JG; Natelson, BH. Decreased vagal power during treadmill walking in patients with chronic fatigue syndrome. Clin Auton Res, 19966, 329-33.

[16] Costa, DC; Tannock, C; Brostoff, J. Brainstem perfusion is impaired in chronic fatigue syndrome. Q J Med, 1995, 88, 767-773.

[17] Dampney, RA; Coleman, MJ; Fontes, MA; Hirooka, Y; Horiuchi, J; Li, YW; Polson, JW; Potts, PD; Tagawa, T. Central mechanisms underlying short- and long-term regulation of the cardiovascular system. *Clin Exp Pharmacol Physiol,* 2002, 29, 261-268.

[18] Dampney, RA; Coleman, MJ; Fontes, MA; Hirooka, Y; Horiuchi, J; Li, YW; Polson, JW; Potts, PD; Tagawa, T. Central mechanisms underlying short- and long-term regulation of the cardiovascular system. *Clin Exp Pharmacol Physiol,* 2002 , 29, 261-268.

[19] De Becker, P; McGregor, N; de Meirleir, K. Possible triggers and mode of onset of chronic fatigue syndrome, *J Chronic Fatigue Syndr,* 2002, 10, 3–18.

[20] De Lange, FP; Kalkman, JS; Bleijenberg, G; Hagoort, P; vander Werf, SP; van der Meer, JW; Toni, I. Neural correlates of the chronic fatigue syndrome: an fMRI study, *Brain,* 2004, 127, 1948–1957.

[21] De Lange, FP; Kalkman, JS; Bleijenberg, G; Hagoort, P; van der Meer, JWM; Toni, I. Grey matter volume reduction in chronic fatigue syndrome. *Neuroimage* (in press).

[22] Deguchi, K; Sasaki, I; Tsukaguchi, M; Kamoda, M; Touge, T; Takeuchi, H; Kuriyama, S. Abnormalities of rate-corrected QT intervals in Parkinson's disease – a comparisonwith multiple system atrophy and progressive supranuclear palsy. *J Neurol Sci,* 2002, 199, 31-37.

[23] Di Girolano, E; Di Iorno, C; Sabatini, P; Leonzio, L; Barbone, C; Barsotti, A. Effects of paroxetine hydrochloride, a selective serotonin reuptake inhibitor, on refractory vasovagal syncope. A randomized double blind placebo-controlled study. J Am Coll *Cardiol,* 1999, 33, 1227-1230.

[24] Duprez, DA; De Buyzere, ML; Drieghe, B; Vanhaverbeke, F; Taes, Y; Michielsen, W; Clement, DL. Long and short-term blood pressure and RR-interval variability and psychosomatic distress in chronic fatigue syndrome. *Clin Sci (Lond),* 1998, 94, 57-63.

[25] Eckman, JP; Kamphorts, SO; Ruelle, R. Recurrence plots of dynamical systems. *Europhys Lett,* 1987, 4, 973-977.

[26] Ewing, DJ; Nellson, JM. QT interval length and diabetic autonomic neuropathy. *Diabet Med,* 1990, 7, 23-26.

[27] Fang, H; Xie, Q; Boneva, R; Fostel, J; Perkins, R; Tong, W. Gene expression profile exploration of a large dataset on chronic fatigue syndrome. *Pharmacogenomics.* 2006 Apr, 7, 429-40.

[28] Freeman, R; Komaroff, AL. Does the chronic fatigue syndrome involve the autonomic nervous system? *Am J Med,* 1997, 102, 357-64.

[29] Fukuda, K; Straus, SE; Hickie, I; Sharpe, MC; Dobbins, JG; Komaroff, A. The chronicfatigue syndrome: a comprehensive approach to its definition and study. International Study Group. *Ann Intern Med,* 1994, 121, 953-9.

[30] Gaab, J; Engert, V; Heitz, V; Schad, T; Schurmeyer, TH; Ehlert, U. Associations between neuroendocrine response to insulin tolerance test and patient characteristics in chronic fatigue syndrome, *J Psychosom Res* 2004, 56, 419–424.

[31] Hadler, NM. Fibromyalgia: La maladie est morte. Vive le malade. *J Rheumatol,* 1997, 24, 1250-1251.

[32] Hatcher, S; House, A. Life events, difficulties and dilemmas in the onset of chronic fatigue syndrome: a case-control study, *Psychol Med,* 2003, 33, 1185–1192.

[33] Heijmans, JWM. Coping and adaptive outcome in chronic fatigue syndrome: importance of illness cognitions, *J Psychosom Res,* 1998, 45, 39–51.

[34] Hickie, IB; Bansal, AS; Kirk, KM; Lloyd, AR; Martin, NG. A twin study of the etiology of prolonged fatigue and immune activation. *Twin Res,* 2001, 4, 94–102.

[35] Hoogveld, S; Prins, J; de Jong, L. Personality characteristics and the chronic fatigue syndrome: a review of the literature, *Gedragstherapie,* 2001, 34, 275–305.

[36] Imrich, R. The role of neuroendocrine system in the pathogenesis of rheumatic diseases (minireview). *Endocrine Regulations,* 2002, 36, 95-106.

[37] Izzo, JL. Stress responses and blood pressure reactivity. In: JL Izzo and Black HR. *Hypertension Primer,* 3d edition, Lippinmcott, Williand & Wilkins, Dallas, 2003, 126-129.

[38] Jason, LA; Richman, JA; Rademaker, AW. et al., A community-based study of chronic fatigue syndrome, *Arch Intern Med,* 1999, 159, 2129–2137.

[39] Jason, LA; Taylor, RR; Kennedy, CL. Chronic fatigue syndrome: comorbidity with fibromyalgia and psychiatric illness. *Medicine and Psychiatry,* 2001, 4, 29 -34.

[40] Joyce, J; Hotopf, M; Wessely, S. The prognosis of chronic fatigue and chronic fatigue syndrome: a systematic review, *QJM,* 1997, 90, 223–233.

[41] Keller, RH; Lane, JL; Klimas, N; Reiter, WM; Fletcher, MA; van Riel, F; Morgan, R. Association between HLA class II antigens and the chronic fatigue immune dysfunction. *Clin Infect Dis,* 1994, 18 (suppl 1), S154–56.

[42] Koelle, DM; Barcy, S; Huang, ML; Ashley, RL; Zeh, J; Ashton, S; Buchwald, D. Markers of viral infection in monozygotic twins discordant for chronic fatigue syndrome. *Clin Infect Dis,* 2002, 35, 518–525.

[43] Larkins, RG; Molesworth, SR. Chronic fatigue syndrome - *Clinical practice guidelines,* 2002. MJA 6 May 2002, 176 (8 Suppl), S17-S55.

[44] Lloyd, AR. Postinfective fatigue. In: LA Jason, PA Fennell and RR Taylor, Editors, *Handbook of chronic fatigue syndrome,* John Wiley & Sons, Hoboken, New Jersey, 2003, 108–123.

[45] Lyall, M; Peakman, M; Wessely, S. A systematic review and critical evaluation of the immunology of chronic fatigue syndrome, *J Psychosom Res,* 2003, 55, 79–90.

[46] Manetti, C; Ceruso, MA; Giuliani, A; Webber, CL; Zbilut, JP. Recurrence quantification analysis in molecular dynamics. *Ann New York Acad Sci,* 1999, 879, 258-266.

[47] Martinez-Lavin, M; Hermosillo, AG. Autonomic nervous system dysfunction may explain the multisystem features of fibromyalgia. *Semin Arthritis Rheum.,* 2000, 29, 197–199.

[48] Martinez-Lavin, M; Hermosillo, AG. Dysautonomia in Gulf War syndrome and in fibromyalgia. *Am J Med.,* 2005, 118, 446.

[49] Mercader, MA; Varghese, PJ; Potolicchio, SJ; Venkatraman, GK; Lee, SW. New insights into the mechanism of neurally mediated syncope. *Heart,* 2002, 88, 217-221.

[50] Michiels, V; Cluydis, R. Neuropsychological functioning in chronic fatigue syndrome: a review. *Acta Psychiatr Scand,* 2001, 103, 84–93.

[51] Middleton, D; Savage, D; Smith, D. No association of HLA class II antigens in chronic fatigue syndrome. *Dis Markers,* 1991, 9, 47–49.

[52] Milne, JR; Camm, AT; Ward, DE; Spurrll, RA. Effect of intravenous propranolol on QT interval: a new method of assessment. *Br Heart J,* 1980, 43, 1-6.

[53] Montague, TJ; Marrie, TJ; Klassen, GA; Bewick, DJ; Horacek, BM. Cardiac function at rest and with exercise in chronic fatigue syndrome. *Chest,* 1989, 95, 779-784.

[54] Mulrow, CD; Ramirez, G; Cornell, JE; Allsup, K. Defining and managing chronic fatigue syndrome. Evidence Report/Technology Assessment No. 42 (Prepared by San Antonio Evidence-based Practice Centre at The University of Texas Health Science Center at San Antonio). AHRQ Publication No. 02-E001. Rockville (MD): *Agency for Healthcare Research and Quality,* October 2001.

[55] Kennedy, G; Abbot, NC; Spence, V; Underwood, C; Belch, JJ. The specificity of theCDC-1994 criteria for chronic fatigue syndrome: comparison of health status in threegroups of patients who fulfill the criteria. *Ann Epidemiol.* 2004, 14, 95-100.

[56] Naschitz, J; Dreyfuss, D; Yeshurun, D; Rosner, I. Midodrine treatment for chronic fatigue syndrome. *Postgrad Med J.,* 2004, 80, 230-232.

[57] Naschitz, JE; Fields, M; Isseroff, H; Sharif, D; Sabo, E; Rosner, I. Shortened QT interval: a distinctive feature of the dysautonomia of chronic fatigue syndrome. *J Electrocardiology,* 2006 (in press).

[58] Naschitz, JE; Gaitini, L; Lowenstein, L; Keren, D; Tamir, A; Yeshurun, D. Rapid, estimation of automatic blood pressure measuring devices (READ). *J Human Hypertension,* 1999, 13, 443-447.

[59] Naschitz, JE; Gaitini, L; Lowenstein, L; Keren, D; Tamir, A; Yeshurun, D. In field validation of automatic blood pressure measuring devices. *J Human Hypertension,* 2000, 14, 37-42.

[60] Naschitz, JE; Rosner, I; Rozenbaum, M; Fields, M; Isseroff, H; Babich, JP; Zuckerman, E; Elias, N; Yeshurun, D; Naschitz, S; Sabo, E. Disease-related phenotypes of cardiovascular reactivity as assessed by fractal and recurrence quantitative analysis of the heart rate and pulse transit time. *Q J Med,* 2004, 97, 141-151.

[61] Naschitz, JE; Rosner, I; Rozenbaum, M; Musafia-Priselac, R; Sabo, E; Gaitini, L; Eldar, S; Zukerman, E; Yeshurun, D. Successful treatment of chronic fatigue syndrome with midodrine: a pilot study. *Clin Exp Rheumatol,* 2003, 21, 416-417.

[62] Naschitz, JE; Rosner, I; Rozenbaum, M; Naschitz, S; Musafia-Priselac, R; Shaviv, N; Isseroff, H; Zukerman, E; Yeshurun, D; Sabo, E. The head-up tilt test with hemodynamic instability score in diagnosing chronic fatigue syndrome. *Quat J Med,* 2003, 96, 133-142.

[63] Naschitz, JE; Rozenbaum, M; Fields, MC; Enis, S; Manor, H; Dreyfuss, D; Peck, S; Peck, ER; Babich, JP; Mintz, EP; Sabo, E; Slobodin, G; Rosner, I. Cardiovascular reactivity in fibromyalgia: evidence for pathogenic heterogeneity. *J Rheumatol,* 2005 32, 335-339.

[64] Naschitz, JE; Sabo, E; Dreyfuss, D; Yeshurun, D; Rosner, I. The head-up tilt test in the diagnosis and management of chronic fatigue syndrome. *Isr Med Assoc J.,* 2003, 5, 807-811.

[65] Naschitz, JE; Sabo, E; Gaitini, L; Ahdoot, A; Ahddot, M; Shaviv, N; Mussafia-Priselac, R; Rosner, I; Eldar, S; Yehurun, D. The hemodynamic instability score (HIS) for assessment of cardiovascular reactivity in hypertensive and normotensive patients. *J Human Hypertension,* 2001, 15, 177-184.

[66] Naschitz, JE; Sabo, E; Naschitz, S; Rosner, I; Rozenbaum, M; Priselac, MR; Gaitini, L; Zukerman, E; Yeshurun, D. Fractal Analysis and Recurrence Quantification Analysis of Heart Rate and Pulse Transit Time for Diagnosing Chronic Fatigue Syndrome. *Clin Autonomic Res,* 2002, 12, 262-274.

[67] Naschitz, JE; Sabo, E; Naschitz, S; Shaviv, N; Rosner, I; Rozenbaum, M; Gaitini, L; Ahdoot, A; Ahdoot, M; Priselac, RM; Eldar, S; Zukerman, E; Yeshurun, D. Hemodynamic instability in chronic fatigue syndrome: indices and diagnostic significance. *Semin Arthritis Rheum,* 2001, 31, 199-208.

[68] Natelson, BH; Cohen, JM; Brassloff, I; Lee, HJ. A controlled study of brain magnetic resonance imaging in patients with the chronic fatigue syndrome. *J Neurol Sci,* 1993, 120, 213-217.

[69] O'Brien, E; Petrie, J; Littler, WA; de Swiet, M; Padfield, PL; O'Malley, K; Jamieson, M; Altman, D; Bland, M; Atkins, N. British hypertension protocol: evaluation of automated and semi-automated blood pressure measuring devices with special reference to ambulatory systems. *J Hypertens,* 1990, 8, 607-619.

[70] Okada, T; Tanaka, M; Kuratsune, H; Watanabe, Y; Sadato, N. Mechanisms underlying fatigue: a voxel-based morphometric study of chronic fatigue syndrome, *BMC Neurol* 2004, 4, 14.

[71] Prins, JB; van der Meer, JW; Bleijberg, G. Chronic fatigue syndrome. *Lancet,* 2006, 367, 346-355.

[72] Rau, CL; Russell, IJ. Is fibromyalgia a distinct clinical syndrome? *Curr Rev Pain,* 2000, 4, 287-294.

[73] Rau, CL; Russell, IJ. Is fibromyalgia a distinct clinical syndrome? *Curr Rev Pain,* 2000, 4, 287-294.

[74] Rautaharju, PM; Warren, JW; Calhoun, HP. Estimation of QT prolongation. A persistent, avoidable error in computer electrocardiography. *J Electrocardiol,* 1990, 23 Suppl, 111-117.

[75] Reeves, WC; Lloyd, A; Vernon, SD; Klimas, N; Jason, LA; Bleijberg, G; Evengard, B; White, PD; Nisenbaum, R; Unger, ER. International Chronic Fatigue Syndrome Study Group. Identification of ambiguities in the 1994 chronic fatigue syndrome research case definition and recommendations for solution, *BMC Health Serv Res,* 2003, 3, 25.

[76] Reid, S; Chalder, T; Cleare, A; Hotopf, M; Wesseley, S. Chronic fatigue syndrome. *BMJ,* 2000, 320, 292-296.

[77] Reyes, M; Nisenbaum, R; Hoaglin, DC; et al., Prevalence and incidence of chronic fatigue syndrome in Wichita, Kansas, *Arch Intern Med,* 2003, 163, 1530–1536.

[78] Robertson, D; Convertino, VA; Vernikos, J. The sympathetic nervous system and the physiologic consequences of spaceflight: a hypothesis. *Am J Med Sci,* 1994, 308, 126-132.

[79] Romans, S; Belaise, C; Martin, J; Morris, E; Raffi, A. Childhood abuse and later medical disorders in women: an epidemiological study. *Psychotherapy and Psychosomatics*, 2002, 71, 141-150.

[80] Rowe, PC; Bou-Holaigah, I; Kan, JS. Is neurally mediated hypotension an unrecognized cause of chronic fatigue? *Lancet,* 1995, 345:623-624.

[81] Russell, IJ. Is fibromyalgia a distinct clinical entity? The clinical investigator's evidence. *Baillieres Best Pract Res Clin Rheumatol,* 1999, 13, 445-454.

[82] Sabath, DE; Barcy, S; Koelle, DM; Zeh, J; Ashton, S; Buchwald, D. Cellular immunity in monozygotic twins discordant for chronic fatigue syndrome. *J Infect Dis*, 2002, 185, 828–832.

[83] Salit, IE. Precipitating factors for the chronic fatigue syndrome, *J Psychiatr Res*, 1997, 31, 59–65.

[84] Schluederberg, A; Straus, SE; Peterson, P; Blumenthal, S; Komaroff, AL; Spring, SB; Landay, A; Buchwald, D. Chronic fatigue syndrome research. Definition and medical outcome assessment. *Ann Intern Med*, 1992, 117, 325-331.

[85] Schondorf, R; Freeman, R. The importance of orthostatic intolerance in the chronic fatigue syndrome. *Am J Med Sci,* 1999, 317, 117-123.

[86] Shen, WK; Hammil, SC; Munger, TM; Stanton, MS; Packer, DL; Osboren, MJ. Adenosine: potential modulator for vasovagal syncope. *J Am Coll Cardiol,* 1996, 28, 146-154.

[87] Shuler, C; Allison, N; Holcomb, S; Harlan, M; McNeill, J; Robinett, G; Bagby, SP. Accuracy of an automated blood pressure device in stable inpatients. *Arch Intern Med,* 1998, 158, 714-721.

[88] Smith, J; Fritz, EL; Kerr, JR; Cleare, AJ; Wessely, S; Mattey, DL. Association of chronic fatigue syndrome with human leucocyte antigen class II alleles. *J Clin Pathol,* 2005, 58, 860–863.

[89] Smith, OA; DeVito, JL. Central nervous integration for the control of autonomic responses associated with emotion. *Annu Rev Neurosci,* 1984, 7, 43-65.

[90] Suys, BE; Huybrechts, SJ; De Wolf, D; Op De Beeck, L; Matthys, D; Van Overmeire, B; Du Caju, MV; Rooman, RP. QTc interval prolongation and QTc dispersion in children and adolescents with type 1 diabetes. *J Pediatr,* 2002, 141, 59-63.

[91] Suys, BE; Huybrechts, SJ; De Wolf, D; Op De Beeck, L; Matthys, D; Van Overmeire, B; Du Caju, MV; Rooman, RP. QTc interval prolongation and QTc dispersion in children and adolescents with type 1 diabetes. *J Pediatr,* 2002, 141, 59-63.

[92] Theorell, T; Blomkvist, V; Lindh, G; Evengard, B. Critical life events, infections, and symptoms during the year preceding chronic fatigue syndrome (CFS): an examination of CFS patients and subjects with a nonspecific life crisis, *Psychosom Med,* 1999, 61, 304–310.

[93] Toussirot, E; Bahjaoui-Bouhaddi, M; Poncet, JC; Cappelle, S; Henriet, MT; Wendling, D; Regnard, J. Abnormal autonomic cardiovascular control in ankylosing spondylitis. *Ann Rheum Dis,* 1999, 58, 481-487.

[94] Training and certification of blood pressure observers. *Hypertension,* 1983, 5, 610-614.

[95] Underhill, JA; Mahalingam, M; Peakman, M; Wessely, S. Lack of association between HLA genotype and chronic fatigue syndrome. *Eur J Immunogenet,* 2001, 28, 425–428.

[96] Van der Greef, J; Stroobant, P; van der Heijden, R. The role of analytical sciences in medical systems biology, *Curr Opin Chem Biol,* 2004, 8, 559–565.

[97] Vercoulen, JHMM; Swanink, CMA; Galama, JMD. The persistence of fatigue in chronic fatigue syndrome and multiple sclerosis: the development of a model, *J Psychosom Res.* 1998, 45, 507–517.

[98] Vernon, SD; Whistler, T; Aslakson, E; Rajeevan, M; Reeves, WC. Challenges for molecular profiling of chronic fatigue syndrome. *Pharmacogenomics*, 2006, 7, 211-218.

[99] Viner, R; Hotopf, M. Childhood predictors of self reported chronic fatigue syndrome/myalgic encephalomyelitis in adults: national birth cohort study, *BMJ,* 2004, 329, 941.

[100] Wang, Q; Curran, ME; Splawski, I; Burn, TC; Millholland, JM; Van Raay, TJ. Positional cloning of a novel potassium channel gene: KVLQT1 mutations cause cardiac arrhythmias. *Nature Genetics*, 1996, 12, 17-23.

[101] Wessely, S; White, PD. There is only one functional somatic syndrome. British J *Psychiatry*, 2004, 185, 95-96.

[102] Whistler, T; Taylor, R; Craddock, RC; Broderick, G; Klimas, N; Unger, ER. Gene expression correlates of unexplained fatigue. *Pharmacogenomics*, 2006, 7, 395-405.

[103] White, PD; Thomas, JM; Kangro, HO; Bruce-Jones, WD; Amess, J; Crawford, DH; Grover, SA; Clare, AW. Predictions and associations of fatigue syndromes and mood disorders that occur after infectious mononucleosis, *Lancet*, 2001, 358, 1946–1954.

[104] White, PD. What causes chronic fatigue syndrome? *BMJ*, 2004, 329, 928–929.

[105] Whitehead, WE; Palsson, O; Jones, KR. Systematic review of the comorbidity of irritable bowel syndrome with other disorders: what are the causes and implications? *Gastroenterology*, 2002, 22, 1140-56.

[106] Whiting, P; Bagnall, A; Sowden, A; Cornell, JE; Mulrow, CD; Ramirez, G. Interventions for the treatment and management of the chronic fatigue syndrome. *JAMA*, 2001, 286, 1360-1368.

[107] Wilson, A; Hickie, I; Hadzi-Pavlovic, D; Wakefield, D. Parker, G; Straus, SD; Dale, J; McCluskey, D; Hinds, G; Brickman, A; Goldenberg, D; Demitrack, M; Blakey, T; Wessely, S; Sharpe, M, Lloyd, A. What is chronic fatigue syndrome? Heterogeneity within an international multicentre study, *Aust N Z J Psychiatry*, 2001, 35, 520–527.

[108] Wolfe, F; Smythe, A; Yunus, MB; Bennett, RM; Bombardier, C; Goldenberg, DL. The American College of Rheumatology 1990 criteria for the classification of fibromyalgia: Report of the Multicenter Criteria Committee. *Arthritis Rheum,* 1990, 33, 160-172.

[109] Yoshiuchi, K; Farkas, J; Natelson, BH. Patients with chronic fatigue syndrome have reduced absolute cortical blood flow. *Clin Physiol Funct Imaging*, 2006, 26, 83-86.

In: Chronic Fatigue Syndrome: Symptoms, Causes & Prevention   ISBN: 978-1-60741-493-3
Editor: E. Svoboda and K. Zelenjcik, pp. 125-141   © 2010 Nova Science Publishers, Inc.

Chapter 6

The Role of Stress in Chronic Fatigue Syndrome

Urs M. Nater[*1] *and Christine Heim*[2]
[1]University of Zurich, Switzerland
[2]Emory University School of Medicine, Atlanta, GA, USA

Abstract

Chronic fatigue syndrome (CFS) is an important public health problem with unique diagnostic and management challenges. Insight into the pathophysiology of CFS is elusive and treatment options are limited. With the advent of the biopsychosocial model in medicine, more recent research efforts have focused on interactions of biological and psychological factors in the development and maintenance of CFS. Stressful experiences have been identified as important risk factors of CFS, particularly when experienced early in life. In addition, psychobiological processes that may translate stress into CFS risk have been considered. In this chapter, we will summarize the current state of research on the role of stress in CFS. We propose that CFS reflects a disorder of adaptation of neural and regulatory physiological systems in response to challenge. Stress likely interacts with other vulnerability factors in determining CFS risk. Understanding the role of stress in CFS may lead towards novel strategies for prevention and treatment of this debilitating disorder.

1. CFS Definition

The definition of CFS according to the International CFS Research Case Definition requires the presence of chronic fatigue of at least 6-months duration. Such fatigue cannot be substantially alleviated by rest, is not the result of ongoing exertion, and is associated with

---

[*] Correspondence Urs M. Nater, PhD, Institute of Psychology, Dept. of Clinical Psychology and Psychotherapy, Binzmuehlestr. 14/ Box 26, 8050 Zurich, Switzerland, Email: u.nater@psychologie.uzh.ch

substantial reductions in occupational, social, and personal activities. In addition, at least 4 out of 8 of the following symptoms must occur with fatigue in a 6-months period: prolonged extraordinary postexertional fatigue, impaired memory or concentration, unrefreshing sleep, aching or stiff muscles, multijoint pain, sore throat, tender glands, and new headaches (Fukuda et al., 1994). There are no known characteristic physical signs or diagnostic laboratory abnormalities to diagnose CFS. Thus, diagnosis depends on evaluation of self-reported symptoms and ruling out a number of medical and psychiatric conditions that may account for the illness.

Thus, the Research Case Definition precludes classification as CFS if a person has an identifiable medical cause of the fatigue. Similarly, subjects with certain psychiatric conditions cannot be classified as CFS cases in research studies. Exclusionary psychiatric conditions include schizophrenia, bipolar disorder or melancholic major depression, substance abuse within 2 years and eating disorders within 5 years. It has been suggested that in clinical practice, however, patients with CFS-like illness but various conditions that would exclude them as a research case may be diagnosed and managed as CFS patients, based on the physician's medical opinion (Jones et al., in press).

In 2003, the International Chronic Fatigue Syndrome Study Group published recommendations concerning standardized application of the 1994 case definition in research studies (Reeves et al., 2003). In order to increase methodological consistency across studies, the Group recommended the use of validated instruments to obtain standardized measures of the major symptom domains of the illness. This is of major importance because the CFS case definition was devised for research purposes and the concept of standardized assessment of criteria and exclusionary conditions is critical to avoid inconsistencies between research studies and confounding of CFS with other disorders.

Despite several decades of research and virtually thousands of published articles, the etiology of CFS remains unclear (Nater, Heim, & Raison, in press; Prins, van der Meer, & Bleijenberg, 2006). A plethora of studies has scrutinized the role of psychosocial and biological factors in the pathophysiology and maintenance of CFS. The following sections will describe the current state of research regarding the role of stress in CFS. Findings will be considered from a developmental perspective, as results from developmental neuroscience have shown that the impact of stress might vary depending on when it has occurred during the life span. In addition to discussing the role of adulthood stress, we will also focus on findings of stress in childhood in this book chapter.

2. Stress in Adulthood and CFS

A variety of studies on the role of stress in CFS have focused on the occurrence of adulthood life events that are considered as stressful. In these studies, investigators have measured burden through such life events (i.e., number, severity) during a defined period of time using different approaches, such as lists of life events or interviews. Uniformly, studies reported that people with CFS experienced significantly more stressful life events than a control group in the year before being examined (Faulkner & Smith, 2008; Masuda, Munemoto, Yamanaka, Takei, & Tei, 2002; Masuda, Nozoe, Matsuyama, & Tanaka, 1994;

Reyes et al., 1996). While these studies have been retrospective in nature, the question of whether stressful life events might be associated with the *onset* or *maintenance* of CFS cannot be readily answered. A longitudinal study found that in patients initially diagnosed with CFS, lower levels of life stress were reported by those who recovered after one year than by those who did not recover (Lim et al., 2003). However, most studies did not examine the relationship between stress and specific CFS symptoms. One available study showed that the physical symptoms of CFS were exacerbated by the stress inflicted on people by Hurricane Andrew (Lutgendorf et al., 1995), whereas another study suggests that negative life events did not predict CFS symptoms (Ray, Jefferies, & Weir, 1995). Finally, a third study reports that high levels of psychological stress were related to increased severity of reported CFS symptoms over a five-week period (Faulkner & Smith, 2008).

In sum, numbers of stressful life events and overall stress levels appear to be increased in persons with CFS. The above studies have focused on whether stress is more prevalent in CFS compared to healthy control groups. However, due to the cross-sectional nature of these examinations, the question remains whether life events might be actually triggering CFS or whether they occur more often as a consequence of the illness.

A number of studies sought to address this question by specifically asking subjects to recall whether they had experienced stressful life events *before* the onset of CFS. Indeed, most studies found that CFS patients reported significantly more stress during the time preceding the illness compared to a control group (Hatcher & House, 2003; Salit, 1997; Stricklin, Sewell, & Austad, 1990). However, the findings are not unequivocal. Some studies found no increased prevalence of stress when compared to control groups (Lewis, Cooper, & Bennett, 1994; MacDonald et al., 1996; Theorell, Blomkvist, Lindh, & Evengard, 1999). Clearly, these studies suffer from the fact that the retrospective nature of the life events assessment was prone to recall biases. Recall bias in turn might be influenced by factors such as emotional state, simple forgetting, and illness duration among others. We are aware of only two studies that investigated whether new onset of CFS was preceded by stress. One study indicated that stress levels prior to manifestation of CFS predicted the risk for developing CFS (Kato, Sullivan, Evengard, & Pedersen, 2006). In this analysis from the Swedish Twin Registry, almost 20,000 participants were asked about self-reported stress levels (via one question) between 1972 and 1973 and fatiguing illnesses (via telephone interview) between 1998 and 2002. Self-reported stress increased the risk of developing a fatiguing illness. This association was even stronger in twins compared to non-twins. In the other study (Kerr & Mattey, 2008), the authors computed a stress index (consisting of responses regarding both stressful life events and perceived stress levels) which was significantly associated with development of fatigue during the acute phase of parvovirus B19 infection and also with chronic fatigue and arthritis occurring 1–3 years following acute parvovirus B19 infection. However, only 5 out of initially 39 subjects eventually developed full CFS. These results are supplemented by studies investigating the role of stress in CFS-like symptom development in occupational groups at high risk for stress, including Gulf War veterans (Kang, Natelson, Mahan, Lee, & Murphy, 2003; L. A. McCauley et al., 2002; Nisenbaum, Barrett, Reyes, & Reeves, 2000) and nurses (Jason et al., 1998) who show higher rates of CFS than the general population.

Another question that arises is whether individuals with CFS not only are exposed to more stressors, but whether they might be more sensitive to subjectively experience stress and thus report more stress. Few laboratory studies have investigated this question. One early study found that subjects with chronic fatigue exhibit exaggerated psychological and physiological responses to a psychological stressor (i.e. anagram test) in comparison to a group with patients suffering from muscular dystrophy and a group with psychiatric patients (Wood, Bentall, Gopfert, Dewey, & Edwards, 1994). Another study, though, used a cognitive stressor, during which CFS patients showed no changes in psychological stress (LaManca et al., 2001).

Taken together, stressful life events are frequent in CFS. There seems to be an association with CFS or CFS-like symptoms, but the nature of this relationship cannot be elucidated based on the results of the aforementioned studies. The inconclusive findings might be due to some limitations. First, quantitative counting of life events is not sufficient. Stress research has repeatedly shown that the qualitative evaluation of a life event as negative is crucial in its subsequent effect on health. Only very studies have actually measured subjective evaluation of stressors. Second, most studies have been cross-sectional. Only using a longitudinal design the temporal relationship of stressor and illness manifestation can be explored adequately. It should be noted that, despite of increased occurrence of stress in the lives of CFS patients, not all CFS patients actually experience stress and, conversely, not all people exposed to stress develop CFS. Based on the latter, clearly, the examination of additional factors that might add risk or resilience to the equation is warranted. Finally, the few studies that subjected CFS patients to a laboratory psychological stressor found altered responses in comparison to control groups. This finding may indicate that general stress responsiveness in everyday life might be altered in individuals with CFS.

3. Stress Early in Life and CFS

Several studies have now provided compelling evidence that exposure to severe stress early in life may be a particularly important risk factor for the development of CFS later in life. In a questionnaire-based study in 1931 women, a history of childhood sexual or physical abuse was associated with increased levels of fatigue and pain in adulthood (J. McCauley et al., 1997). A similar study found that a variety of medical problems, chronic fatigue among them, were highly associated with one or more types of childhood abuse (Romans, Belaise, Martin, Morris, & Raffi, 2002). Whereas these studies were investigating the association of early life stress and states of fatigue, only very few studies have examined the relationship between early experience and syndromal CFS. In these studies, a similar pattern has been found, with higher prevalence rates of emotional neglect and abuse, as well as physical abuse (Van Houdenhove et al., 2001) and increased reports of sexual assault or physical battery as children or teenagers in tertiary care CFS patients compared to controls (Sundbom, Henningsson, Holm, Soderbergh, & Evengard, 2002). Of note, because these studies recruited treatment seeking patients, the associations between early life stress and CFS might be artificially increased because early adversity is associated with higher health care seeking (Arnow, 2004). Of note, one community study in Chicago did not find an association between child abuse and CFS; however, child abuse was assessed in 2 questions only and cases with PTSD were excluded (Taylor & Jason, 2001). A subsequent report from the same sample revealed an association between childhood abuse and PTSD in chronically fatigued subjects (Taylor & Jason, 2002). In a population-based survey in Wichita, KS, a wide range of early experiences (i.e. sexual, physical, emotional abuse, and sexual and physical neglect) were assessed using validated dimensional rating scales and using standard criteria to define CFS cases (Heim et al., 2006). This study identified childhood trauma as a major risk factor of CFS. Any exposure was associated with 6-fold increased risk for CFS. Specifically, childhood emotional maltreatment and sexual abuse were identified as best predictors of CFS when controlling for intercorrelations between different types of abuse. In addition, there was a graded dose-response relationship between exposure levels and increasing risk for CFS. Childhood trauma was associated with symptoms of depression, anxiety, and PTSD in CFS. Childhood trauma remained a significant risk factor for CFS, even in the face of low levels of psychopathology. Recently, these findings were replicated and extended in an independent larger study conducted in metropolitan, urban, and rural regions of Georgia (Heim et al., 2009). Of note, this study included assessment of morning cortisol levels which are discussed to be altered in CFS. In the total CFS group, cortisol responses to awakening were flattened, in accordance with the literature (see below). However, when stratifying groups based on exposure to childhood trauma, only those individuals with CFS who reported exposure to childhood trauma exhibited low cortisol responses to awakening, but not individuals with CFS without such exposure. Implications of this finding are discussed below.

In sum, there now is strong evidence suggesting that stress during development plays an important role in the pathophysiology of CFS. Stress likely interacts with other vulnerability factors in inducing CFS risk. Ongoing or acute stressors might elicit physiological changes in the predisposed individual, ultimately leading to the pathophysiological changes that are associated with CFS (see 5.).

4. Stress Coping in CFS

A broad literature on dysfunctional coping styles in CFS patients exists, with several studies documenting maladaptive coping styles in CFS (Ax, Gregg, & Jones, 2002). Patients with CFS were shown to use significantly more escape-avoidance strategies than healthy controls (Blakely et al., 1991; Cope, Mann, Pelosi, & David, 1996). Escape-avoidance strategies involve disengaging or staying away from a stressful situation and its behavioral and cognitive/emotional consequences. In accordance with this finding, Afari and colleagues (2000) observed that twins with CFS or other chronic fatigue utilized more avoidance strategies than their non-fatigued siblings. Another study showed that CFS patients more frequently employed defensive coping styles than did healthy controls or patients with other chronic illness (Creswell & Chalder, 2001), and a recent population-based study found that CFS cases used escape-avoidance coping strategies significantly more frequently than non-ill controls (Nater et al., 2006). Interestingly, cognitive appraisals and maladaptive coping styles were associated with clinical features of CFS (e.g. severity of fatigue, impairment, illness burden, psychosocial problems, and psychiatric comorbidity) (Antoni et al., 1994), with another study in a population-based sample of CFS cases showing specifically that escape-avoidance coping was related to fatigue severity, pain, and disability (Nater et al., 2006). Despite this relative convergence of results, another community-based study of chronic fatigue showed no differences with regard to coping styles between individuals with CFS and healthy controls (Jason, Witter, & Torres-Harding, 2003).

Taken together, these studies indicate that CFS is associated with maladaptive coping strategies, potentially resulting in inadequate treatment efforts and regulatory adaptation to challenge, with the consequence of persistent fatigue and other related symptoms. Identification of cognitive-behavioral factors might ultimately lead to the further development of intervention strategies based on cognitive and behavioral changes

5. Biological Stress Response Systems in CFS

The physiological stress response comprises a complex physiological system, which is located in both the central nervous system (CNS) and the periphery of the body. The peripheral components include outflow from the hypothalamic-pituitary-adrenal (HPA) axis, the efferent sympathetic-adrenomedullary (SAM) system, and components of the parasympathetic system (Campeau, Day, Helmreich, Kollack-Walker, & Watson, 1998; Huether, 1996; Pacak & Palkovits, 2001; Stratakis & Chrousos, 1995), with the latter two forming the autonomic nervous system (ANS). These systems closely interact with the immune system (Sternberg, 2006). These systems are affected by stress in a top-down (and bottom-up) manner. E.g., the hypothalamic level of the HPA axis is activated through pathways that involve cortico-limbic and brain stem circuits. The central control of the HPA axis is governed by the hypothalamic paraventricular nucleus (PVN). The PVN receives input from stress-excitatory and -inhibitory circuits (Herman & Cullinan, 1997). The purpose of these circuits is to evaluate the importance of a stimulus to survival, and to use the resulting information to elicit an appropriate hormonal response (Gaab, Rohleder, Nater, & Ehlert, 2005; Herman et al., 2003). In the brain, glucocorticoids - in concert with neurotransmitters - modulate vigilance, alertness, sleep, cognition, and affect. Thus, alterations of the HPA axis may represent a common pathway linking precipitating factors, such as stress, with symptoms of CFS. Because the HPA axis plays a fundamental role in regulating other homeostatic systems, including the ANS and the immune system, it may be that dysregulation of these systems contributes to CFS expression. For example, glucocorticoids exert inhibitory control over CRH-induced activation of the locus coeruleus in the brain stem, the main origin of noradrenergic projections to the forebrain (Koob, 1999). Therefore, reduced glucocorticoid levels may sensitize the central noradrenergic system. Increased locus coeruleus responses to stress might in turn contribute to affective symptoms in CFS (Heim & Nater, 2007). Moreover, since cortisol exerts inhibitory effects on the secretion of pro-inflammatory cytokines, including interleukin (IL)-6, and helps return these cytokines to baseline levels after stress, alterations in cortisol secretion may be associated with disinhibition of immune mediators in CFS. Of note, inflammatory cytokines have been shown to induce many of the features of CFS, including fatigue, cognitive dysfunction, sleep disturbance, and affect impairment. It should be noted that increased sympathetic responses may mediate increased immune responses especially during stress. Thus, altered HPA axis regulation of sympathetic responses may further contribute to an inflammatory diathesis (Heim, Ehlert, & Hellhammer, 2000; Raison & Miller, 2003). Taken together, the HPA axis likely influences ANS and immune responses in CFS patients. Stress-induced alterations in these regulatory systems may also plausibly contribute to other functional somatic and emotional disorders, which often coincide with CFS.

Previous research has focused on individual consideration of these systems in CFS. A wealth of information has accumulated on both basal and challenge outcomes of HPA axis functioning in CFS (Cleare, 2003, 2004; Van Den Eede, Moorkens, Van Houdenhove, Cosyns, & Claes, 2007). In an early and seminal study by Demitrack and colleagues, low levels of cortisol in 24-hour urine of CFS patients were found in comparison to healthy controls (Demitrack et al., 1991). These findings were among the first to suggest hypoactivity of this axis in CFS. Subsequent studies of basal HPA axis found similar results. Some studies reported on lower cortisol levels after awakening in comparison to healthy controls (Jerjes, Cleare, Wessely, Wood, & Taylor, 2005; Nater, Maloney et al., 2008; Roberts, Wessely, Chalder, Papadopoulos, & Cleare, 2004; Strickland, Morriss, Wearden, & Deakin, 1998). Altered awakening cortisol levels are associated with increased stress (Pruessner, Hellhammer, & Kirschbaum, 1999; Schlotz, Hellhammer, Schulz, & Stone, 2004; Steptoe, Cropley, Griffith, & Kirschbaum, 2000). Furthermore, a generally reduced diurnal fluctuation of salivary cortisol in CFS compared to healthy controls was observed (Jerjes et al., 2005; Nater, Youngblood et al., 2008). However, other studies found no difference in salivary cortisol concentrations between CFS and healthy controls (Gaab, Huster, Peisen, Engert, Schad et al., 2002; Young et al., 1998). Insight from pharmacological challenge studies testing specific levels of HPA axis regulation indicates enhanced feedback sensitivity (Gaab, Huster, Peisen, Engert, Schad et al., 2002; Jerjes, Taylor, Wood, & Cleare, 2007; Segal, Hindmarsh, & Viner, 2005), increased adrenocortical sensitivity to adrenocorticotropic hormone (ACTH), and a reduced maximal cortisol response compared to normal subjects (Demitrack et al., 1991; Scott, Medbak, & Dinan, 1998), with non-significant findings being reported also (Gaab et al., 2003; Hudson & Cleare, 1999). Only one study so far has investigated central levels of the HPA axis responsivity using a psychological stressor, but no conclusive cortisol findings were reported (Gaab, Huster, Peisen, Engert, Heitz et al., 2002).

A number of studies have examined the involvement of the ANS in the pathophysiology of CFS based on the observation that many CFS symptoms are also observed in conditions of known dysautonomia, including disabling fatigue, dizziness, diminished concentration, tremulousness, and nausea (Komaroff & Buchwald, 1991). Numerous studies have found evidence of increased occurrence of orthostatic intolerance, which includes development of symptoms upon assuming and maintaining upright posture (De Lorenzo, Hargreaves, & Kakkar, 1996; Schondorf, Benoit, Wein, & Phaneuf, 1999; J. Stewart, Weldon, Arlievsky, Li, & Munoz, 1998; J. M. Stewart, Gewitz, Weldon, & Munoz, 1999; Tanaka, Matsushima, Tamai, & Kajimoto, 2002; Yataco et al., 1997). However, results are not consistent, with some studies finding no differences between CFS and control groups regarding orthostatic symptoms (Duprez et al., 1998; Jones et al., 2005; LaManca et al., 1999; Poole, Herrell, Ashton, Goldberg, & Buchwald, 2000). Another line of research in the study of ANS alterations in CFS has focused on cardiovascular autonomic measures. Many studies have found increased heart rate measures in CFS both at rest and due to challenge (Duprez et al., 1998; Freeman & Komaroff, 1997; Karas, Grubb, Boehm, & Kip, 2000; Naschitz et al., 2001; Streeten, Thomas, & Bell, 2000; van de Luit, van der Meulen, Cleophas, & Zwinderman, 1998; Winkler et al., 2004). This is in accordance with other studies showing low vagal tone (Cordero et al., 1996; Freeman & Komaroff, 1997; Sisto et al., 1995; J. M. Stewart, 2000) and a general sympathetic overactivity (De Becker et al., 1998; Pagani, Lucini, Mela, Langewitz, & Malliani, 1994; J. Stewart et al., 1998). However, there are also reports on decreased heart rate in response to exercise (Montague, Marrie, Klassen, Bewick, & Horacek, 1989) or mental stress (Soetekouw, Lenders, Bleijenberg, Thien, & van der Meer, 1999), or no differences between CFS and healthy controls at all (De Becker et al., 1998; Soetekouw et al., 1999; Yataco et al., 1997).

Other studies have indicated signs of immune disturbance in patients with CFS, especially in the form of elevated proinflammatory cytokine levels (Patarca-Montero, Antoni, Fletcher, & Klimas, 2001; Patarca, 2001), such as IL-6 and tumor necrosis factor (TNF)-alpha (Borish et al., 1998; Kruesi, Dale, & Straus, 1989; Nater, Youngblood et al., 2008). Consistent with these findings, increased *in vitro* inflammatory cytokine release has been reported in stimulated peripheral blood mononuclear cells of CFS patients (Cannon et al., 1997). Other indices of cytokine-mediated immune alterations that have been reported in patients with CFS include increased levels of autoantibodies, decreased natural killer cell activity, high levels of type 2 cytokine-producing cells, activated T lymphocytes, CD19+ B cells, neopterin (a marker of activated cell-mediated immunity) and activated complement (Mawle et al., 1997; Skowera et al., 2004; von Mikecz, Konstantinov, Buchwald, Gerace, & Tan, 1997; Whiteside & Friberg, 1998). In addition, alterations in the gene expression involved in immunity have been detected (Steinau, Unger, Vernon, Jones, & Rajeevan, 2004).

Despite the wealth of data on physiological alterations in stress systems in CFS patients, only few consistent findings may be summarized. The above reported inconsistencies might be attributed to the substantial differences in methodology, recruitment, and analysis strategies. There seems to be a relative hypoactivity of the HPA axis, an increased ANS, and increased immune activity in CFS patients. These alterations might potentially be able to explain at least some of CFS symptomatology. However, inconsistent results might also be found if biological changes are not present in all cases with CFS. In fact, some of the variation may be explained because these changes might be associated with a particular illness feature or even a risk factor of CFS, rather than with having the illness itself. As of yet, only one study has examined an association between stress as a risk factor for CFS and biological stress system alterations (Heim et al., 2009). In this study, the authors found decreased morning cortisol concentrations in only those CFS cases that also reported high levels of childhood trauma. This might suggest that biological stress system alterations are only observed in individuals with CFS that is preceded by high levels of stress. Whether these findings can be extended to ANS and immune system alterations needs to be investigated. As of now, no CFS study has been concomitantly measuring parameters from multiple stress systems. Clearly, research is needed incorporating a multidimensional measurement approach.

6. Integration

Exposure to stressors is more prevalent in individuals with CFS compared to controls, and CFS cases often report experiencing high levels of psychological distress. Based on the above findings that suggest that childhood adversity is a risk factor of CFS that is associated with changes in stress regulatory systems, it has been suggested that CFS may be a disorder of adaptation and failure to compensate in response to psychological challenge (Heim et al., 2009; Heim et al., 2006). Such failure may be reflected in dysfunctional regulatory outflow systems, i.e. neuroendocrine, autonomic, and immune systems. Alterations in brain systems involved in cognitive-emotional processing and processing of somatic stimuli might in part underlie alterations in peripheral outflow systems in CFS. One factor that is well known to directly program central nervous system, physiological and behavioral response to subsequent stress is early adverse experience (Heim, Plotsky, & Nemeroff, 2004; Meaney & Szyf, 2005; Plotsky, Sanchez, & Levine, 2001). Early adverse experience in animal models has been shown to induce a phenotype with neurobiological vulnerability to the effects of stress. Upon additional challenge, e.g. by the experience of negative life events, neuroendocrine alterations, such as low cortisol availability, might lead to disinhibition of central nervous and peripheral immune and autonomic responses (see e.g. Heim et al., 2009). Such maladaptive responses might ultimately evolve into the characteristic symptom pattern of CFS (Clauw & Chrousos, 1997). The effects of early experience and experience of stress in adulthood on illness manifestation are likely moderated by genetic factors at the neuronal and peripheral physiological levels as well as coping strategies.

Although this book chapter documents findings of increased occurrence of stressors both early and later in life, it needs to be critically noted that this phenomenon is not specific for CFS. Apart from CFS, the importance of psychological stress as a potential risk factor in the manifestation and maintenance of a variety of other functional somatic syndromes (FSS) has been recognized in recent years, and the psychobiological processes assumed to play a role in the translation of stress into functional symptoms and syndromes has been examined in numerous studies. Among the convergent findings in the literature are increased prevalence of early life stress (Nater & Heim, in press) and decreased responsivity of the HPA axis (Heim & Nater, 2007) in FSS, such as irritable bowel syndrome, fibromyalgia, and others.

Based on the finding that HPA axis dysfunctions are mainly observed in CFS cases reporting high levels of early life stress, it might be proposed that alterations in biological stress systems are only observed in a sub-group of individuals with CFS. The possibility of different subtypes of CFS with different pathogenetic pathways bears important consequences for further research on pathophysiology and, ultimately, treatment options. It might also be important to further scrutinize CFS patients that did not report higher prevalence rates of stressful experiences and/or alterations in physiological stress systems. Clearly, future research is needed in this area.

Numerous treatments have been applied to CFS patients with various results. Those with the best experimental data to support efficacy include graded exercise training and cognitive behavioral therapy (CBT). CBT strategies for CFS typically involve organizing activity and rest cycles, initiating graded increases in activity, establishing a consistent sleep regimen, attempting to restructure beliefs around self, as well as disease attributions, and stress management (Malouff, Thorsteinsson, Rooke, Bhullar, & Schutte, 2008). The latter employs stress reducing strategies and improves coping behavior. It seems critical to devote research resources to a detailed understanding of the processes that lead from stress to CFS in order to improve current treatment strategies. Given the above described biological alterations of the stress system in CFS, interactions of treatment intervention and biological outcome variables seem to be very promising (Roberts, Papadopoulos, Wessely, Chalder, & Cleare, 2008).

References

Afari, N., Schmaling, K. B., Herrell, R., Hartman, S., Goldberg, J. & Buchwald, D. S. (2000). Coping strategies in twins with chronic fatigue and chronic fatigue syndrome. *J Psychosom Res, 48*(6), 547-554.

Antoni, M. H., Brickman, A., Lutgendorf, S., Klimas, N., Imia-Fins, A. & Ironson, G. (1994). Psychosocial correlates of illness burden in chronic fatigue syndrome. *Clin Infect Dis, 18 Suppl 1*, S73-78.

Arnow, B. A. (2004). Relationships between childhood maltreatment, adult health and psychiatric outcomes, and medical utilization. *J Clin Psychiatry, 65 Suppl 12*, 10-15.

Ax, S., Gregg, V. H. & Jones, D. (2002). Caring for a relative with chronic fatigue syndrome: difficulties, cognition and acceptance over time. *J R Soc Health, 122*(1), 35-42.

Blakely, A. A., Howard, R. C., Sosich, R. M., Murdoch, J. C., Menkes, D. B. & Spears, G. F. (1991). Psychiatric symptoms, personality and ways of coping in chronic fatigue syndrome. *Psychol Med, 21*(2), 347-362.

Borish, L., Schmaling, K., DiClementi, J. D., Streib, J., Negri, J. & Jones, J. F. (1998). Chronic fatigue syndrome: identification of distinct subgroups on the basis of allergy and psychologic variables. *J Allergy Clin Immunol, 102*(2), 222-230.

Campeau, S., Day, H. E., Helmreich, D. L., Kollack-Walker, S. & Watson, S. J. (1998). Principles of psychoneuroendocrinology. *Psychiatr Clin North Am, 21*(2), 259-276.

Cannon, J. G., Angel, J. B., Abad, L. W., Vannier, E., Mileno, M. D., Fagioli, L., et al. (1997). Interleukin-1 beta, interleukin-1 receptor antagonist, and soluble interleukin-1 receptor type II secretion in chronic fatigue syndrome. *J Clin Immunol, 17*(3), 253-261.

Clauw, D. J. & Chrousos, G. P. (1997). Chronic pain and fatigue syndromes: overlapping clinical and neuroendocrine features and potential pathogenic mechanisms. *Neuroimmunomodulation, 4*(3), 134-153.

Cleare, A. J. (2003). The neuroendocrinology of chronic fatigue syndrome. *Endocr Rev, 24*(2), 236-252.

Cleare, A. J. (2004). The HPA axis and the genesis of chronic fatigue syndrome. *Trends Endocrinol Metab, 15*(2), 55-59.

Cope, H., Mann, A., Pelosi, A. & David, A. (1996). Psychosocial risk factors for chronic fatigue and chronic fatigue syndrome following presumed viral illness: a case-control study. *Psychol Med, 26*(6), 1197-1209.

Cordero, D. L., Sisto, S. A., Tapp, W. N., LaManca, J. J., Pareja, J. G. & Natelson, B. H. (1996). Decreased vagal power during treadmill walking in patients with chronic fatigue syndrome. *Clin Auton Res, 6*(6), 329-333.

Creswell, C. & Chalder, T. (2001). Defensive coping styles in chronic fatigue syndrome. *J Psychosom Res, 51*(4), 607-610.

De Becker, P., Dendale, P., De Meirleir, K., Campine, I., Vandenborne, K. & Hagers, Y. (1998). Autonomic testing in patients with chronic fatigue syndrome. *Am J Med, 105*(3A), 22S-26S.

De Lorenzo, F., Hargreaves, J. & Kakkar, V. V. (1996). Possible relationship between chronic fatigue and postural tachycardia syndromes. *Clin Auton Res, 6*(5), 263-264.

Demitrack, M. A., Dale, J. K., Straus, S. E., Laue, L., Listwak, S. J., Kruesi, M. J., et al. (1991). Evidence for impaired activation of the hypothalamic-pituitary-adrenal axis in patients with chronic fatigue syndrome. *J Clin Endocrinol Metab, 73*(6), 1224-1234.

Duprez, D. A., De Buyzere, M. L., Drieghe, B., Vanhaverbeke, F., Taes, Y., Michielsen, W., et al. (1998). Long- and short-term blood pressure and RR-interval variability and psychosomatic distress in chronic fatigue syndrome. *Clin Sci (Lond), 94*(1), 57-63.

Faulkner, S. & Smith, A. (2008). A longitudinal study of the relationship between psychological distress and recurrence of upper respiratory tract infections in chronic fatigue syndrome. *Br J Health Psychol, 13*(Pt 1), 177-186.

Freeman, R. & Komaroff, A. L. (1997). Does the chronic fatigue syndrome involve the autonomic nervous system? *Am J Med, 102*(4), 357-364.

Fukuda, K., Straus, S. E., Hickie, I., Sharpe, M. C., Dobbins, J. G. & Komaroff, A. (1994). The chronic fatigue syndrome: a comprehensive approach to its definition and study. International Chronic Fatigue Syndrome Study Group. *Ann Intern Med, 121*(12), 953-959.

Gaab, J., Huster, D., Peisen, R., Engert, V., Heitz, V., Schad, T., et al. (2003). Assessment of cortisol response with low-dose and high-dose ACTH in patients with chronic fatigue syndrome and healthy comparison subjects. *Psychosomatics, 44*(2), 113-119.

Gaab, J., Huster, D., Peisen, R., Engert, V., Heitz, V., Schad, T., et al. (2002). Hypothalamic-pituitary-adrenal axis reactivity in chronic fatigue syndrome and health under psychological, physiological, and pharmacological stimulation. *Psychosom Med, 64*(6), 951-962.

Gaab, J., Huster, D., Peisen, R., Engert, V., Schad, T., Schurmeyer, T. H., et al. (2002). Low-dose dexamethasone suppression test in chronic fatigue syndrome and health. *Psychosom Med, 64*(2), 311-318.

Gaab, J., Rohleder, N., Nater, U. M. & Ehlert, U. (2005). Psychological determinants of the cortisol stress response: the role of anticipatory cognitive appraisal. *Psychoneuroendocrinology, 30*(6), 599-610.

Hatcher, S. & House, A. (2003). Life events, difficulties and dilemmas in the onset of chronic fatigue syndrome: a case-control study. *Psychol Med, 33*(7), 1185-1192.

Heim, C., Ehlert, U. & Hellhammer, D. H. (2000). The potential role of hypocortisolism in the pathophysiology of stress-related bodily disorders. *Psychoneuroendocrinology, 25*(1), 1-35.

Heim, C., Nater, U. M., Maloney, E., Boneva, R., Jones, J. F. & Reeves, W. C. (2009). Childhood trauma and risk for chronic fatigue syndrome: association with neuroendocrine dysfunction. *Arch Gen Psychiatry, 66*(1), 72-80.

Heim, C., Plotsky, P. M. & Nemeroff, C. B. (2004). Importance of studying the contributions of early adverse experience to neurobiological findings in depression. *Neuropsychopharmacology, 29*(4), 641-648.

Heim, C., Wagner, D., Maloney, E., Papanicolaou, D. A., Solomon, L., Jones, J. F., et al. (2006). Early adverse experience and risk for chronic fatigue syndrome: results from a population-based study. *Arch Gen Psychiatry, 63*(11), 1258-1266.

Heim, C. M. & Nater, U. M. (2007). Hypocortisolism and stress. In G. Fink (Ed.), *Encyclopedia of stress* (2nd ed., pp. 400-407). Oxford: Academic Press.

Herman, J. P. & Cullinan, W. E. (1997). Neurocircuitry of stress: central control of the hypothalamo-pituitary-adrenocortical axis. *Trends Neurosci, 20*(2), 78-84.

Herman, J. P., Figueiredo, H., Mueller, N. K., Ulrich-Lai, Y., Ostrander, M. M., Choi, D. C., et al. (2003). Central mechanisms of stress integration: hierarchical circuitry controlling hypothalamo-pituitary-adrenocortical responsiveness. *Front Neuroendocrinol, 24*(3), 151-180.

Hudson, M. & Cleare, A. J. (1999). The 1microg short Synacthen test in chronic fatigue syndrome. *Clin Endocrinol (Oxf), 51*(5), 625-630.

Huether, G. (1996). The central adaptation syndrome: psychosocial stress as a trigger for adaptive modifications of brain structure and brain function. *Prog Neurobiol, 48*(6), 569-612.

Jason, L. A., Wagner, L., Rosenthal, S., Goodlatte, J., Lipkin, D., Papernik, M., et al. (1998). Estimating the prevalence of chronic fatigue syndrome among nurses. *Am J Med, 105*(3A), 91S-93S.

Jason, L. A., Witter, E. & Torres-Harding, S. (2003). Chronic fatigue syndrome, coping, optimism and social support. *Journal of Mental Health, 12*(2), 109-118.

Jerjes, W. K., Cleare, A. J., Wessely, S., Wood, P. J. & Taylor, N. F. (2005). Diurnal patterns of salivary cortisol and cortisone output in chronic fatigue syndrome. *J Affect Disord.*

Jerjes, W. K., Taylor, N. F., Wood, P. J. & Cleare, A. J. (2007). Enhanced feedback sensitivity to prednisolone in chronic fatigue syndrome. *Psychoneuroendocrinology, 32*(2), 192-198.

Jones, J. F., Lin, J.-M., Maloney, E. M., Boneva, R. S., Unger, E. R., Nater, U. M., et al. (in press). Exploration of exclusionary criteria in chronic fatigue syndrome: to exclude or not to exclude. *BMC Medicine.*

Jones, J. F., Nicholson, A., Nisenbaum, R., Papanicolaou, D. A., Solomon, L., Boneva, R., et al. (2005). Orthostatic instability in a population-based study of chronic fatigue syndrome. *Am J Med, 118*(12), 1415.

Kang, H. K., Natelson, B. H., Mahan, C. M., Lee, K. Y. & Murphy, F. M. (2003). Post-traumatic stress disorder and chronic fatigue syndrome-like illness among Gulf War veterans: a population-based survey of 30,000 veterans. *Am J Epidemiol, 157*(2), 141-148.

Karas, B., Grubb, B. P., Boehm, K. & Kip, K. (2000). The postural orthostatic tachycardia syndrome: a potentially treatable cause of chronic fatigue, exercise intolerance, and cognitive impairment in adolescents. *Pacing Clin Electrophysiol, 23*(3), 344-351.

Kato, K., Sullivan, P. F., Evengard, B. & Pedersen, N. L. (2006). Premorbid predictors of chronic fatigue. *Arch Gen Psychiatry, 63*(11), 1267-1272.

Kerr, J. R. & Mattey, D. L. (2008). Preexisting psychological stress predicts acute and chronic fatigue and arthritis following symptomatic parvovirus B19 infection. *Clin Infect Dis, 46*(9), e83-87.

Komaroff, A. L. & Buchwald, D. (1991). Symptoms and signs of chronic fatigue syndrome. *Rev Infect Dis, 13 Suppl 1*, S8-11.

Koob, G. F. (1999). Corticotropin-releasing factor, norepinephrine, and stress. *Biol Psychiatry, 46*(9), 1167-1180.

Kruesi, M. J., Dale, J. & Straus, S. E. (1989). Psychiatric diagnoses in patients who have chronic fatigue syndrome. *J Clin Psychiatry, 50*(2), 53-56.

LaManca, J. J., Peckerman, A., Sisto, S. A., DeLuca, J., Cook, S. & Natelson, B. H. (2001). Cardiovascular responses of women with chronic fatigue syndrome to stressful cognitive testing before and after strenuous exercise. *Psychosom Med, 63*(5), 756-764.

LaManca, J. J., Peckerman, A., Walker, J., Kesil, W., Cook, S., Taylor, A., et al. (1999). Cardiovascular response during head-up tilt in chronic fatigue syndrome. *Clin Physiol, 19*(2), 111-120.

Lewis, S., Cooper, C. L. & Bennett, D. (1994). Psychosocial factors and chronic fatigue syndrome. *Psychol Med, 24*(3), 661-671.

Lim, B. R., Tan, S. Y., Zheng, Y. P., Lin, K. M., Park, B. C. & Turk, A. A. (2003). Psychosocial factors in chronic fatigue syndrome among Chinese Americans: a longitudinal community-based study. *Transcult Psychiatry, 40*(3), 429-441.

Lutgendorf, S. K., Antoni, M. H., Ironson, G., Fletcher, M. A., Penedo, F., Baum, A., et al. (1995). Physical symptoms of chronic fatigue syndrome are exacerbated by the stress of Hurricane Andrew. *Psychosom Med, 57*(4), 310-323.

MacDonald, K. L., Osterholm, M. T., LeDell, K. H., White, K. E., Schenck, C. H., Chao, C. C., et al. (1996). A case-control study to assess possible triggers and cofactors in chronic fatigue syndrome. *Am J Med, 100*(5), 548-554.

Malouff, J. M., Thorsteinsson, E. B., Rooke, S. E., Bhullar, N. & Schutte, N. S. (2008). Efficacy of cognitive behavioral therapy for chronic fatigue syndrome: A meta-analysis. *Clinical Psychology Review, 28*, 736–745.

Masuda, A., Munemoto, T., Yamanaka, T., Takei, M. & Tei, C. (2002). Psychosocial characteristics and immunological functions in patients with postinfectious chronic fatigue syndrome and noninfectious chronic fatigue syndrome. *J Behav Med, 25*(5), 477-485.

Masuda, A., Nozoe, S. I., Matsuyama, T. & Tanaka, H. (1994). Psychobehavioral and immunological characteristics of adult people with chronic fatigue and patients with chronic fatigue syndrome. *Psychosom Med, 56*(6), 512-518.

Mawle, A. C., Nisenbaum, R., Dobbins, J. G., Gary, H. E., Jr., Stewart, J. A., Reyes, M., et al. (1997). Immune responses associated with chronic fatigue syndrome: a case-control study. *J Infect Dis, 175*(1), 136-141.

McCauley, J., Kern, D. E., Kolodner, K., Dill, L., Schroeder, A. F., DeChant, H. K., et al. (1997). Clinical characteristics of women with a history of childhood abuse: unhealed wounds. *Jama, 277*(17), 1362-1368.

McCauley, L. A., Joos, S. K., Barkhuizen, A., Shuell, T., Tyree, W. A. & Bourdette, D. N. (2002). Chronic fatigue in a population-based study of Gulf War veterans. *Arch Environ Health, 57*(4), 340-348.

Meaney, M. J. & Szyf, M. (2005). Environmental programming of stress responses through DNA methylation: life at the interface between a dynamic environment and a fixed genome. *Dialogues Clin Neurosci, 7*(2), 103-123.

Montague, T. J., Marrie, T. J., Klassen, G. A., Bewick, D. J. & Horacek, B. M. (1989). Cardiac function at rest and with exercise in the chronic fatigue syndrome. *Chest, 95*(4), 779-784.

Naschitz, J. E., Rozenbaum, M., Rosner, I., Sabo, E., Priselac, R. M., Shaviv, N., et al. (2001). Cardiovascular response to upright tilt in fibromyalgia differs from that in chronic fatigue syndrome. *J Rheumatol, 28*(6), 1356-1360.

Nater, U. M. & Heim, C. (in press). Childhood trauma and functional somatic syndromes. In C. M. Worthman, P. M. Plotsky, D. S. Schechter & C. Cummings (Eds.), *Formative experiences: The interaction of caregiving, culture, and developmental psychobiology*. Cambridge: University Press.

Nater, U. M., Heim, C. & Raison, C. (in press). Chronic fatigue syndrome. In M. J. Aminoff, F. Boller & D. F. Swaab (Eds.), *Handbook of Clinical Neurology 3rd Series*.

Nater, U. M., Maloney, E., Boneva, R. S., Gurbaxani, B. M., Lin, J. M., Jones, J. F., et al. (2008). Attenuated morning salivary cortisol concentrations in a population-based study of persons with chronic fatigue syndrome and well controls. *J Clin Endocrinol Metab, 93*(3), 703-709.

Nater, U. M., Wagner, D., Solomon, L., Jones, J. F., Unger, E. R., Papanicolaou, D. A., et al. (2006). Coping styles in people with chronic fatigue syndrome identified from the general population of Wichita, KS. *J Psychosom Res, 60*(6), 567-573.

Nater, U. M., Youngblood, L. S., Jones, J. F., Unger, E. R., Miller, A. H., Reeves, W. C., et al. (2008). Alterations in diurnal salivary cortisol rhythm in a population-based sample of cases with chronic fatigue syndrome. *Psychosomatic Medicine, 70*, 298–305.

Nisenbaum, R., Barrett, D. H., Reyes, M. & Reeves, W. C. (2000). Deployment stressors and a chronic multisymptom illness among Gulf War veterans. *J Nerv Ment Dis, 188*(5), 259-266.

Pacak, K. & Palkovits, M. (2001). Stressor specificity of central neuroendocrine responses: implications for stress-related disorders. *Endocr Rev, 22*(4), 502-548.

Pagani, M., Lucini, D., Mela, G. S., Langewitz, W. & Malliani, A. (1994). Sympathetic overactivity in subjects complaining of unexplained fatigue. *Clin Sci (Lond), 87*(6), 655-661.

Patarca-Montero, R., Antoni, M., Fletcher, M. A. & Klimas, N. G. (2001). Cytokine and other immunologic markers in chronic fatigue syndrome and their relation to neuropsychological factors. *Appl Neuropsychol, 8*(1), 51-64.

Patarca, R. (2001). Cytokines and chronic fatigue syndrome. *Ann N Y Acad Sci, 933*, 185-200.

Plotsky, P. M., Sanchez, M. M. & Levine, S. (2001). Intrinsic and extrinsic factors modulating physiological coping systems during development. In D. M. Broom (Ed.), *Coping with challenge* (pp. 169-196). Berlin Dahlem University Press.

Poole, J., Herrell, R., Ashton, S., Goldberg, J. & Buchwald, D. (2000). Results of isoproterenol tilt table testing in monozygotic twins discordant for chronic fatigue syndrome. *Arch Intern Med, 160*(22), 3461-3468.

Prins, J. B., van der Meer, J. W. & Bleijenberg, G. (2006). Chronic fatigue syndrome. *Lancet, 367*(9507), 346-355.

Pruessner, J. C., Hellhammer, D. H. & Kirschbaum, C. (1999). Burnout, perceived stress, and cortisol responses to awakening. *Psychosom Med, 61*(2), 197-204.

Raison, C. L. & Miller, A. H. (2003). When not enough is too much: the role of insufficient glucocorticoid signaling in the pathophysiology of stress-related disorders. *American Journal of Psychiatry, 160*, 1554-1565.

Ray, C., Jefferies, S. & Weir, W. R. (1995). Life-events and the course of chronic fatigue syndrome. *Br J Med Psychol, 68 (Pt 4)*, 323-331.

Reeves, W. C., Lloyd, A., Vernon, S. D., Klimas, N., Jason, L. A., Bleijenberg, G., et al. (2003). Identification of ambiguities in the 1994 chronic fatigue syndrome research case definition and recommendations for resolution. *BMC Health Serv Res, 3*(1), 25.

Reyes, M., Dobbins, J. G., Mawle, A. C., Steele, L., Gary, H. E., Jr., Malani, H., et al. (1996). Risk factors for CFS: a case control study. *Journal of Chronic Fatigue Syndrome, 2*, 17-33.

Roberts, A. D., Papadopoulos, A. S., Wessely, S., Chalder, T. & Cleare, A. J. (2008). Salivary cortisol output before and after cognitive behavioural therapy for chronic fatigue syndrome. *J Affect Disord.*

Roberts, A. D., Wessely, S., Chalder, T., Papadopoulos, A. & Cleare, A. J. (2004). Salivary cortisol response to awakening in chronic fatigue syndrome. *Br J Psychiatry, 184*, 136-141.

Romans, S., Belaise, C., Martin, J., Morris, E. & Raffi, A. (2002). Childhood abuse and later medical disorders in women. An epidemiological study. *Psychother Psychosom, 71*(3), 141-150.

Salit, I. E. (1997). Precipitating factors for the chronic fatigue syndrome. *J Psychiatr Res, 31*(1), 59-65.

Schlotz, W., Hellhammer, J., Schulz, P. & Stone, A. A. (2004). Perceived work overload and chronic worrying predict weekend-weekday differences in the cortisol awakening response. *Psychosom Med, 66*(2), 207-214.

Schondorf, R., Benoit, J., Wein, T. & Phaneuf, D. (1999). Orthostatic intolerance in the chronic fatigue syndrome. *J Auton Nerv Syst, 75*(2-3), 192-201.

Scott, L. V., Medbak, S. & Dinan, T. G. (1998). The low dose ACTH test in chronic fatigue syndrome and in health. *Clin Endocrinol (Oxf), 48*(6), 733-737.

Segal, T. Y., Hindmarsh, P. C. & Viner, R. M. (2005). Disturbed adrenal function in adolescents with chronic fatigue syndrome. *J Pediatr Endocrinol Metab, 18*(3), 295-301.

Sisto, S. A., Tapp, W., Drastal, S., Bergen, M., DeMasi, I., Cordero, D., et al. (1995). Vagal tone is reduced during paced breathing in patients with the chronic fatigue syndrome. *Clin Auton Res, 5*(3), 139-143.

Skowera, A., Cleare, A., Blair, D., Bevis, L., Wessely, S. C. & Peakman, M. (2004). High levels of type 2 cytokine-producing cells in chronic fatigue syndrome. *Clin Exp Immunol, 135*(2), 294-302.

Soetekouw, P. M., Lenders, J. W., Bleijenberg, G., Thien, T. & van der Meer, J. W. (1999). Autonomic function in patients with chronic fatigue syndrome. *Clin Auton Res, 9*(6), 334-340.

Steinau, M., Unger, E. R., Vernon, S. D., Jones, J. F. & Rajeevan, M. S. (2004). Differential-display PCR of peripheral blood for biomarker discovery in chronic fatigue syndrome. *J Mol Med, 82*(11), 750-755.

Steptoe, A., Cropley, M., Griffith, J. & Kirschbaum, C. (2000). Job strain and anger expression predict early morning elevations in salivary cortisol. *Psychosom Med, 62*(2), 286-292.

Sternberg, E. M. (2006). Neural regulation of innate immunity: a coordinated nonspecific host response to pathogens. *Nat Rev Immunol, 6*(4), 318-328.

Stewart, J., Weldon, A., Arlievsky, N., Li, K. & Munoz, J. (1998). Neurally mediated hypotension and autonomic dysfunction measured by heart rate variability during head-up tilt testing in children with chronic fatigue syndrome. *Clin Auton Res, 8*(4), 221-230.

Stewart, J. M. (2000). Autonomic nervous system dysfunction in adolescents with postural orthostatic tachycardia syndrome and chronic fatigue syndrome is characterized by attenuated vagal baroreflex and potentiated sympathetic vasomotion. *Pediatr Res, 48*(2), 218-226.

Stewart, J. M., Gewitz, M. H., Weldon, A. & Munoz, J. (1999). Patterns of orthostatic intolerance: the orthostatic tachycardia syndrome and adolescent chronic fatigue. *J Pediatr, 135*(2 Pt 1), 218-225.

Stratakis, C. A. & Chrousos, G. P. (1995). Neuroendocrinology and pathophysiology of the stress system. *Ann N Y Acad Sci, 771*, 1-18.

Streeten, D. H., Thomas, D. & Bell, D. S. (2000). The roles of orthostatic hypotension, orthostatic tachycardia, and subnormal erythrocyte volume in the pathogenesis of the chronic fatigue syndrome. *Am J Med Sci, 320*(1), 1-8.

Strickland, P., Morriss, R., Wearden, A. & Deakin, B. (1998). A comparison of salivary cortisol in chronic fatigue syndrome, community depression and healthy controls. *J Affect Disord, 47*(1-3), 191-194.

Stricklin, A., Sewell, M. & Austad, C. (1990). Objective measurement of personality variables in epidemic neuromyasthenia patients. *S Afr Med J, 77*(1), 31-34.

Sundbom, E., Henningsson, M., Holm, U., Soderbergh, S. & Evengard, B. (2002). Possible influence of defenses and negative life events on patients with chronic fatigue syndrome: a pilot study. *Psychol Rep, 91*(3 Pt 1), 963-978.

Tanaka, H., Matsushima, R., Tamai, H. & Kajimoto, Y. (2002). Impaired postural cerebral hemodynamics in young patients with chronic fatigue with and without orthostatic intolerance. *J Pediatr, 140*(4), 412-417.

Taylor, R. R. & Jason, L. A. (2001). Sexual abuse, physical abuse, chronic fatigue, and chronic fatigue syndrome: a community-based study. *J Nerv Ment Dis, 189*(10), 709-715.

Taylor, R. R. & Jason, L. A. (2002). Chronic fatigue, abuse-related traumatization, and psychiatric disorders in a community-based sample. *Soc Sci Med, 55*(2), 247-256.

Theorell, T., Blomkvist, V., Lindh, G. & Evengard, B. (1999). Critical life events, infections, and symptoms during the year preceding chronic fatigue syndrome (CFS): an examination of CFS patients and subjects with a nonspecific life crisis. *Psychosom Med,* *61*(3), 304-310.

van de Luit, L., van der Meulen, J., Cleophas, T. J. & Zwinderman, A. H. (1998). Amplified amplitudes of circadian rhythms and nighttime hypotension in patients with chronic fatigue syndrome: improvement by inopamil but not by melatonin. *Angiology, 49*(11), 903-908.

Van Den Eede, F., Moorkens, G., Van Houdenhove, B., Cosyns, P. & Claes, S. J. (2007). Hypothalamic-pituitary-adrenal axis function in chronic fatigue syndrome. *Neuropsychobiology, 55*(2), 112-120.

Van Houdenhove, B., Neerinckx, E., Lysens, R., Vertommen, H., Van Houdenhove, L., Onghena, P., et al. (2001). Victimization in chronic fatigue syndrome and fibromyalgia in tertiary care: a controlled study on prevalence and characteristics. *Psychosomatics, 42*(1), 21-28.

von Mikecz, A., Konstantinov, K., Buchwald, D. S., Gerace, L. & Tan, E. M. (1997). High frequency of autoantibodies to insoluble cellular antigens in patients with chronic fatigue syndrome. *Arthritis Rheum, 40*(2), 295-305.

Whiteside, T. L. & Friberg, D. (1998). Natural killer cells and natural killer cell activity in chronic fatigue syndrome. *Am J Med, 105*(3A), 27S-34S.

Winkler, A. S., Blair, D., Marsden, J. T., Peters, T. J., Wessely, S. & Cleare, A. J. (2004). Autonomic function and serum erythropoietin levels in chronic fatigue syndrome. *J Psychosom Res, 56*(2), 179-183.

Wood, G. C., Bentall, R. P., Gopfert, M., Dewey, M. E. & Edwards, R. H. (1994). The differential response of chronic fatigue, neurotic and muscular dystrophy patients to experimental psychological stress. *Psychol Med, 24*(2), 357-364.

Yataco, A., Talo, H., Rowe, P., Kass, D. A., Berger, R. D. & Calkins, H. (1997). Comparison of heart rate variability in patients with chronic fatigue syndrome and controls. *Clin Auton Res, 7*(6), 293-297.

Young, A. H., Sharpe, M., Clements, A., Dowling, B., Hawton, K. E. & Cowen, P. J. (1998). Basal activity of the hypothalamic-pituitary-adrenal axis in patients with the chronic fatigue syndrome (neurasthenia). *Biol Psychiatry, 43*(3), 236-237.

In: Chronic Fatigue Syndrome: Symptoms, Causes & Prevention   ISBN: 978-1-60741-493-3
Editor: E. Svoboda and K. Zelenjcik, pp. 143-163   © 2010 Nova Science Publishers, Inc.

Chapter 7

Patterns of Cardiovascular Reactivity and Electrocardiographic QT Intervals Distinguish Fibromyalgia from Chronic Fatigue Syndrome

Jochanan Naschitz[1], Gleb Slobodin[1],
Michael Rozenbaum[2] and Itzhak Rosner[2]
Departments of Internal Medicine A[1] and Rheumatology[2]
Bnai Zion Medical Center and Ruth and Bruce Rappaport Faculty of Medicine,
Technion-Israel Institute of Technology, Haifa, Israel

Fibromyalgia and Chronic Fatigue Syndrome

Fibromyalgia (FM) is a clinical syndrome characterized by widespread pain and abnormal sensitivity on palpation of specific tender points [1]. The pathogenesis of FM has been elusive, made difficult by the absence of distinctive biochemical or histological abnormalities. There is much debate and controversy about this condition. On the one side are those who deny the existence of fibromyalgia as a nosologic entity and consider it an artificial summation of unrelated symptoms [2, 3]. A consequence of the view that FM is but an expression of low self-esteem and unhappiness may to change our approach to this condition and deal with these patients in psychological and sociological terms. On the other side are clinicians and researchers who define fibromyalgia as a distinct clinico-pathologic disorder and suggest that it is a genetically based disease with autosomal-dominant transmission [4]. Much of the evidence that FM is the projection of an underlying physiologic disturbance relates to studies describing autonomic system dysfunction in FM patients [5-13].

A point of obfuscation in classifying patients with FM lies in the overlap of this syndrome with other functional somatic and pain syndromes: chronic fatigue syndrome, irritable bowel syndrome, Gulf War syndrome, migraine, etc [14-17]. Studies have documented common risk factors operating at the background of these syndromes as well as the presence of autonomic nervous dysfunction (Figure 1). The clinical overlap of FM and chronic fatigue syndrome (CFS) is particularly prominent and the two are mentioned frequently as a single disorder [14-16]. In a study of 163 women with primary CFS, 43% also met criteria for FM [15] and in another study, 18% of patients with FM had also been diagnosed with CFS [16].

Proposed pathophysiology and overlap of functional somatic syndromes

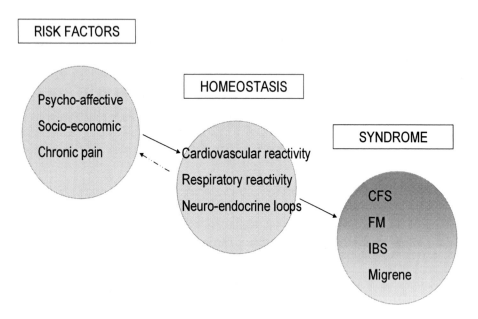

Figure 1. The conundrum of functional somatic syndromes

Clinically evaluated, medically unexplained fatigue of at least six months duration, that is of new onset, is not a result of ongoing exertion, not substantially alleviated by rest, and considerably reducing previous levels of activity is called chronic fatigue syndrome (CFS) [18]. Previous studies have documented a close connection between impairment of autonomic nervous functions, i.e. dysautonomia, and CFS [19-28]. Abnormalities of central nervous system on magnetic resonance imaging [29] and single photon emission tomography (30), as well as disruption of the hypothalamic-pituitary-adrenal axis and serotoninergic and noradrenergic pathways have been demonstrated [31,32], and a 'distal dysautonomia' has been described in CFS patients [33]. Further, evidence for this comes from overlapping symptoms between autonomic disorders and CFS, the common occurrence of neurally mediated hypotension during head-up tilt (HUTT) in patients with CFS, and the improvement of symptoms of CFS following therapy directed at neurally mediated hypotension [19-21, 34]. Also, the postural tachycardia syndrome, which has been attributed to a partial dysautonomia involving the vasculature of the legs, has also been described in CFS [22, 27, 28].

Our studies of the past decade began with attempts to clarify the dysautonomia of CFS. We proceded thereafter by focusing on cardiovascular reactivity as a reflection of automic nervous activity in CFS. These studies lead to the description of a characteristic pattern of cardiovascular reactivity in CFS, which is specific to CFS [16]. As part of the efforts to define FM more closely, studies were carried out to assess whether the cardiovascular reactivity patterns of CFS were present in FM as well.

Autonomic Nervous System Activity

In the clinical setting, autonomic nervous system activity is assessed by surrogate methods, chiefly cardiovascular reactivity (CVR). The fast response of the blood pressure (BP) and heart rate (HR) to acute stimuli is under autonomic nervous control. Therefore, BP and HR measurements during orthostatic challenge on head-up tilt testing (HUTT) can be used as one measure of cardiovascular autonomic activity, providing there is no evidence of organic heart disease, venous insufficiency, hypovolemia or pharmacological interference [35]. Classical pathological reactions to the HUTT are: vasodepressor reaction, cardioinhibitory reaction, orthostatic hypotension and postural tachycardia syndrome. In studies utilizing these outcome measures, evidence for abnormal cardiovascular reactivity was found in up to 60% FM patients [36, 37] and roughly one half of CFS patients [20, 33]. However, these aberrations of CVR are considered to be nonspecific since the same reactions occur in a large variety of conditions associated with autonomic dysfunction [38]. HR variability during the HUTT is another measure applied to the study of the CVR in FM and CFS. FM patients had significantly more low-frequency (LF) and less high-frequency (HF) components of the power spectra than controls [9, 10]. CFS patients had significantly less low-frequency and high-frequency variances at baseline than healthy subjects, however the differences disappeared in the standing position [39]. We could not find in the literature a direct comparison of the HR variability in patients with FM versus CFS.

In fact, autonomic cardiovascular modulation is characterized by a considerable non-linearity between external stimuli and cardiovascular response [40]. A number of methods have been proposed in an attempt to address the issue of non-linear dynamics of the cardiovascular responses. These include fractal analysis [39, 41], recurrence quantification analysis [42, 43] and multivariate models that consider the relationship between two or more cardiovascular signals [40]. It has been suggested that joint quantification of BP and HR fluctuations and utilization of non-Euclidian mathematic analysis may provide more reliable information on CVR [40]. This approach was utilized in two methodologies recently proposed by us for the assessment of cardiovascular reactivity, the 'hemodynamic instability score' (HIS) and the 'Fractal and Recurrence Analysis-based Score' (FRAS).

Our studies received a further impetus a few years back with the exciting finding of a specific cardiovascular reactivity (CVR) pattern in patients with CFS [44]. This observation was validated in 5 studies using different methodologies [45-50].

The Hemodynamic Instability Score (HIS)

The HIS involves computing BP- and HR- changes during the course of a head-up tilt test, followed by processing the data curves generated by utilizing image analysis techniques [44].

In a first study, patients with CFS (n = 25) and their age and sex-matched healthy controls (n = 37) as well as patients with fibromyalgia (n= 30), generalized anxiety disorder (n = 15) and essential hypertension (n = 20) were evaluated with the aid of a head-up tilt test (HUTT). The protocol of the HUTT was based on the 10-minute supine/30 minute head-up tilt test as previously described [41, 44]. Testing was conducted from 8:00 to 11:00 a.m., in a quiet environment, and at constant room temperature of 22-25° C. The patients maintained a regular meal schedule, but were restricted from smoking and caffeine ingestion for 6 hours prior to the examination. Intake of food products and medications with sympathomimetic activity prior to the study was prohibited. Manual BP readings were taken by a physician certified in the BP measurement technique according to American Heart Association recommendations [51]. We favored the mercury column sphygmomanometer (Bauman ometer, standby model 0661-0250), since this is the standard non-invasive method for BP measurement, and is the most accurate for evaluation of BP at rest [52, 53] and during HUTT [54, 55]. The HR measurements were recorded on an electrocardiographic monitor. The patient lay in a supine position on the tilt table, secured to the table at the chest, hips and knees with adhesive girdles. The cuff of the BP recording device was attached to the left arm, which was supported at heart level at all times during the study. Three measurements in the supine position were recorded at 5-minute intervals. The table was then gently tilted head-up to an angle of 70°. The duration of the tilt was 30 minutes. During the initial 5 minutes of tilt, measurements were obtained at one-minute intervals, followed by readings every 5 minutes. When dizziness or faintness occurred, repeated measurements were taken at 30-second intervals. In the event of a loss of consciousness the test was discontinued.

Parameters The 'BP-change' and 'HR-change' were computed.

a). Systolic and diastolic BP-changes were defined as the differences between individual BP values measured during HUTT and the last recumbent BP value, and divided by the last recumbent BP value. The result is BP change, expressed as a relative value by comparison to the last supine measurement, and calculated according to the following equation:

$$BP \text{ change} = BP_{(n1....n13)} - BP_{n3}/BP_{n3}). \qquad \text{Equation 1}$$

The averages and SD of the current values of the systolic and diastolic BP changes was calculated for each subject and labeled SYST-AVG.cur, DIAST-AVG.cur, SYST-SD.cur and DIAST SD.cur, respectively (Figure 1).

The BP changes were also represented graphically in time-curves (Figure 2). These figures were constructed in a fixed template on Microsoft Excel graphics. The frame measured 2 standard rectangles on the horizontal axis (72 pixels width each) and 12 rectangles on the vertical axis (21 pixels height each). The X-axis was calibrated from 1 to 13 representing the sequentially fixed measurements. The Y-axis was calibrated from 0 to 0.6 representing the amplitude of the BP change. The default of the time-curves was set such as to modify BP changes < 0.02 to be represented $= 0.02$, and BP changes > 0.6 to be represented $= 0.6$. The time-curves were depicted as continuous, thin, black lines on white background. Subsequently, the time-curves were loaded on the MS Windows Paintbrush program. The field size was 320 x 320 pixels. The original colors were inverted to white line on black background. The images were saved as 24-bit Bitmap image format. The images were loaded in the computerized image analyzer Benoit Version 1.3 (Trusoft Int'l, Inc, 1999, St. Petersburg, Florida). The time-curve's fractal dimension (FD) was automatically assessed by using the box counting method. FD represents a 'self-similarity' in dynamic behavior over multiple scales of time. FD is calculated:

$$FD = \log \text{ (number of self-similar pieces)} / \log \text{ (magnification factor)}$$

The side length of the largest box of the grid was 80 pixels. The coefficient of box size decrease was 1.3. The number of box sizes used was 17. The increment of grid rotation was 15 degrees. The length of the time-curve outlines was automatically measured. The outline ratio (OR) was calculated by dividing the length of the outline curve by the length of a straight line on the horizontal axis from intervals 1 to 13.

b). 'Absolute systolic and diastolic BP changes' were computed by transforming positive and negative BP changes into positive values. The relative values of BP changes were calculated as above. Subsequently, the average, SD, OR and FD of the absolute BP changes were calculated and labeled SYST-AVG.abs, SYST-SD.abs, SYST-OR.abs, SYST-FD.abs, DIAST-AVG.abs, DIAST-SD.abs, DIAST-OR.abs and DIAST-FD.abs.

c). 'Heart rate change' was defined as the difference between successive HR values and the last recumbent HR value, and divided by the last recumbent HR value:

$$\text{HR change} = HR_{(n1....n13)} - HR_{n3} / HR_{n3} \qquad\qquad \text{Equation 2}$$

The HR changes average, SD, OR and FD were calculated and labeled HR-AVG.cur, HR-SD.cur, HR-OR.cur, and HR-FD.cur.

d). Absolute HR changes were derived from the transformation of positive and negative HR change values into positive numbers. The absolute HR changes average, SD, OR and FD were calculated: HR-AVG.abs, HR-SD.abs, HR-OR.abs, HR-FD.abs.

Overall, 24 variables were defined and collectively called 'cardiovascular instability indices'. A multivariate analysis of all 24 parameters was conducted, evaluating independent predictors of CFS versus healthies. Results of multivariate analysis identified the best predictors for the assessment of CFS versus healthy to be SYST-FD.abs, SYST-SD.cur and HR-SD.cur. Based on the regression coefficients (slopes and intercept) of these predictors, a linear discriminant score was computed for each subject. This discriminant score was called 'hemodynamic instability score' (HIS).

$$HIS = 64.3303 + (SYST\text{-}FD.abs \times -68.0135) + (SYST\text{-}SD.cur \times 111.3726) \quad \text{Equation 3}$$
$$+ HR\text{-}SD.cur \times 60.4164$$

In this equation, SYST-FD.abs = the fractal dimension of absolute values of the systolic BP changes, SYST-SD.cur = the standard deviation of the current values of the systolic BP changes, and HR-SD.cur = the standard deviation of the current values of the heart rate changes. Group averages (SD) of HIS were: CFS = +3.72 (SD 5.02) and healthy = -4.62 (SD 2.26). The best cut-off differentiating CFS from healthy was HIS −0.98. HIS values >-0.98 was associated with CFS (sensitivity 97% specificity 96.6%).

A

	syst	diast	HR	syst.difs.cur	syst.difs.abs	HR.difs.cur
supine 1	122	70	52	0.109	0.109	0.106
supine 5	116	72	42	0.055	0.055	-0.106
supine10	110	70	47	0.000	0.002	0.000
tilt 1	94	76	82	-0.145	0.145	0.745
tilt 2	100	76	84	-0.091	0.091	0.787
tilt 3	102	74	84	-0.073	0.073	0.787
tilt 4	102	78	84	-0.073	0.073	0.787
tilt 5	102	76	82	-0.073	0.073	0.745
tilt 10	106	76	87	-0.036	0.036	0.851
tilt 15	106	78	88	-0.036	0.036	0.872
tilt 20	104	78	90	-0.055	0.055	0.915
tilt 25	100	76	89	-0.091	0.091	0.894
tilt 30	106	76	86	-0.036	0.036	0.830

B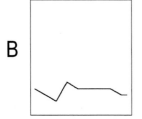

C	
SYST-SD.cur	0.062
HR-SD.cur	0.366
SYST-FD.cur	1.132
HIS	16.48

Figure 2. Processing the HIS (Reference 44, with permission). Systolic, diastolic BP, and HR values of a CFS patient, taken throughout the HUTT are represented in Figure 1A. From the measured values, the relative changes of BP and HR were calculated, according to the equation: BP difference = BP (n1....n13) - BP$_{n3}$/BP$_{n3}$. Absolute values were then obtained by converting all results to positive numbers. Shown in the table are systolic BP differences as current (c) and absolute (a) values, as well as HR differences in current values (c). The BP and HR changes were utilized to calculate the SYS-DIF-c-SD and HR-DIF-c-SD (Figure 1C), which are independent predictors of the HIS. The third independent predictor of HIS is the SYS-DIF-a-FD, and it was processed from the time-curve of the systolic BP differences (Figure 1B) by a fractal analysis program. Finally, the three independent predictors were applied to compute the HIS (Figure 1C). In this specific case, HIS +5.137 is typical for a CFS patient

**Table 1. HIS values in CFS compared with other groups of subjects
(From 44, with permission)**

Group (No Cases)	HIS avg (SD), 95% CI of avg	P value – CFS
CFS (n = 25)	+3.72 (5.02), +1.65 to +5.8	
Generalized anxiety disorder (n = 15)	+1.08 (5.2), -1.81 to +3.97	NS
Fibromyalgia (n = 25)	-3.27 (2.63), -4.14 to -2.41	<0.0001
Healthy (n = 37)	-4.62 (2.26), -5.37 to -3.86	<0.0001
Hypertension (n = 20)	-5.53 (2.24), -6.58 to -4.48	<0.0001

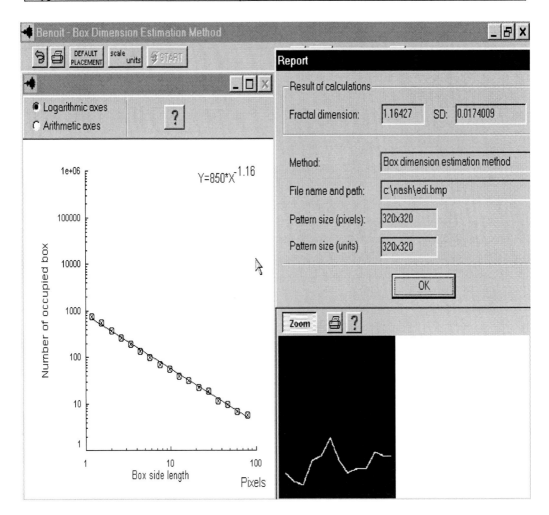

Figure 3. Computation of the fractal dimension of the heart rate by the box method method

With the aid of Equation 3, HIS values were calculated in the other groups (Table 1 and Figure 3). Comparison of HIS values showed significant differences (p < 0.0001) between CFS and healthy, hypertensives and FM groups, but not versus generalized anxiety disorder.

In a second study, the specificity of the proposed HIS threshold of -0.98 for CFS was evaluated comparing patients with CFS and non-CFS chronic fatigue and patients with recurrent syncope [45]. These groups were chosen for their clinical similarity to CFS and possible dysautonomic background. In this second study, the HIS threshold -0.98 differentiated between CFS patients (HIS = +2.02 (SD 4.07)) and healthy subjects (HIS = -2.48 (SD 4.07)) as well other groups. Subsequent studies confirmed thses observations [37, 46, 47]. The overall specificity of the HIS for the diagnosis of CFS was 85.1%.

Thus, in the appropriate clinical context, a HIS value greater than −0.98 is consistent with a diagnosis of CFS, providing certain confounding conditions are excluded. As a general rule, patients with any other medical or psychiatric illness should not be diagnosed with CFS [18]. In particular, patients with generalized anxiety disorder were found to have comparable HIS values to CFS patients. Pathologically elevated HIS may be expected to occur in cardiovascular deconditioning following prolonged bed rest or under zero-gravity [57, 58], in autonomic dysfunction associated with neurological or chronic inflammatory disorders [59, 60], or as result of drug effects on the autonomic nervous system, though no systematical studies have appraised the effects of any of these conditions on the HIS. From the clinician's point of view, differentiation of these disorders from CFS is usually simple. Overall, the potential utility of the HIS for diagnostic purposes can be assumed from the data presented in this study. The HIS can reinforce the clinician's diagnosis by providing objective criteria to the assessment of CFS, which until now, could only be subjectively inferred.

Distinguishing CFS from FM may be difficult on clinical grounds since FM shares many features with CFS [10, 11]. By applying the HIS methodology, dissimilar cardiovascular responses to postural challenge were observed in CFS (HIS = +3.72 (SD 5.02)) and FM (HIS = -3.25 (SD 2.63)) (p <0.0001) (44). This was again demoinstrated in another study: in CFS, HIS = +2.14(SD 4.67) and in FM HIS = -2.81(SD 2.62) [46]. The unique features to the CFS dysautonomia phenotype were not observed in FM patients, supporting the separation of FM from CFS in terms of autonomic nervous activity.

The 'Fractal and Recurrence Analysis-Based Score' (FRAS)

To further support the prospect of defining a characteristic dysautonomia in CFS patients, an additional technique was proposed to assess the cardiovascular reactivity during the HUTT.

The protocol of the tilt test and PTT (pulse transit time) recordings were also based on the 10-minute supine - 30 minute head-up tilt test as previously described (37). In a first study [48], patients with CFS (n=23), familial Mediterranean fever (n=15), psoriatic arthritis (n=10), generalized anxiety disorder (n=12), neurally mediated syncope (n=20), and healthy subjects (n=20) were evaluated. The patient lay in a supine position on the tilt table, secured to the table at the chest, hips and knees with adhesive girdles. The cuff of the BP recording device was attached to the left arm, which was supported at heart level at all times during the study. The right forearm and hand were supported by a cast, and suspended with a sling to the patient's neck. The fingers pointed to the mid-axillary line at the level of the fourth intercostal space. The photoelectric sensor of the photoplethysmograph (PPG) was placed on the distal phalanx of the second or third finger. The hand was held in a relaxed semi-open position, with the palm turned downward and fixed with adhesive strips, taking care not to apply pressure to the PPG transducer [48]. The electrocardiogram (ECG) and PPG were recorded on a Datex-Engstrom Cardiocap™ II instrument (Datex Instrumentation Corporation, Helsinki, Finland), connected to the Biopac MP 100 data acquisition system (Biopac,Santa Barbara, California). The PTT was automatically computed on the AcqKnowledge software, and the tracings were continuously displayed on the computer screen. The computer program identified the PTT as the time interval between the peak of the electrocardiographic R wave and the peak of the pressure wave at the finger, as measured by the pulse plethysmograph. A sample rate of 500 samples per second provided 1/500 Hz resolution for the HR and PTT measurements. Measurements were acquisitioned in the supine position over a 10-minute period. The table was then gently tilted head-up to an angle of 70° and the acquisition continued for a total of 600 cardiac cycles (usually 5 to 10 minutes).

Data processing The RR intervals on ECG recordings and the corresponding PTT values were automatically computed with the AcqKnowledge software. Four sets of values were obtained each comprising approximately 600 measurements – the HR supine, PTT supine, HR tilt, and PTT tilt. Later the measurements were reviewed and edited. For this purpose, the computer program signaled HR values less than 45 bpm or in excess of 110 bpm, and PTT values less than 0.2 sec or longer than 0.4 sec. For each of the aberrant measurements the investigator decided whether or not it was likely in the context of 30-40 contiguous measurements. PTT measurements less than 0.2 sec were considered to be artifacts, based on our experience that such values occurred only upon movement of the transducer. PTT values greater than 0.4 seconds were considered artifacts when occurring alone or as couples, but when clustering in series of 3 or more spikes the occurrence was considered to be authentic. Suspicious HR values were deleted together with the concomitant PTT measurements, and suspicious PTT values were deleted together with the concomitant HR measurements. After editing, the data were advanced to mathematical analysis.

Mathematical processing of data Three mathematical methods were applied: general statistics, recurrence plot analysis, and fractal analysis.

Fractal analysis: For fractal analysis, time series of 500-600 consecutive edited measurements, either HR or PTT, were loaded into the Benoit Version 1.3 analyzer (Trusoft Int'l, Inc, 1999, St. Petersburg, Florida). Time curves were constructed. The fractal dimension of the time curve (FD) was calculated with the aid of four different methods: R/S, roughness-length, variogram, and wavelets analysis. Typical tracings are shown in Figure 4.

Recurrence Quantitative Analysis (RQA): In our study, we utilized the Visual Recurrence Analysis computer program version 4.2 developed by Eugene Kononov, 1999. Recurrence plot analysis is a relatively new technique for the qualitative assessment of time series [42, 43]. Technically, this method expands a one-dimensional time series into a higher dimensional space. This is done by using a "delayed coordinate embedding", which creates a phase space portrait (recurrence plot) of the system. To start RQA calculations, 500-600 consecutive edited HR or PTT measurements were loaded in the computer program. The embedding dimension, time delay and false nearest neighbor were determined. On this basis, the RQA variables were computed: recurrence, determinism, ratio, entropy, maxline, trend, and spatio-temporal entropy. Figure 5 illustrates the recurrence plot of the HR in a patient with CFS. A 'structured pattern' is seen on gross. Besides the global impression given by the appearance of the recurrent plot, quantitative descriptors were developed and are included in the recurrence quantification analysis method (RQA). These are: recurrence, determinism, ratio, entropy, maxline, trend, and spatio-temporal entropy [42, 43]. Recurrence quantifies the percentage of the plot occupied by recurrent points. Determinism is the percentage of recurrent points that appear in sequence, forming diagonal line structures in the distance matrix. Entropy, measures the richness of deterministic structuring of the series. Trend is the regression coefficient of the relation between time and the amount of recurrence.

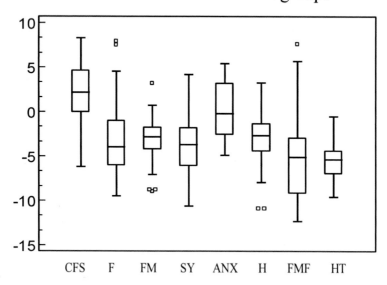

Figure 4. HIS values in different disorders (From 46, with permission). The HIS in CFS patients differs significantly from other patients groups, except for patients with anxiety disorder. CFS = chronic fatigue syndrome, F = non-CFS fatigue, FM = fibromyalgia, SY = neuraly mediated syncope, ANX = generalized anxiety disorder, H = healthy, FMF = familial Mediterranean fever, HT = essential hypertension

On collecting all computed variables derived by analysis of time series measurements, thirteen variables were obtained. By summarizing the four data sets in each patient, including HR and PTT in supine and tilt positions, a total of 52 variables of cardiovascular reactivity were obtained.

Study phases I and II Phase I of the study ('training phase') compared the data of CFS patients with data of a heterogenous control population. This data was tailored to differentiate the phenotype of cardiovascular reactivity in CFS patients versus a spectrum of other clinical entities, some with an exaggerated reactivity and others with a normal cardiovascular reactivity. For this purpose, in the control group patients with syncope and patients with FMF were included. Patients with recurrent syncope often have increased cardiovascular reactivity and may show overlapping features with CFS patients, while FMF patients usually have normal reactivity (Naschitz et al, personal communication).

Fractal dimension of the HR by different methods

R/S analysis   Roughness-Length

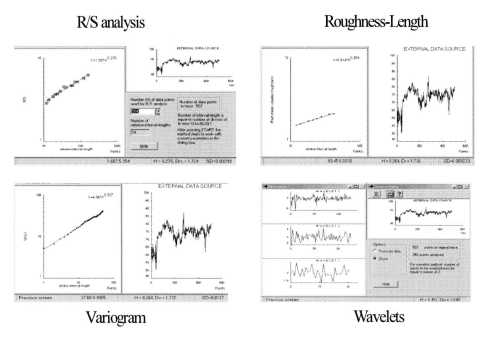

Variogram   Wavelets

Figure 5. Computation of the heart rate fractal dimension based on a time series of 500 continuous cardiac cycles (From 47, with permission).. Four different methods are implemented

In study phase I, means and SDs of all 52 cardiovascular reactivity variables were calculated and comparisons between the data of CFS patients and controls were performed. A multivariate analysis was conducted, evaluating independent predictors of CFS. Based on the regression coefficients (slopes and intercept) of these predictors, a linear discriminant score was computed for each subject. This discriminant score was called 'Fractal and Recurrence Analysis-based Score' (FRAS). The best cut-off between the FRAS of patients and controls was established. In CFS patients and the mixed control group including patients with neurally mediated syncope and patients with FMF, the average and SD of the 52 variables of cardiovascular reactivity were calculated and group comparisons were performed. On univariate analysis, 13 variables showed significant differences between CFS and controls. These included 6 fractal parameters, 5 RQA parameters and 2 parameters derived from summary statistic analysis.

The multivariate model identified the best predictors for the assessment of CFS versus mixed control patients to be: 1. HR on tilt - fractal dimension by roughness-length analysis (HR-tilt-R/L) (p = 0.0063), 2. PTT on tilt - fractal dimension by roughness-length analysis (PTT-tilt-R/L) (p = 0.0035), 3. HR supine – determinism on recurrence quantification analysis (HR-supine-DET) (p = 0.0009), 4. PTT on tilt - fractal dimension by wavelets analysis (PTT-tilt-WAVE) (p = 0.0003), and 5. HR on tilt standard deviation (HR-tilt-SD) (p = 0.0001). Based on the regression coefficients (slopes and intercept) of these predictors, a linear discriminant score was computed for each subject, called FRAS.

FRAS = 76.2 + 0.04*HR-supine-DET − 12.9*HR-tilt-R/L −   Equation 1
0.31*HR-tilt-SD - 19.27*PTT-tilt-R/L − 9.42* PTT-tilt-WAVE

The best cut-off differentiating CFS from the control population was FRAS = +0.22.

With the aid of Equation 1, FRAS values were calculated in study phase II in the other patient groups. Comparison of FRAS values in CFS patients and in the other groups showed significant differences compared to healthy subjects (p <0.0001), FMF patients (p <0.0001), psoriatic arthritis (0.03), syncope (p <0.0001), but not between CFS and generalized anxiety disorder. FRAS >0.22 was associated with CFS (sensitivity 70% and specificity 88%). A subsequent study [48] confirmed these observations.

Recurrence Quantitative Analysis of the HR

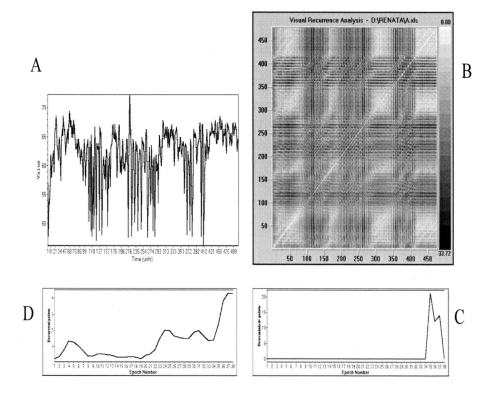

Figure 6. Steps in processing the heart rate recurrence plot (From 47, with permission). Time series of the HR are displayed in A. The visual recurrence plot in shown in B, recurrence points in C, and deterministic points in D

Based on the method of the FRAS we conducted a study to evaluate cardiovascular reactivity in fibromyalgia [50]. The study group included 30 women with FM, average age of 46.7 years (SD 7.03). An age matched group of 30 women with other rheumatic disorders or having a dysautonomic background - chronic fatigue syndrome (CFS), non-CFS fatigue, neurally mediated syncope and psoriatic arthritis − served as controls. Variables acting as independent predictors of the cardiovascular reactivity in FM patients versus the comparison group were identified. By univariate analysis comparing variables of the cardiovascular reactivity in FM patients against control patients, no statistically significant differences were found between the groups. This is illustrated in Figure 6 by the fractal dimensions of the heart rate in FM vs. controls.

Thus, study of the cardiovascular reactivity utilizing a head-up tilt test and processing the data with the method of the 'Fractal and Recurrence Analysis Score' did not reveal a specific, FM-associated abnormality. These data confirmed prior studies that utilized a variety of other methodologies and reached similar conclusions. FM patients represent a heterogenic group with respect to their pattern of cardiovascular reactivity. These findings appear consistent with the concept that fibromyalgia is a common symptomatic framework, rather than a separate disease entity [2, 3], and therefore patients' cardiovascular reactivity patterns are accordingly, heterogenic. Thus, a distinctive cardiovascular reactivity was identified in CFS patients but not in FM.

Mechanisms Involved in Disease-Related Cardiovascular Reactivity Patterns

The mechanisms putatively involved in disease-related cardiovascular reactivity patterns may be speculated upon. The conventional understanding that cardiovascular reactivity is merely the result of arterial baroreflexes is simplistic and no longer tenable. Indeed, numerous factors modulate the response to baroreflex activation apart from strength of the activating stimulus. These include the set point of the reflex, neuronal input from hypothalamus, cortical centers, brainstem centers, the responsiveness of cardiovascular receptors and structures, interactions of aortocarotid with chemoreflex arcs, as well as modulatory influences of neuro-humoral and vasoactive substances [60-66]. Serotonin, adenosine and opioids are additional triggers of the Betzold-Jarisch reflex; peripheral sympathetic afferents are directly activated by circulating mediators; and higher nervous centers modulate the cardiovascular reflexes. Disease-specific cardiovascular reactivity patterns may be explained by the existence of unique permutations in the cardiovascular, neuro-endocrine and paracrine changes present in certain disorders.

In applying the FRAS to the study of cardiovascular reactivity in healthy subjects, no specific reactivity pattern was observed [49]. We speculate that CVR in healthy individuals is heterogenic, not modulated by a specific pathologic mechanism into uniformity. The present study conducted in patients with FM did not disclose a specific CVR pattern. These findings appear consistent with the concept that fibromyalgia is a common symptomatic framework, rather than a separate disease entity [2, 3, 67], and therefore patients' cardiovascular reactivity patterns are, accordingly, heterogenic.

Shortened Electrocardiographic QT Interval

It is known that QT interval on the electrocardiogram is influenced among others by autonomic nervous function. Since a specificity of cardiovascular reactivity, as an expression of autonomic dysfunction, had been noted in CFS, it was elected to examine the QT interval in this disorder as well.

The QT interval on the surface electrocardiogram (ECG) reflects depolarization and repolarization of myocardial cells. A variety of factors may influence the QT interval, including heart rate, genetic abnormalities of the potassium channel, electrolyte disturbances, myocardial ischemia, drugs, and sympathetic and parasympathetic tone [68-72]. Changes in autonomic tone may condition the QT interval directly by altering repolarization kinetics of myocardial cells through influences on ion currents or indirectly by modulating the heart rate (HR)[68]. The effects of the autonomic nervous system on the QT interval have been studied in patients with combined sympathetic and parasympathetic failure, such are patients with idiopathic pure autonomic failure, familial dysautonomia, multiple system atrophy and Parkinson's disease as well as patients with diabetic autonomic neuropathy and chronic liver disease [73-75]. The above conditions often are associated with abnormally prolonged QT intervals. In contrast, patients with isolated sympathetic failure, such as subjects with congenital deficiency of dopamine-beta-hydroxylase, have a normal duration of the QT interval [73].

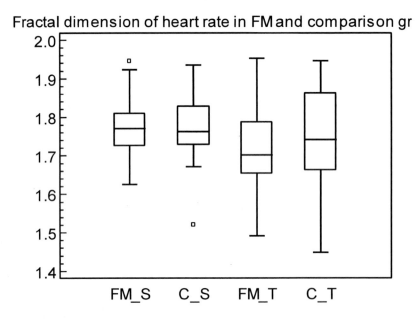

Figure 7. Fractal analysis of the heart rate in FM vs. control patients (From 50, with permission). The fractal dimensions in both groups are similar

We examined whether the corrected QT interval (QTc) in CFS differs from QTc in other populations [76]. On search of the literature no previous publications on QT interval in patients with CFS were found. The QTc was calculated at the end of 10 minutes of recumbence and the end of 10 minutes of head-up tilt. In a pilot study, groups of 15 subjects, CFS and controls matched for age and gender, were investigated. In a second phase of the study, the QTc was measured in larger groups of CFS (n=30) and control patients (n=96), not matched for demographic features. In the pilot study, the average supine QTc in CFS was

0.371 ± 0.02 sec and QTc on tilt 0.385 ± 0.02 sec, significantly shorter than in controls (p = 0.0002 and 0.0003, respectively). Results of phase II confirmed this data (Figure 7). Thus, relative short QTc intervals are features of the CFS-related dysautonomia.

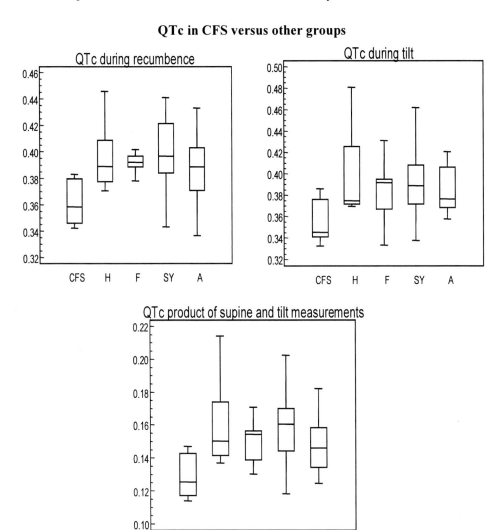

Figure 8. QTc values in five groups matched for age and gender (From 46, with permission). QTc in CFS differs significantly from QTc in each control group. CFS = chronic fatigue syndrome, H = healthy subjects, F = non-CFS fatigue, SY = neurally mediated syncope, A = psoriatic arthritis. The boxes contain the 50% of values falling between the 25th and 75th percentiles, the horizontal line within the box represents the median value, and the "whiskers" are the lines that extend from the box to the highest and lowest values, excluding the outliers

In a follow-up study, we evaluated whether FM and CFS can be distinguished by QTc (Naschitz et al, personal communication). The study groups were comprised of women with FM (n = 30) and with CFS (n = 28). The patients were evaluated with a 10 minute supine-30 minute head-up tilt test. The electrocardiographic QT interval was corrected for heart rate (HR) according to Fridericia's equation (QTc). In addition, cardiovascular reactivity was assessed based on blood pressure and HR changes and was expressed as the 'hemodynamic instability score' (HIS)(Figure 8).

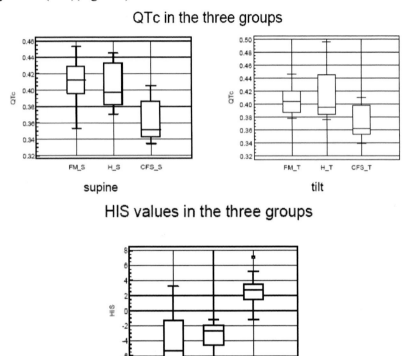

Figure 9. QTc in FM vs. CFS. The QTc in CFS differs significantly from QTc in FM. FM_S = fibromyalgia patient measurements at the end of the supine phase, CFS_S = CFS patient measurements at the end of the supine phase; FM_T = FM patient measurements at 10 minutes of tilt; CFS_T = CFS patient measurements at 10 minutes of tilt. The boxes contain the 50% of values falling between the 25th and 75th percentiles; the horizontal line within the box represents the median value; the 'whiskers' are the lines that extend from the box to the highest and lowest values excluding the outliers

The average supine QTc in FM was 0.417 ± 0.025 sec versus 0.372 ± 0.022 sec in CFS (p <0.0001); the supine QTc cut-off <0.385.7 sec was 79% sensitive and 87% specific for CFS vs. FM. The average QTc at the 10th minute of tilt was 0.409 ± 0.018 sec in FM versus 0.367 ± 0.021 in CFS (p <0.0001); the tilt QTc cut-off <383.3 msec was 71% sensitive and 91% specific for CFS vs. FM. In this study, the average HIS in FM patients was -3.52 ± 1.96 vs. +3.21 ± 2.43 in CFS (p <0.0001). Thus, the QTc and HIS were within the normal range in the large majority of FM patients. In contrast, a short QTc interval and increased HIS characterized CFS patients.

Combined evaluation of the cardiovascular reactivity and cardiac depolarisation-repolarisation may provide objective measures distinguishing between FM and CFS. Both HIS and QTc are influenced by autonomic nervous activity. Thus, an alteration in autonomic function which is operative in CFS but not in FM may explain the differences in QTc and

HIS. The mechanisms underlying the relatively short QTc in CFS have not been investigated. Prior studies in CFS, based on spectral analysis of HR and BP, showed that the vagal tone is reduced in these patients [78, 79]. Decreased vagal tone may provide the mechanism for QTc shortening in CFS; however, it should be noted that not all studies have confirmed that vagal tone is diminished in CFS [80].

Conclusion

The pathogenesis of FM is elusive. An important step in furthering the understanding of FM is to separate it from other similar and overlapping functional somatic syndromes, particularly CFS. To this end, we proceded by evaluating dysautonomia in CFS especially in terms of cardiovascular reactivity. A specific cardiovascular reactivity pattern was defined in CFS utilizing both the HIS and FRAS methodologies. Thereafter, a unique finding of the electrocardiographic QTc interval in CFS was established. Subsequently, the above described methodologies were applied to FM in direct comparison to CFS. Our findings of a relatively short QTc interval and positive HIS as features of CFS-related dysautonomia were not present in the large majority of FM patients. These data support the contention that FM and CFS are distinct disorders.

References

[1]   Wolfe, F; Smythe, A; Yunus, MB; Bennett, RM; Bombardier, C; Goldenberg, DL. et al. The American College of Rheumatology 1990 criteria for the classification of fibromyalgia: Report of the Multicenter Criteria Committee. *Arthritis Rheum* 1990, 33, 160-172.

[2]   Rau, CL; Russell, IJ. Is fibromyalgia a distinct clinical syndrome? *Curr Rev Pain* 2000, 4, 287-294.

[3]   Hadler, NM. Fibromyalgia: La maladie est morte. Vive le malade. *J Rheumatol* 1997, 24, 1250 - 1251.

[4]   Buskila, D; Neumann, L. Fibromyalgia syndrome (FM) and nonarticular tenderness in relatives of patients with FM. *J Rheumatol* 1997, 24, 941– 944.

[5]   Martinez-Lavin, M; Hermosillo, AG; Rosas, M; Soto, ME. Circadian studies of autonomic nervous balance in patients with fibromyalgia: a heart rate variability analysis. *Arthritis Rheum.* 1998, 42, 1966 –1971.

[6]   Martinez-Lavin, M; Hermosillo, AG; Mendoza, C. Orthostatic sympathetic derangement in subjects with fibromyalgia. *J Rheumatol.* 1997, 24, 714 –718.

[7]   Bou-Holaigah, I; Calkins, H; Flynn, JA. Provocation of hypotension and pain during upright tilt table testing in adults with fibromyalgia. *Clin Exp Rheumatol.* 1997, 15, 239 -246.

[8]   Kelemen, J; Lang, E; Balint, G. Orthostatic sympathetic derangement of baroreflex in patients with fibromyalgia. *J Rheumatol.* 1998, 25, 823– 825.

[9]   Raj, RR; Brouillard, D; Simpson, CS. Dysautonomia among patients with fibromyalgia: a noninasive assessment. *J Rheumatol.* 2000, 27, 2660 –2665.

[10]   Cohen, H; Neumann, L; Shore, M. Autonomic dysfunction in patients with fibromyalgia: application of power spectral analysis of heart rate variability. *Semin Arthritis Rheum.* 2000, 29, 217–227.

[11]   Martinez-Lavin, M; Hermosillo, AG. Autonomic nervous system dysfunction may explain the multisystem features of fibromyalgia. *Semin Arthritis Rheum.* 2000, 29, 197–199.

[12]   Martinez-Lavin, M. Fibromyalgia as a sympathetically maintained pain syndrome. *Curr Headache Pain Rep.* 2004, 5, 385–389.

[13]   Ulas, UH; Unlu, E. Hamamcioglu K; Odabasi Z; Cakci A; Vural O. Dysautonomia in fibromyalgia syndrome: sympathetic skin responses and RR Interval analysis. *Rheumatol Int.* 2005 Jun 30, 1-5.

[14]   Ciccone, DS; Natelson, BH. Comorbid illness in women with chronic fatigue syndrome: a test of the single syndrome hypothesis. *Psychosom Med.* 2003, 65, 268-275.

[15]   Wessely, S; Chalder, T; Hirsch, S; Wallace, P; Wright, D. Psychological symptoms, somatic symptoms; and psychiatric disorder in chronic fatigue and chronic fatigue syndrome: a prospective study in the primary care setting. *Am J Psychiatry* 1996; 153; 1050–1059.

[16]   Aaron, LA; Burke, MM; Buchwald, D. Overlapping conditions among patients with chronic fatigue syndrome, fibromyalgia and temporomandibular disorder. *Arch Intern Med.* 2000, 160, 221-227.

[17]   Martinez-Lavin, M; Hermosillo, AG. Dysautonomia in Gulf War syndrome and in fibromyalgia. *Am J Med.* 2005, 118, 446.

[18]   Fukuda, K; Straus, SE; Mickie, I. The chronic fatigue syndrome: a comprehensive approach to its definition and study. International Study Group. *Ann Intern Med* 1994, 121, 953-9.

[19]   Rowe, PC; Bou-Holaigah, I; Kan, JS. Is neurally mediated hypotension an unrecognized cause of chronic fatigue? *Lancet* 1995, 345, 623-4.

[20]   Bou-Holaigah, I; Rowe, PC; Kan, J; Calkins, H. The relationship between neurally mediated hypotension and the chronic fatigue syndrome. *JAMA* 1995, 274, 961-967.

[21]   Montague, TJ; Marrie, TJ; Klassen, GA; Bewick, DJ; Horacek, BM. Cardiac function at rest and with exercise in chronic fatigue syndrome. *Chest* 1989, 95, 779-784.

[22]   Freeman, R; Komaroff, AL. Does the chronic fatigue syndrome involve the autonomic nervous system? *Am J Med* 1997, 102, 357-64.

[23]   Evengard, B; Schachterle, RS; Komaroff, AL. Chronic fatigue syndrome: new insights and old ignorance. *J Internal Med* 1999, 246, 455-469.

[24]   Rowe, PC; Bou-Holaigah, I; Kan, JS. Is neurally mediated hypotension an unrecognized cause of chronic fatigue? *Lancet* 1995, 345, 623-4.

[25]   Bou-Holaigah, I; Rowe, PC; Kan, J; Calkins, H. The relationship between neurally mediated hypotension and the chronic fatigue syndrome. *JAMA* 1995, 274, 961-7.

[26]   Freeman, R; Komaroff, AL. Does the chronic fatigue syndrome involve the autonomic nervous system? *Am J Med* 1997, 102, 357-64.

[27]   Schondorf, R; Freeman, R. The importance of orthostatic intolerance in the chronic fatigue syndrome. *Am J Med Sci* 1999, 317, 117-123.

[28] DeLorenzo, F; Hargraves, J; Kakkar, VV. Possible relationship between chronic fatigue and postural tachycardia syndromes. *Clin Autonom Res* 1996, 6, 263-4.

[29] Natelson, BH; Cohen, JM; Brassloff, I; Lee, HJ. A controlled study of brain magnetic resonance imaging in patients with the chronic fatigue syndrome. *J Neurol Sci* 1993, 120, 213-217.

[30] Costa, DC; Tannock, C; Brostoff, J. Brainstem perfusion is impaired in chronic fatigue syndrome. *Q J Med* 1995, 88, 767-773.

[31] Demitrack, MA; Dale, JK; Straus, SE; Laue, L; Listwak, SJ; Kruesi, MJ; Chrousos GP; Gold PW. Evidence for impaired activation of the hypothalamic-pituitary axis in patients with the chronic fatigue syndrome. *J Clin Endocrinol Metab* 1991, 73, 1224-1234.

[32] Cleare, AJ; Bearn, J; Allain, T; McGregor, A; Wessely, S; Murray, RM; O'Keane V. Contrasting neuroendocrine responses in depression and chronic fatigue syndrome. *J Affect Disord* 1995, 35, 283-289.

[33] Streeten, DH; Anderson, GH Jr. The role of delayed orthostatic hypotension in the pathogenesis of chronic fatigue. *Clin Auton Res* 1998, 8, 119-124.

[34] Naschitz, J; Dreyfuss, D; Yeshurun, D; Rosner, I. Midodrine treatment for chronic fatigue syndrome. *Postgrad Med J.* 2004, 80, 230-232.

[35] Fealey, RD; Robertson, D. Management of orthostatic hypotension. In: PL Low: Clinical autonomic disorders. *Evaluation and Management.* Second Edition. Lippincott - Raven Publishers, Philadelphia 1997, 763-775.

[36] Bou-Holaigah, I; Calkins, H; Flynn, JA; Tunin, C; Chang, HC; Kan, JS. Provocation of hypotension and pain during upright tilt table testing in adults with fibromyalgia. *Clin Exp Rheumatol* 1997, 15, 239-246.

[37] Naschitz, JE; Rozenbaum, M; Rosner, I; Sabo, E; Musafia-Priselac, R; Shaviv, N; Ahdoot, A; Ahdoot, M; Gaitini, L; Eldar, S; Yeshurun, D. Cardiovascular response to upright tilt in fibromyalgia differs from that in chronic fatigue syndrome. *J Rheumatol* 2001, 28, 1356-1360.

[38] Wieling. W; Karemaker. JM. Measurement of heart rate and blood pressure to evaluate disturbances in neurocardiovascular control. In: Ch. J. Mathias: *Autonomic failure. A textbook of clinical disorders of the autonomic nervous system.* Fourth edition. Oxford Univeristy Press, 1999:198-210.

[39] Iyengar. N; Peng. CK; Morin. R; Goldberger. AL; Lipsitz. LA. Age-related alterations of the fractal scaling of cardiac interbeat interval dynamics. *Am J Physiol* 1996, 271:R1078-1084.

[40] Parati. G; DiRienzo. M; Omboni. S; Mancia. G. Computer analysis of blood pressure and heart rate variability in subjects with normal and abnormal autonomic cardiovascular control. In: Matias CJ; Bannister R; *Autonomic failure. A textbook of clinical disorders of the autonomic nervous system.* Fourth edition, Oxford Univervity Press, 1999:211-223.

[41] Naschitz. JE; Sabo. E; Gaitini. L; Ahdoot. A. The hemodynamic instability score (HIS) for assessment of cardiovascular reactivity in hypertensive and normotensive patients. *J Human Hypertension* 2001, 15, 177-184.

[42] Eckman, JP; Kamphorts, SO; Ruelle, R. Recurrence plots of dynamical systems. *Europhys Lett* 1987; 4, 973-977.

[43] Manetti, C; Ceruso, MA; Giuliani, A; Webber, CL; Zbilut, JP. Recurrence quantification analysis in molecular dynamics. *Ann New York Acad Sci* 1999, 879, 258-266.

[44] Naschitz, JE; Sabo, E; Naschitz, S. Hemodynamic instability in chronic fatigue syndrome: indices and diagnostic significance. *Semin Arthritis Rheum*, 2001, 31, 199-208.

[45] Naschitz, JE; Sabo, E; Naschitz, S. Hemodynamic Instability Score in Chronic Fatigue Syndrome (CFS) and non-CFS Chronic Fatigue. *Semin Arthritis Rheum*, 2002, 32, 141-148.

[46] Naschitz, JE; Rosner, I; Rozenbaum, M. The head-up tilt test with hemodynamic instability score in diagnosing chronic fatigue syndrome. *Quat J Med* 2003, 96, 133-142.

[47] Naschitz, JE; Sabo, E; Dreyfuss, D; Yeshurun, D; Rosner, I. The head-up tilt test in the diagnosis and management of chronic fatigue syndrome. *Isr Med Assoc J.* 2003, 5, 807-811.

[48] Naschitz, JE; Sabo, E; Naschitz, S. Fractal Analysis and Recurrence Quantification Analysis of Heart Rate and Pulse Transit Time for Diagnosing Chronic Fatigue Syndrome. *Clin Autonomic Res* 2002, 12, 262-274.

[49] Naschitz, JE; Rosner, I; Rozenbaum, M; Fields, M; Isseroff, H; Babich, JP; Zuckerman, E; Elias, N; Yeshurun, D; Naschitz, S; Sabo, E. Disease-related phenotypes of cardiovascular reactivity as assessed by fractal and recurrence quantitative analysis of the heart rate and pulse transit time. *Q J Med*, 2004, 97, 141-151.

[50] Naschitz, JE; Rozenbaum, M; Fields, MC; Enis, S; Manor, H; Dreyfuss, D; Peck, S; Peck, ER; Babich, JP; Mintz, EP; Sabo, E; Slobodin, G; Rosner, I. Cardiovascular reactivity in fibromyalgia, evidence for pathogenic heterogeneity. *J Rheumatol.* 2005 32, 335-339.

[51] Training and certification of blood pressure observers. *Hypertension* 1983, 5, 610-614.

[52] O'Brien, E; Petrie, J; Littler, WA; de Swiet, M; Padfield, PL; O'Malley, K; Jamieson, M; Altman, D; Bland, M; Atkins, N. British hypertension protocol: evaluation of automated and semi-automated blood pressure measuring devices with special reference to ambulatory systems. *J Hypertens* 1990, 8, 607-619.

[53] Shuler, C; Allison, N; Holcomb, S; Harlan, M; McNeill, J; Robinett, G; Bagby, SP. Accuracy of an automated blood pressure device in stable inpatients. *Arch Intern Med*,1998, 158, 714-721.

[54] Naschitz, JE; Gaitini, L; Lowenstein, L; Keren, D; Tamir, A; Yeshurun, D. Rapid estimation of automatic blood pressure measuring devices (READ). *J Human Hypertension* 1999, 13, 443-447.

[55] Naschitz, JE; Gaitini, L; Lowenstein, L; Keren, D; Tamir, A; Yeshurun, D. In field validation of automatic blood pressure measuring devices. *J Human Hypertension*, 2000, 14, 37-42.

[56] Pavy-Le Traon, A; Sigaudo, D; Vasseur, P; Fortat, JO; Guell, A; Hughes, RL; Gharib, C. Orthostatic tests after a 4-day confinement or simulated weightlessness. *Clin Physiol* 1997, 17, 41-55.

[57] Robertson, D; Convertino, VA; Vernikos, J. The sympathetic nervous system and the physiologic consequences of spaceflight: a hypothesis. *Am J Med Sci* 1994, 308, 126-132.

[58] Toussirot, E; Bahjaoui-Bouhaddi, M; Poncet, JC; Cappelle, S; Henriet, MT; Wendling, D; Regnard, J. Abnormal autonomic cardiovascular control in ankylosing spondylitis. *Ann Rheum Dis* 1999, 58, 481-487.

[59] Schluederberg, A; Straus, SE; Peterson, P. Chronic fatigue syndrome research. Definition and medical outcome assessment. *Ann Intern Med* 1992, 117, 325-331.

[60] Dampney, RA; Coleman, MJ; Fontes, MA; Hirooka, Y; Horiuchi, J; Li, YW; Polson, JW; Potts, PD; Tagawa, T. Central mechanisms underlying short- and long-term regulation of the cardiovascular system. *Clin Exp Pharmacol Physiol.* 2002 , 29, 261-268.

[61] Di Girolano, E; Di Iorno, C; Sabatini, P; Leonzio, L; Barbone, C; Barsotti, A. Effects of paroxetine hydrochloride, a selective serotonin reuptake inhibitor, on refractory vasovagal syncope. A randomized double blind placebo-controlled study. *J Am Coll Cardiol* 1999, 33, 1227-1230.

[62] Shen, WK; Hammil, SC; Munger, TM; Stanton, MS; Packer, DL; Osboren, MJ. Adenosine: potential modulator for vasovagal syncope. *J Am Coll Cardiol* 1996, 28, 146-154.

[63] Barraco, RA; Janusz, CJ; Polasek, PM; Parizon, M; Roberts, PA; Cardiovascular effects of microinjection of adenosine into the nucleus tractus solitarius. *Brain Res Bull* 1988, 20, 129-132.

[64] Smith, OA; DeVito, JL. Central nervous integration for the control of autonomic responses associated with emotion. *Annu Rev Neurosci* 1984, 7, 43-65.

[65] Mercader, MA; Varghese, PJ; Potolicchio, SJ; Venkatraman, GK; Lee, SW. New insights into the mechanism of neurally mediated syncope. *Heart* 2002, 88, 217-221.

[66] Imrich, R. The role of neuroendocrine system in the pathogenesis of rheumatic diseases (minireview). *Endocrine Regulations* 2002, 36, 95-106.

[67] Russell, IJ. Is fibromyalgia a distinct clinical entity? The clinical investigator's evidence. *Baillieres Best Pract Res Clin Rheumatol* 1999, 13, 445-454.

[68] Rautaharju, PM; Warren, JW; Calhoun, HP. Estimation of QT prolongation. A persistent, avoidable error in computer electrocardiography. *J Electrocardiol* 1990, 23 Suppl, 111-117.

[69] Ewing, DJ; Nellson, JM. QT interval length and diabetic autonomic neuropathy. *Diabet Med* 1990, 7, 23-26.

[70] Wang Q; Curran, ME; Splawski, I; Burn, TC; Millholland, JM; Van Raay, TJ;. Positional cloning of a novel potassium channel gene: KVLQT1 mutations cause cardiac arrhythmias. *Nature Genetics* 1996, 12, 17-23.

[71] Milne, JR; Camm, AT; Ward, DE; Spurrll, RA. Effect of intravenous propranolol on QT interval: a new method of assessment. *Br Heart J* 1980, 43, 1-6.

[72] Browne, KF; Zipes, DP; Heger, JJ; Prystowsky, EN. Influence of the autonomous nervous system on the QT interval in man. *Am J Cardiol* 1982, 50, 1099-1103.

[73] Choy, AMJ; Lang, CJ; Roden, DM; Robertson, D; Wood, AJJ; Robertson, RM; Biaggioni, I. Abnormalities of the QT in primary disorders of autonomic failure. *Am Heart J* 1998, 136, 664-671.

[74] Deguchi, K; Sasaki, I; Tsukaguchi, M; Kamoda, M; Touge, T; Takeuchi, H; Kuriyama, S. Abnormalities of rate-corrected QT intervals in Parkinson's disease – a comparison with multiple system atrophy and progressive supranuclear palsy. *J Neurol Sci* 2002, 199, 31-37.

[75] Suys, BE; Huybrechts, SJ; De Wolf, D; Op De Beeck, L; Matthys, D; Van Overmeire, B; Du Caju, MV; Rooman, RP. QTc interval prolongation and QTc dispersion in children and adolescents with type 1 diabetes. *J Pediatr* 2002, 141, 59-63.

[76] Naschitz, JE; Fields, M; Isseroff, H; Sharif, D; Sabo, E; Rosner, I. Shortened, QT. interval: a distinctive feature of the dysautonomia of chronic fatigue syndrome. *J Electrocardiology*, in press.

[77] Somberg, JC; Molnar, J. Usefulness of QT dispersion as an electrocardiographically derived index. *Am J Cardiol* 2002, 89, 291-294.

[78] Suys, BE; Huybrechts, SJ; De Wolf, D; Op De Beeck, L; Matthys, D; Van Overmeire, B; Du Caju, MV; Rooman, RP. QTc interval prolongation and QTc dispersion in children and adolescents with type 1 diabetes. *J Pediatr* 2002, 141, 59-63.

[79] Cordero, DL; Sisto, SA; Tapp, WN; LaManca, JJ; Pareja, JG; Natelson, BH. Decreased vagal power during treadmill walking in patients with chronic fatigue syndrome. *Clin Auton Res* 1996 Dec, 6(6), 329-33

[80] Duprez, DA; De Buyzere, ML; Drieghe, B; Vanhaverbeke, F; Taes Y; Michielsen, W; Clement, DL. Long- and short-term blood pressure and RR-interval variability and psychosomatic distress in chronic fatigue syndrome. *Clin Sci* (Lond) 1998, 94, 57-63.

In: Chronic Fatigue Syndrome: Symptoms, Causes & Prevention   ISBN: 978-1-60741-493-3
Editor: E. Svoboda and K. Zelenjcik, pp. 167-173   © 2010 Nova Science Publishers, Inc.

Chapter 8

The Burden of Chronic Fatigue Syndrome (CFS) in Canada

Frank Mo,[*1,2]*, Heidi Liepold*[1]*, Michelle Bishop*[1]*,
Lianne Vardy*[1] *and Howard Morrison*[1]

[1]Division for Chronic Disease Management, Centre for Chronic Disease
Prevention and Control, Public Health Agency of Canada
[2]The R Samuel McLaughlin Centre, Institute of Population Health,
University of Ottawa, Ottawa, Canada

Abstract

Chronic fatigue syndrome (CFS) poses many socioeconomic, psychosocial, disability and quality of life difficulties for people with CFS in Canada. The self-reported prevalence of CFS was 0.78%, 1.22% and about 201,900, 331,500 Canadians have reported having CFS in 2000 and 2005 respectively. Canadians aged 40-64 years old (57.87% in 2000, and 58.59% in 2005) were the most frequently infected. More female Canadians (71.41% in 2000, and 68.44% in 2005) were affected than males (28.59% and 31.56%). Both physical and mental fatigue caused by CFS cost the Canadian economy an estimated $3.5 billion per year, and the annual lost productivity in Canada is estimated at $2.5 billion in 2003. However, the capacity in Canada for prevention and management of CFS is limited. Currently, there are only few medical doctors using the Clinical Working Case Definition, diagnostic and treatment protocols. Therefore, we need more research in the surveillance, diagnosis, treatment, and evaluation of CFS management in Canada.

Keywords: Chronic fatigue syndrome, lifestyle, socioeconomic status, burden, disability, CCHS, Canada.

* **Correspondence:** Frank Mo, MD, PhD, Medical Research Scientist, Chronic Disease Management Division, Centre for Chronic Disease Prevention and Control, Health Promotion and Chronic Disease Prevention Branch, Public Health Agency of Canada, 785 Carling Avenue, Ottawa, Ontario K1A 0K9, Canada. Tel: 613-946-2616; Fax: 613-954-8631; E-mail: frank_mo@phac-aspc.gc.ca

Introduction

Chronic fatigue syndrome (CFS) is an illness, which is characterized by long term debilitating fatigue that lasts for more than six months. Patients experience a substantial reduction in their ability to participate in occupational, socially or physically demanding activities. Patients with CFS do not recover from their fatigue with rest (1). CFS is prevalent in the Canadian community and it is costly to the health care system. Without treatment, the symptom of CFS worsens with time. Its causes are not fully understood; however, multiple risk factors have been suggested to influence the occurrence, some of the factors include over 40 years of age, being female, having a sedentary or unhealthy lifestyle. The capacity in Canada to accurately monitor and forecast trends or evaluate the effects of interventions is evidently limited (2). At present Canada does not have a CFS surveillance system. For this reason, this nation is not able to accurately measure the potential associations of this syndrome's prevalence, incidence, hospitalization, disability, mortality and economic burden.

Many individuals who suffer from CFS experience financial hardship and psychosocial problems, which reduces their quality of life. The self-reported prevalence of CFS in Canada increased from 0.78% in 2000 (201,940), to 1.22% in 2005 (331,530 cases) (3). Canadians aged 40 years and over were the most frequently affected with CFS compared to other age groups. More females reported having CFS than males. A recent study from the United Kingdom estimated the cost of CFS at 3.46 billion pounds per year. To crudely convert to Canadian dollars and adjust for size of this nation's economy (just under half of the British one) and currency exchange (just over double), the physical and mental fatigue caused by CFS cost the Canadian economy would be about $3.5 billion per year, and the annual lost productivity in Canada due to CFS is estimated at $2.5 billion in 2003 (4). The second study was done through the Center for Disease Control and Prevention in the US. It focuses on calculation of the loss of productivity of just over $20,000 US dollars per CFS patient each year, and there is in total a productivity loss of $9.1 billion US, which has been converted to the Canadian context (adjusting for GDP and exchange rates). This would be about $1 billion in Canadian economic loss (5). However, the capacity in Canada to prevent and manage CFS is limited. Currently, there are few medical doctors working on the clinical case definition, diagnostic and treatment protocols, and research. Furthermore, there is no gold standard laboratory or a specific diagnostic test available in Canada. Presently, there is no consensus among Canadian doctors as to the clinical definition of CFS. Medical training program related to the syndrome do not exist. Furthermore, there is no financial support for research projects relating to CFS (6). Therefore, we need more research in the surveillance, diagnosis, treatment, and evaluation of CFS management in Canada.

Risk factors and diagnosis

The causes of CFS remain unknown. Clinicians have proposed one or more risk factors, which might trigger the occurrence of CFS. These may include viral infection, injury, psychological depression, profound stress or exposure to toxins (7). While a single cause for CFS may yet be identified, another possibility is that CFS represents a common endpoint of disease resulting from multiple precipitating causes (8). In Canada and worldwide, researchers continue to explore possible causes, risk factors and triggering factors for the condition. However, many questions still remain about diagnosis since there is no treatment guideline or CFS case definition. The idea that CFS is an illness that primarily affects white, middle-class, well-educated, professional women still needs to be verified (2).

Methods

The Canadian Community Health Survey (CCHS) (9) is a collaborative effort between Statistics Canada, Health Canada, Public Health Agency of Canada and the Canadian Institute for Health Information. This national household cross-sectional survey was created to gather national health-related data to provide timely estimates of Canadians demographic information, lifestyle, risk factors, and socioeconomic status. The CCHS began collecting its first cycle of data in September of 2000, and subsequent data collection is based on a two-year collection cycle. Data from CCHS Cycle 1.1 (2000) to 3.1 (2005) were used in this analysis. The survey excluded individuals living on crown or reserve land, in institutions, members of the Canadian Armed Forces, and in certain remote areas of the country; but it still represents ~98% of the Canadian population over 12 years of age (10). A multistage stratified cluster design combined with random sampling methods was used to select the sample (10).

Sampling

The CCHS is scheduled to collect data every month from that point forward. Each two-year collection cycle comprises two distinct surveys: a health region-level survey in the first year with a total sample of 130,000, and a provincial-level survey in the second year with a total sample of 30,000. Sample sizes in any particular month or year can increase from provincial or health region-level buy-ins. Both computer-assisted personal and telephone interviews are planned (9). There was one randomly selected respondent per household. Eligibility for the first collection cycle were limited to only those 12 years of age and over; although it is expected that in future cycles, child-specific content will be included.

Definition of covariates

The self-reported covariates in the analysis are age, gender, living area (province/territories, urban/rural) lifestyle (smoking status, frequency of alcohol use, and physical activity) and socioeconomic status (education, income, immigration status). The level of education achieved by all members of the household was grouped into three categories (less than secondary, secondary, postsecondary school or more). Family income was classified on the basis of total household annual income and the number of household members into low (<$30,000 CAD) or middle (>=$30,000 to $59,999 CAD) and high ($60,000 CAD and over) level. Immigration status includes participants that were either born in Canada or were born elsewhere. Other variables were included in the analysis: physical activities were categorized as active, moderate, and inactive, based on kilo-calories per kilogram of body weight per day expended (KKD). Physically active is defined as an energy expenditure of at least 3 KKD; moderately active corresponds to energy expenditure between 1.5 and 3 KKD; physically in-active is defined as less than 1.5 KKD. The highest level of physical activity can be achieved by playing team sports for an hour or a half an hour of running, combined with an accumulated hour of walking throughout the day (11,12). Cigarette smoking was evaluated by three different methods: 1) patients were asked if they had ever smoked a whole cigarette (yes, no)? 2) if they were a 'current smoker' (daily, occasionally, not at all); 3) or a 'former smoker' (stopped smoke meanwhile survey was started). Patients were asked on a questionnaire how often they drank alcohol. They were asked to categorize their drinking habits as being "a regular drinker", "a former regular drinker(one who used to drink regularly, but no longer does)", or "a non-drinker" (a person who does not drink alcohol). The occurrence of CFS related to risk factors or socioeconomic status were calculated for total population and compared in proportions in people with or without CFS, where statistical significance was conducted by Odds Ratio and P values.

Data analysis

A descriptive model has been used to examine demographics, lifestyle, and socio-economic factors that could influence the occurrence of CFS. Multivariate logistic regression was then employed to determine independent factors associated with CFS, with Odds Ratio (OR) and P values calculated for each model. The logistic regression models were bootstrapped to take the design effects of the CCHS into account. Data was analysed using the SAS version 9.1 (SAS Institute, Cary, NC) (13).

Results

The adjusted prevalence of CFS increased from 0.78% to 1.22% from 2000 to 2005 in Canada. Individuals aged 40-64 years were more likely to report having CFS compared to other age groups in both 2000 (OR, 1.51; P<0.005) and in 2005 (OR, 2.67; P<0.001). Females made up more than two-thirds of reported cases in both 2000 and 2005 (see table 1). There are no significant statistical differences between current smoking and former smoking (OR from 0.51 to 0.86, P>0.05). However, the differences for CFS patients with less than secondary school education level (OR, 1.24 in 2000 and OR, 1.25 in 2005, P<0.01), and secondary school level (OR, 1.14 in 2000 and OR, 1.08 in 2005, P<0.05) are significant in comparison to post-secondary school educated individuals. Regular alcohol users (OR, 1.11, P<0.05 in 2000 and OR, 1.27, P<0.01 in 2005) have higher occurrences than non-alcohol users, but former regular alcohol users (OR from 0.66 to 0.96, P>0.05 in 2000 and in 2005) had no significant differences compared to non-drinking individuals. Moreover, non-immigrant Canadians (OR from 0.83 to 0.89, P>0.05) who live in the urban area (OR from 1.21 to 1.28, P<0.01), who have low family income level (OR,1.37, P<0.01 in 2000 and OR,1.18, P<0.05 in 2005), middle family income (OR, 2.48, P<0.001 in 2000, OR,1.06,

P>0.05 in 2005), those who were physical inactive (OR from 1.33, P<0.01 to 1.55, P<0.005) were exposed to more risk of CFS than others.

The prevalence of CFS is higher in Nunavut (1.09%), Nova Scotia (0.90%), Quebec (0.90%), Alberta (0.80%), and Ontario (0.79%) in 2000; however, this prevalence in Nova Scotia (1.47%), Quebec (1.38%), and Ontario (1.29%) in 2005 is higher than Canadian nation level (1.22%) (see table 1).

Table 1. Adjusted self-reported prevalence of Chronic Fatigue Syndrome (CFS) by age, sex, lifestyle, socioeconomic status and geographic in the CCHS, Canada, 2000-2005

Chronic Fatigue Syndrome	2000		2005	
	Cases of CFS	Prevalence (%)	Cases of CFS	Prevalence (%)
Cases of CFS	201,938	0.78	331,526	1.22
Non-CFS	25,597,000	99.17	27,057,000	98.48
Missing cases	12,131	0.05	82,510	0.30
Total	25,811,069	100.00	27,471,036	100.00
Provinces & Territories				
Newfoundland & Labrador	1,636	0.36	3,197	0.71
PEI	469	0.40	445	0.38
Nova Scotia	7,067	0.90	11,711	1.47
New Brunswick	4,815	0.76	5,838	0.91
Quebec	55,898	0.90	89,317	1.38
Ontario	78,206	0.79	136,457	1.29
Manitoba	3,780	0.42	7,521	0.81
Saskatchewan	4,330	0.54	6,554	0.83
Alberta	19,896	0.80	31,194	1.16
British Columbia	25,502	0.75	38,900	1.08
YUKON	39	0.16	173	0.64
NWT	86	0.27	205	0.59
NUNAVUT	212	1.09	10	0.07
Total	201,938	0.78	331,526	1.22
Age (year)	Cases of CFS	Percent (%)	Cases of CFS	Percent (%)
12-19	8,303	4.11	6,586	1.99
20-39	51,226	25.37	63,731	19.22
40-64	116,864	57.87	194,235	58.59
65 & over	25,544	12.65	66,974	20.20
Total	201,937	100.00	331,526	100.00
Sex				
Males	57,736	28.59	104,639	31.56
Females	144,402	71.41	226,886	68.44
Total	201,938	100.00	331,526	100.00
Smoking status				
Non-smoker	55,180	27.40	86,142	26.00
Chronic Fatigue Syndrome	2000		2005	

Table 1. (Continued)

	Cases of CFS	Prevalence %)	Cases of CFS	Prevalence (%)
Current smoker	65,792	32.68	112,439	33.93
Former smoker	80,381	39.92	132,760	40.07
Total	201,353	100.00	331,341	100.00
Education levels				
Less than secondary school	30,941	15.77	34,624	11.70
Secondary school	27,969	14.26	29,808	10.07
Post-secondary school	137,248	69.97	231,577	78.23
Total	196,159	100.00	296,009	100.00
Alcohol drinker				
Regularly drinker	137,659	68.34	228,633	70.00
Former drinker	43,954	21.82	79,040	24.20
Non-drinker	19,823	9.84	18,957	5.80
Total	201,436	100.00	326,630	100.00
Living area				
Urban	170,171	84.27	278,304	83.95
Rural	31,767	15.73	53,221	16.05
Total	201,938	100.00	331,526	100.00
Immigrant status				
Immigrant	38,874	19.36	72,108	22.40
Non immigrant	161,959	80.64	249,789	77.60
Total	200,833	100.00	321,897	100.00
Total yearly family income				
Less than $29,999	48,595	25.99	99,505	36.47
$30,000 - $59,999	108,969	58.28	88,992	32.62
$60,000 & over	29,421	15.73	84,322	30.91
Total	186,985	100.00	272,818	100.00
Physical activity				
Active	29,641	16.14	54,614	17.16
Moderate	31,178	16.98	70,092	22.02
Inactive	122,818	66.88	193,619	60.82
Total	183,637	100.00	318,325	100.00

Discussion

Chronic fatigue syndrome (CFS) is one of a group of illnesses which have unexplained and unknown causes; others include fibromyalgia, diffuse pain and irritable bowel syndrome (14). However, these do not necessary have the same causes and symptoms. For example, patients may sleep poorly and thus develop fatigue, whereas people who have disturbed sleep and inactivity may have different conditions (15). The exact risk factors and causes of CFS have not been identified yet. Researches have theorized that this syndrome may be related to infectious and immunologic, psychiatric, behaivioral, socioeconomic and environmental factors (16).

Table 2. Adjusted Odds Ratio and 95% confidence interval between age, gender, lifestyle, and socioeconomic status for CFS in the CCHS, Canada, 2000-2005

Chronic Fatigue Syndrome	2000		2005	
	Percent(%)	Odds Ratio (OR) and P-Value	Percent (%)	Odds Ratio (OR) and P-Value
[a] Age (year)				
<40 and 65+	42.13	*1.00*	41.41	*1.00*
40 – 64	57.87	1.51; P<0.005	58.59	2.67; P<0.001
[b] Gender				
Males	28.59	*1.00*	31.56	*1.00*
Females	71.41	2.49; P<0.001	68.44	2.46; P<0.001
[c] Risk factors and socioeconomic status				
Smoking status				
Non-smoker	27.40	*1.00*	26.00	*1.00*
Current smoker	32.68	0.51; P>0.05	33.93	0.58; P>0.05
Former smoker	39.92	0.71; P>0.05	40.07	0.86; P>0.05
Education levels				
Post-secondary school	69.97	*1.00*	78.23	*1.00*
Less than secondary school	15.77	1.24; P<0.01	11.70	1.25; P<0.01
Secondary school	14.26	1.14; P<0.05	10.07	1.08; P>0.05
Alcohol drinker				
Non-drinker	9.84	*1.00*	5.80	*1.00*
Regularly drinker	68.34	1.11; P<0.05	70.00	1.27; P<0.01
Former drinker	21.82	0.66; P>0.05	24.20	0.96; P>0.05
Living area				
Rural	15.73	*1.00*	16.05	*1.00*
Urban	84.27	1.28; P<0.01	83.95	1.21; P<0.01
Immigrant status				
Immigrant	19.36	*1.00*	22.40	*1.00*
Non immigrant	80.64	0.89; P>0.05	77.60	0.83; P>0.05
$60,000 & over	15.73	*1.00*	30.91	*1.00*
Less than $29,999	25.99	1.37; P<0.01	36.47	1.18; P<0.05
$30,000 - $59,999	58.28	2.48; P<0.001	32.62	1.06; P>0.05
Physical activity				
Active	16.14	*1.00*	17.16	*1.00*
Moderate	16.98	0.88; P>0.05	22.02	1.01; P>0.05
Inactive	66.88	1.33; P<0.01	60.82	1.55; P<0.005

a. Adjusted Odds Ratio were controlled by gender, risk factors and socioeconomic status.
b. Adjusted Odds Ratio were controlled by age, risk factors and socioeconomic status.
c. Adjusted Odds Ratio were controlled by age and gender.

Studies have found that there is a high economic and disability burden associated with CFS, for the families and society as a whole. A conservative estimate of the direct economic impact of CFS and the huge health care expenditure in Canada is about $3.5 billion per year. The cost to governments in Canada is about $2.2 billion per year in 2002 (4). At a personal level, economic losses caused by absenteeism can have a substantial long-term impact on CFS patients' quality of life. With high unemployment rates among individuals with CFS, there is a surcharged cost of medical services that could become even more problematic to CFS patients and their families, due to a loss of health insurance benefits, and thus, increases in out-of-pocket medical expenses (17). Bombardier and Buchwald (18) estimated an average annual medical expenditure of $1,031 CAD per CFS patient. Lloyd and Pender (19) and McCrone et al (20) also used samples from Australia and the United Kingdom respectively, to estimate the same situation.

The study results in table 1-2 revealed that CFS aflicts people in the age group (40-64 years) at twice the rate of other age groups. The occurrence of CFS in females is also more common than in males. Regular alcohol use, people have a low education level (less than secondary schooling), being a non-immigrant status, being a Canadian living in an urban area, physical inactivity, and having lower annual family income (less than $29,999 CAD) have a higher prevalence and burden.

Conclusions

CFS is a chronic, severely disabling medical disorder. It is problematic to the patients socioeconomic and psychosocial status.It can be more accurately diagnosed and treated symptomatically with improved surveillance, research, and management. Further developing funded knowledge exchange, health education, and research may reduce the burden and result in better outcomes for CFS patient treatment and management.

References

[1]   US Department of Health and Human Services Centers for Disease Control and Prevention 2008. URL: http://www.cdc.gov/cfs.

[2]   Carruthers BM. Definitions and aetiology of myalgic encephalomyelitis (ME): How the Canadian consensus clinical definition of ME works. J Clin Pathol 2007;60(2):117-9.

[3]   Statistics Canada. Canadian Community Health Survey (CCHS), 2000-2005.

[4]   The economic impact of ME/CFS. Sheffield Hallam University on behalf of Action for ME, a UK charity. 2003 May 12. http://www.shu.ac.uk/cgi-bin/news_full. pl?id_num=PR405anddb=03.

[5]   Reynolds KJ, Vernon SD, Bouchery E, Reeves WC. The economic impact of chronic fatigue syndrome. Cost Eff Resour Alloc 2004; 2(1):4.

[6]   Logan AC, Bested AC, Lowe R, Logan A, Howe R. Hope and help for chronic fatigue syndrome and fibromyalgia. Nasville, TN: Cumberland House Publ, 2008.

[7]   Chronic fatigue syndrome. Connecticut Centre for Health 2008. http://www. Connecticut centerfor health.com/chronic-fatigue-syndrome.html.

[8]   Fact sheet. Chronic fatigue syndrome. Pamphlet by: National Institute of Allergy and Infectious Diseases, Health Care Industry, 2000.

[9]   Statistics Canada. Canadian Community Health Survey (CCHS). 2001-2005. http://www.statcan.ca/ english/survey/other/canforgen.htm.

[10] Beland Y. Canadian community health survey—methodological overview. Health Rep 2002;13(3):9-14.

[11] Statistics Canada. National population health survey, 1996-7. Ottawa, ON: Health Stat Div, Public Use Microdata Files, 1997.

[12] Canadian Fitness and Lifestyle Research Institute. Physical activity monitor survey, 1997.

[13] SAS Institute. Statistical Application System (SAS), version 9.1.3. 2005.

[14] Aaron LA, Buchwald D. A review of the evidence for overlap among unexplained clinical conditions. Ann Intern Med 2001; 134:868-81.

[15] Moldofsky H, Scarisbrick P. Induction of neurasthenic musculoskeletal pain syndrome by selective sleep stage deprivation. Psychosom Med 1976;38:35-44.

[16] Natelson BH, Lange G. A status report on chronic fatigue syndrome. Environ Health Perspect 2002;110(Suppl 4).

[17] Jason LA, Benton MC, Valentine L, Johnson A, Torres-Harding S. The economic impact of ME/CFS: Individual and societal costs. Dyn Med 2008;7:6.

[18] Bombardier CH, Buchwald D. Chronic fatigue, chronic fatigue syndrome, and fibromyalgia: Disability and health Care use. Medical Care 1996, 34:924-930.

[19] Lloyd AR, Pender H: The economic impact of chronic fatigue syndrome. Med J Austr 1992;157:599-601.

[20] McCrone P, Darbishire L, Ridsdale L, Seed P. The economic cost of chronic fatigue and chronic fatigue syndrome in UK primary care. Psychol Med 2003;33:253-61.

Submitted: December 05, 2008.
Revised: Decemner 30, 2008
Accepted: January 07, 2009.

In: Chronic Fatigue Syndrome: Symptoms, Causes & Prevention   ISBN: 978-1-60741-493-3
Editor: E. Svoboda and K. Zelenjcik, pp. 175-184   © 2010 Nova Science Publishers, Inc.

Chapter 9

An Innovative Approach in Training Health Care Workers to Diagnose and Manage Patients with CFS

Leonard A. Jason[1][*], *Chuck Lapp*[**],
K. Kimberly Kenney[#] *and Terri Lupton*[#]
*DePaul University
**Hunter-Hopkins Center
[#]The CFIDS Association of America, Inc

Abstract

This study provides a description and evaluation of this innovative Train-the-Trainer approach for training health care workers in the diagnosis and management of patients with CFS. Those who attended this workshop did have significant changes in their understanding of CFS as well as attitudes towards those with this illness. Following the workshops, these trainers went back to their own settings and put on workshops to train others, and through this process, several thousand individuals were presented with information about the diagnosis and management of CFS.

Chronic fatigue syndrome (CFS) is an illness characterized by prolonged, debilitating fatigue and multiple nonspecific symptoms such as headache, recurrent sore throat, muscle and joint pain, and cognitive complaints. Profound fatigue, the hallmark of the disorder, can come on suddenly or gradually and persist or recur throughout the period of illness (Fukuda et al., 1994). Unlike the short-term disability of an acute infection, CFS symptoms by definition linger for at least six months and often for years. The majority of patients report an acute onset, over a period of hours or a few days. Others report a more gradual onset, as if they have a bout of flu from which they do not completely recover. CFS is marked by a dramatic difference in the patient's pre- and

---

[1] Corresponding author: Leonard A. Jason, Ph.D., DePaul University, Center for Community Research, 990 W. Fullerton Ave., Suite 3100, Chicago, Il. 60614.

post-illness activity level and stamina (Jason & Taylor, 2003). Health care professionals play an important role in diagnosing and treating patients with CFS.

Approximately a quarter of all patients seeing general practitioners complain of prolonged and incapacitating fatigue, a symptom common to many illnesses such as cancer, depression, autoimmune diseases, hormonal disorders, and infections (Friedberg & Jason, 1998). The majority of these illnesses are treatable and must be promptly identified so that timely treatment can be started. Therefore, causes of fatigue must be ruled out before a definitive diagnosis of CFS can be considered. Despite more than a decade of extensive research, the cause of CFS remains unknown and no diagnostic tests exist (Jason, Fennell, & Taylor, 2003). However, health care providers must recognize that CFS is a real and debilitating condition that can only be diagnosed through a process of elimination.

CFS is one of the nation's most prevalent, yet misunderstood, chronic illnesses. In a community based epidemiologic study by Jason and colleagues (1999), they found that about 800,000 Americans would meet the case definition for CFS, although only ten percent of those identified as having CFS in their community based sample had actually been diagnosed with this illness. The research group also identified that women, African-Americans, and Hispanics were at a greater risk for developing the illness than men, Whites, or Asian-Americans. Findings from this community-based prevalence study also indicated that rates of CFS were highest in females of lower socioeconomic status, a segment of the population that is less likely to have access to health care providers, and therefore may be less likely to seek and receive care for this disabling illness. Given the high percentage of these patients who go undiagnosed, it is clear that many patients are not receiving appropriate care for this illness. By staying abreast of new information, health care professionals can play an important role in better diagnosing this illness and providing a higher level of care to patients.

Many patients with chronic fatigue syndrome (CFS) have felt stigmatized or misunderstood by medical professionals (Looper & Kirmayer, 2004). For example, Anderson and Ferrans (1997) found that 77percent of individuals with CFS reported past negative experiences with health care providers. Another survey found that 57percent of respondents were treated badly or very badly by their doctors (David, Wessely, and Pelosi, 1991). Green, Romei, and Natelson (1999) also found that 95percent of individuals seeking medical treatment for CFS reported feelings of estrangement, and 70percent believed that others attributed their CFS symptoms to psychological causes. Asbring and Narvanen (2003) found physicians regarded the illness as less serious than the patients, and the physicians characterized the patients with CFS and Fibromyalgia as illness focused, demanding, and medicalising. Twemlow, Bradshaw, Coyne, and Lerma (1997) found that 66percent of individuals with CFS stated that they were made worse by their doctors' care. Clearly, there is a need to help sensitize health care professionals to the unique needs of patients with CFS.

It is possible that negative attitudes toward people with CFS might help explain the consistent finding that patients with CFS have mixed experiences with the health care system. Shlaes, Jason, and Ferrari (1999) developed a CFS Attitudes Test, and found that if someone believes that people with CFS are responsible for their illness, it is likely that they will also believe that people with CFS have negative personality characteristics, such as being compulsive or overly driven. It is possible that negative attitudes might be a function of past negative portrayals of CFS as either non-existent or as a function of a neurotic, overworked, stressed lifestyles (Jason et al., 1997). Any training program for health care professionals will need to deal with the negative stigma that patients with CFS feel, and attempts to change these types of negative attitudes could lead to more positive patient experiences when dealing with the health care system.

Improving patient care through the education of health care professionals has become a major initiative for The CFIDS (Chronic Fatigue Immune Dysfunction Syndrome) Association of America, the largest CFS patient and advocacy organization in the US. A Primary Care Provider Education Project was developed by the CFIDS Association to offer various learning opportunities for providers, including lecture presentations, and print, video- and Web-based self-study courses. Health care providers who were interested in educating other health care providers about CFS were offered the opportunity to attend a two-day Train-the-Trainer workshop, lead by CFS experts. After completion of this workshop, attendees were asked to return to their home regions and present one-to-two hour long programs for at least 40 of their peers, or to students in health care disciplines. Continuing education units were provided and expenses were covered for participants. This study provides a description and evaluation of this innovative Train-the-Trainer approach for training health care workers in the diagnosis and management of patients with CFS.

Method

The objective of the Primary Care Provider Education Project was to expand the knowledge base of health care providers to improve diagnosis and treatment of CFS. In 1999, the Centers for Disease Control and Prevention (CDC), Health Resources and Services Administration, and the Illinois Area Health Education Centers Program jointly agreed to sponsor the project to educate primary care providers about CFS. A group of CFS experts from across the U.S. gathered to develop the project components.

The project was piloted in 2000 and 2001 and funding was renewed by the CDC in 2002 and 2003. The project is currently co-administered by The CFIDS Association of America and the CDC. William Reeves, MD, at the CDC and K. Kimberly Kenney, CEO of The CFIDS Association serve as Project Directors. The Project Coordinator is Terri Lupton, and the Project Administrative assistant is Kasia Faryna, both of The CFIDS Association of America. A multidisciplinary Advisory Committee provides input and direction, along with the administrative team.[2]

The project included print-based self-study, video self-study, Web-based self-study, exhibits at provider conferences, scientific meetings, promotional activities, and Train-the-Trainer. The provider education project was designed to teach health care providers how to better recognize and manage CFS. The self-study courses in three formats were approved for continuing education credits through the CDC, an accredited provider of continuing education for multiple health care disciplines. Print-, video-, and Web-based modules are now available free of charge for health care providers.

All formats were based on the multidisciplinary curriculum developed by a group of CFS experts from across the United States. At completion of this activity, the participants were

---

[2] Advisory Committee members include: William Reeves, MD, CDC; K. Kimberly Kenney, CEO, The CFIDS Association of America, Inc.; Julie Barroso, PhD, MSN, RN, University of North Carolina-Chapel Hill; Kristine Healy, MPH, PA-C, Midwestern University; Joann House, Program Analyst, CDC; Leonard Jason, PhD, DePaul University; James Jones, MD, CDC; Nancy Klimas, MD, University of Miami; Charles Lapp, MD, Hunter-Hopkins Center; Dimitris Papanicolaou, MD, Emory University; John Stewart, MD, CDC; Terri Lupton, RN, BSS, The CFIDS Association of America, Inc.; and Kasia Faryna, BA, The CFIDS Association of America, Inc.

expected to be able to: define CFS and recognize its symptoms, discuss possible etiologies of CFS, based on current research, differentiate CFS from Major Depressive Disorder, use clinical decision-making strategies in forming a diagnosis of CFS, cite various treatment options for CFS, both supportive and symptomatic, and recognize the variability of CFS prognosis, and recognize the variability of CFS levels of severity and disability.

Print-Based Self-Study

Print-based self-study materials were made available as a learning tool for health care providers. This module was approved for continuing education credits through the CDC education and training administrative unit, accredited providers of continuing education for multiple health care disciplines. Continuing education credits are offered for those who complete the requirements.

Web Site Self-Study

CFS materials that are based on the printed curriculum, with case studies included, are available on the medical professionals section of The CFIDS Association's Web site. Continuing education credits, identical to the print-based version have been approved for this format through the CDC, accredited providers of multidisciplinary continuing education credits. The course was free of charge. To access the Web-based curriculum, health care professionals were required to complete the course registration process, which includes their professional licensure information. The site is secure and a privacy policy is in effect. Registered participants have unlimited access to the reading, testing, and evaluation materials. It is not necessary to complete the contents in one setting, enabling course work to be accomplished as participants' schedules permit. Participants need to obtain a score of 70 percent or greater on the post-test to obtain continuing education credits. Two attempts to take the post-test are granted.

Video Self-Study

The video was filmed in 2001 during the first Train-the-Trainer session. Continuing education credits have been approved through the CDC, accredited provider of multidisciplinary continuing education credits, and are based on three hours of instruction.

The video format consists of two tapes that include a 45-minute presentation by Charles Lapp, MD; a 30-minute patient interview section (filmed with two persons with CFIDS and three providers); and a two-part case study assessment facilitated by Dr. Lapp and Dr. Jason. A packet of printed materials, consisting of additional case studies and various other learning resources, accompanied the videotape. The video was intended to reach those persons who did not have Internet access, availability to "live" presentations, or who preferred to learn through this method.

Provider Conference Exhibits

Conference exhibits occurred at the American College of Physicians, American Society of Internal Medicine, American Association of Physician Assistants, and National Medical Association, and various smaller, regional conferences.

Promotional Activities

Promotions that focused on the availability and advantages of the self-study module were developed. Rolodex cards and flyers, for distribution at conferences and meetings, were produced. Web banners and ads for publication in medical Web sites, journals, and newsletters were designed by a graphic artist. Promotional activities were used to generate interest in the exhibit booth, CFS/CFIDS information, and the self-study courses.

Train-the-Trainer

A significant part of the project is the Train-the-Trainer module, in which multidisciplinary professionals from across the U.S. attend a two-day intensive workshop to study the curriculum developed by national CFS experts. These trainers in turn present a one- to two-hour instructional session for providers practicing in their home regions. Each trainer is asked to educate a minimum of 40 professionals. Charles Lapp, MD and Leonard Jason, PhD served as master trainers for these sessions. Attendees at these events received 12 hours of continuing education credits for participating. Fifty-five providers (Level II trainers) from nine states were trained, and they then scheduled presentations in their local regions. The target audiences for presentations by Level II trainers are located in medical schools, medical societies, nursing programs, physician assistant programs, clinics, hospitals, public health agencies, provider conferences and universities. Continuing education credits were approved for presentations given by Level II trainers and were offered to attendees at these events.

Diagnostic Issues Covered in the Train-the-Trainer Sessions

Participants were first familiarized with the 1994 International Case Definition (Fukuda et al., 1994), and they were instructed to exclude other possible diagnoses (e.g., anemia, hypothyroidism, lupus, Lyme disease, MS). Participants also were informed about CFS's widely heterogeneous patient population, and the varying subsets could be grouped, for example, by onset characteristics or symptom patterns, making treatment options even more challenging. There was instruction in addressing symptoms and psychosocial issues comprehensively. Participants were informed that patients with CFS are frequently hypersensitive to medicines, foods, and vaccines, therefore, it was often best to try prescribing a fraction of the usual recommended dosage to start and increase slowly, as necessary, to tolerance and to achieve symptom relief. Participants were informed about the need to stay alert for symptoms of sleep disturbances, as unrefreshing sleep is a nearly universal CFS symptom, and improving sleep can positively impact other symptoms. They were also informed about considering sleep studies and/or referral to a sleep specialist for appropriate patients.

Treatment Issues Covered in the Train-the-Trainer sessions

Participants were told that treating CFS presents a significant challenge for physicians and nurses. Because there is no known cause, cure, or universal treatment for CFS, therapy is based upon helping manage the individual's presenting symptoms. Medications that provide symptom relief are frequently the first line of treatment chosen by primary care providers, and they include medications for pain; sleep disturbances; digestive problems such as nausea; flu-like symptoms and; if present, depression and anxiety. Medications may be supplemented by supportive therapies. In regard to pain, NSAIDS are the first step, and as a last step, long-acting narcotics may be necessary for patients with unrelenting, severe pain. Referral to a chronic pain management program may be helpful as well. Altered digestion, food intolerances, decreased energy, fatigue, cognitive problems, and sleeplessness create the need for revisions in daily living routines. These can include changes in diet; exercise modifications; alterations in activities of daily living according to one's energy level; and sleep/rest management. All may require the assistance of professional clinicians, such as a dietitian, physical and/or occupational therapist, mental health professional, and sleep therapist.

For people who have been diagnosed with an autonomic nervous system abnormality such as orthostatic intolerance, fluid and salt loading may be a treatment of choice. Participants were instructed to treat orthostatic intolerance with fluid management and medications such as beta blockers or alpha agonists.

As many patients with CFS have cognitive problems such as difficulty concentrating and short-term memory deficits, it is important to enhance verbal communication with written instructions and/or tape recorded instructions or consultations.

Therapies that help people to relax and improve coping skills include counseling for emotional and mental health, cognitive behavioral therapy, sleep management therapy, and massage. They were also informed to allow extra time for interaction with patients, and to consider referral to a counselor or other behavioral health professional who is able to extend patient contact to discuss the impact of the illness on the patient, family, finances, etc. Participants were informed about simplified psychological evaluation tools and functional capacity tools to screen for psychological or physical dysfunction. It is not unusual for CFS patients to become depressed or anxious as they try to cope with the complexities of a chronic illness, so participants were provided assessment tools to help in detecting the onset of problems and deterioration or improvement in symptoms. The program stressed the importance of being particularly conscious of one's attitude, as many patients experience skepticism and disbelief from others about their illness. These attitudes can make them sensitive to verbal and non-verbal signs of disrespect and lack of acceptance of their reality in living with CFS. Treating patients with respect and validating their illness may be the single most important therapy primary care providers can provide.

Participants were instructed to work with patients to develop individualized, modest stretching and exercise plans, or consider referral to a physical or occupational therapy program. Participants were also encouraged to recommend a well-balanced diet to prevent nutritional deficiencies or weight fluctuations. Many persons find complementary therapies such as acupuncture, tai chi and alternative food and herbal supplements to be helpful. Participants were informed that adding food and herbal supplements to a therapy regimen needs to be done with care in order to prevent undesirable side effects.

Procedures

Prior to and at the completion of training, the participants in the Train-the-Trainer program were asked to complete a 25-item knowledge of CFS test (that was developed specifically for this program). Participants also filled out at pre and post-point a 19-item Chronic Fatigue Syndrome Attitudes Test (or CAT; Schlaes, Jason & Ferrari, 1999). There are three factors on this CAT scale "Responsibility for CFS" contains items relating to whether or not people with CFS are responsible for getting sick. "Relevance of CFS" contains items relating to the relevance of CFS to society. "Traits of People with CFS" contains items relating to perceptions about personality characteristics of individuals with CFS. The composite scale and factor scores have acceptable internal reliability. Test-retest reliability analysis has indicated that the CAT subscale scores, as well as the CAT composite score, were consistent over a six-week period of time. Lower scores indicate more positive attitudes

Results

Knowledge

Trainers demonstrated significantly improved performance from pretest to posttest on knowledge of CFS. Out of a total of 25 items, trainers averaged 16.4 (or 65percent) correct responses on the pretest and 21.6 (or 86percent) correct responses on the posttest (t-test; $p < .001$). Thus, trainers increased their knowledge of CFS from the pretest to the posttest by five items or approximately 20percent. On the posttest, 93% of trainees correctly answered 20 (80percent) or more of the 25 knowledge questions.

Attitudes-CAT

For the total CAT score, the trainer attitudes improved significantly (Ms from 40.5 to 35.1, with lower scores indicating more positive attitudes, $p < .05$). For the factor Responsibility for CFS, attitudes significantly improved from 7.8 to 6.4 (t-test, $p < .05$).

Discussion

In general, on several domains that were evaluated, including information and attitudes, positive changes were observed over time among the participants in this Train-the-Trainer workshop. These findings suggest that at least in terms of information and attitudes, those who attended this workshop did have significant changes in these self-report indices of understanding about CFS as well as attitudes towards those with this illness. Following the workshops, these trainers went back to their own settings and put on workshops to train others, and through this process, we estimate that several thousand individuals were presented with accurate information about the diagnosis and management of CFS.

There are wide variations in implementation of health care services, as well as how such systems are appreciated by health care workers and patients. We might need a guiding framework for understanding behavior in interaction with its social and cultural contexts (Kelly, 1990). In other words, we need to understand a specific patient's interaction with a particular health care practice and cultural context. If there is a negative set of attitudes toward patients with CFS, these attitudes will have a detrimental effect on patient care. It is important to assess self-report data on attitudes and beliefs, and without such data it would be difficult to understand successes and failures in implementation.

The research to date on physician behavior has often demonstrated small effects at best. For example, Janes, Anderson, and Jenkins (1997) conducted a meta-analytic review of provider office based interventions designed to improve the delivery of preventive services. They concluded that these interventions had only a small effect of providers' adherence to preventive recommendations. It is probably that significant changes in a physician's diagnostic and management behavior in a practice setting as a result of CE is dependent on the following conditions: 1) the CE offered is closely linked to the behavior, 2) the CE offered provides ample opportunities for clinicians to practice the behavior successfully, 3) the practice setting does not present disincentives that discourage the occurrence of the desired behaviors, and 4) the practice setting contains incentives that reinforce and prompt the desired behaviors.

Certainly, the data reviewed in the introduction indicate we need a more positive collaborative relationship between the health practitioners and patients with CFS. In a sense, the collaborative endeavor is a discovery process in which the different parties share the different constructions of their contexts, learn about events and processes that help define their understanding of the contexts, and work together to define the intervention activity (Kelly, 1990). Inappropriate health care can occur when there is a lack of attention to these types of processes. Bottom up type planning might secure the cooperation and motivation of both parties to be committed to change that endures and becomes rooted within the health care delivery system. Variations in health care might be strongly influenced by how well patients and the different players within a region feel their interests, values, and customs have been incorporated into the interventions.

The group that planned this provider education program is currently developing a curriculum for use by ancillary health care provides, such as psychologists, psychiatrists, physical therapists, occupational therapists, social workers, and counselors. Clearly, these types of programs are needed in order to disseminate basic information and skills on the diagnosis and management of patients with CFS. Still, it is important to recognize that changing health practice behaviors among health care professionals was not assessed in this evaluation, and future studies are needed to assess whether these types of programs are able to improve the way patients are both diagnosed and managed.

References

Anderson, J. S. & Ferrans, C. E. (1997). The quality of life of persons with chronic fatigue syndrome. *Journal of Nervous and Mental Disease, 185*, 359-367.

Asbring, P. & Narvanen, A. L. (2003). Ideal versus reality: Physicians perspectives on patients with chronic fatigue syndrome (CFS) and fibromyalgia. *Social Science & Medicine, 57*, 711-720.

David, A. S., Wessely, S. & Pelosi, A. J. (1991). Chronic fatigue syndrome: Signs of a new approach. *British Journal of Hospital Medicine, 45*, 158-163.

Friedberg, F. & Jason, L. A. (1998). *Understanding chronic fatigue syndrome: An empirical guide to assessment and treatment.* Washington, D.C.: American Psychological Association.

Fukuda, K., Straus, S. E., Hickie, I., Sharpe, M. C., Dobbins, J. G. & Komaroff, A. (1994). The chronic fatigue syndrome: A comprehensive approach to its definition and study. *Annals of Internal Medicine, 121*, 953-959.

Green, J., Romei, J. & Natelson, B. J. (1999). Stigma and chronic fatigue syndrome. *Journal of Chronic Fatigue Syndrome, 5,* 63-75.

Janes, G. R., Anderson, L. A. & Jenkins, C. A. (1997). A review and synthesis of provider-based interventions to improve the delivery of preventive services. *Health Services Review, 14*, 281.

Jason, L. A., Fennell, P. & Taylor, R. R. (Editors)(2003). *Handbook of chronic fatigue syndrome & fatiguing illnesses.* New York, N.Y.: John Wiley & Sons, Inc.

Jason, L. A., Richman, J. A., Friedberg, F., Wagner, L., Taylor, R. & Jordan, K.M. (1997). Politics, science, and the emergence of a new disease: The case of Chronic Fatigue Syndrome. *American Psychologist, 52,* 973-983.

Jason, L. A., Richman, J. A., Rademaker, A. W., Jordan, K.M., Plioplys, A. V., Taylor, R. R., McCready, W., Huang, C. & Plioplys, S. (1999). A community-based study of chronic fatigue syndrome. *Archives of Internal Medicine, 159,* 2129- 2137.

Jason, L. A. & Taylor, R. R. (2003). Chronic fatigue syndrome. In A. M. Nezu, C. M. Nezu, & P. A. Geller (Eds.), *Handbook of Psychology, Volume 9: Health Psychology.* (pp. 365-391). Wiley: New York.

Kelly, J. G. (1990). Changing contexts and the field of community psychology. *American Journal of Community Psychology, 18,* 769- 792.

Looper, K. J. & Kirmayer, L. J. (2004). Perceived stigma in functional somatic syndromes and comparable medical conditions. *Journal of Psychosomatic Research, 57,* 373-378.

Shlaes, J. L., Jason, L. A. & Ferrari, J. (1999). The development of the Chronic Fatigue Syndrome Attitudes Test: A psychometric analysis. *Evaluation and the Health Professions, 22,* 442-465.

Twemlow, S. W., Bradshaw, S. L., Jr., Coyne, L. & Lerma, B. H. (1997). Patterns of utilization of medical care and perceptions of the relationship between doctor and patient with chronic illness including chronic fatigue syndrome. *Psychological Reports, 80,* 643-659.

Index